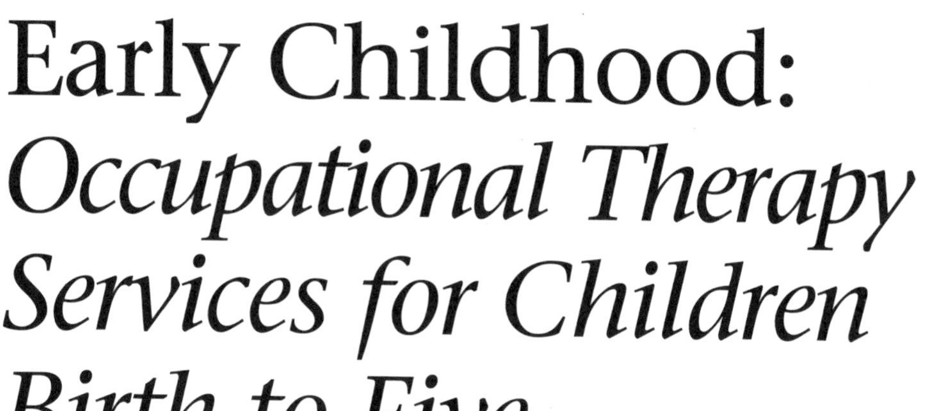

Early Childhood: *Occupational Therapy Services for Children Birth to Five*

Edited by Barbara E. Chandler, PhD, OTR/L, FAOTA

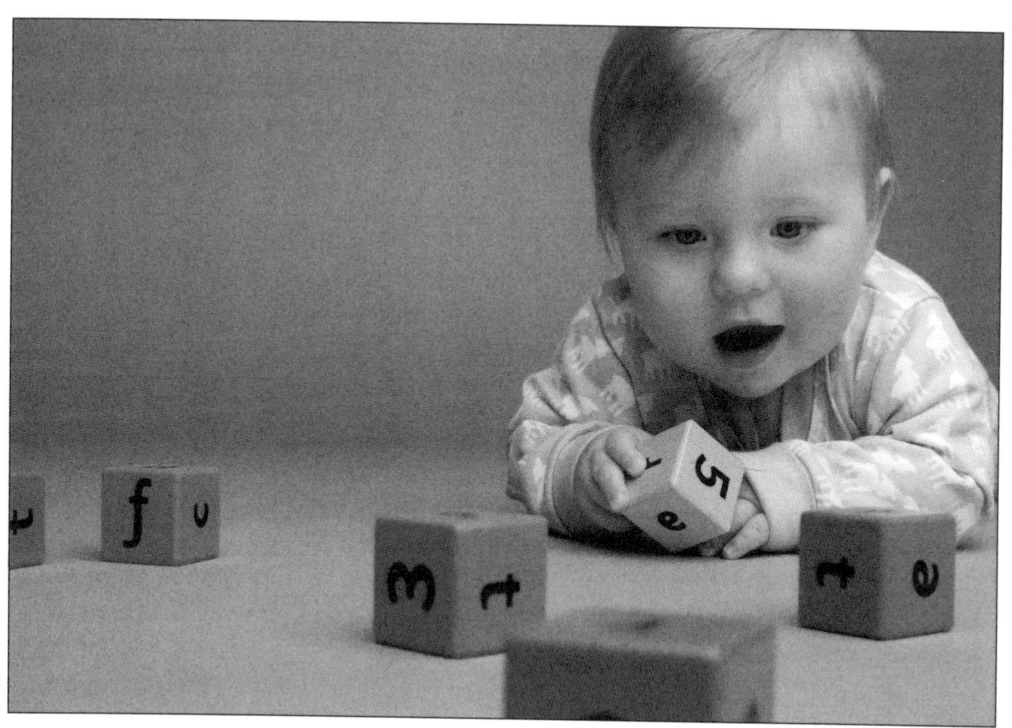

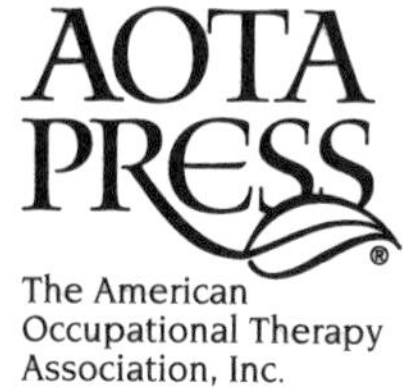

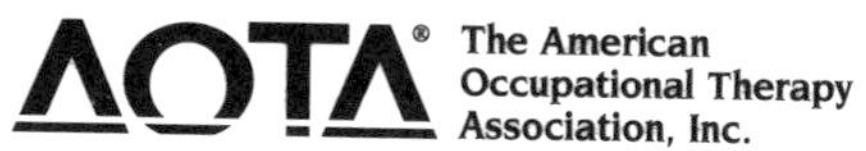

Centennial Vision
We envision that occupational therapy is a powerful, widely recognized, science-driven, and evidence-based profession with a globally connected and diverse workforce meeting society's occupational needs.

Vision Statement
The American Occupational Therapy Association advances occupational therapy as the pre-eminent profession in promoting the health, productivity, and quality of life of individuals and society through the therapeutic application of occupation.

Mission Statement
The American Occupational Therapy Association advances the quality, availability, use, and support of occupational therapy through standard-setting, advocacy, education, and research on behalf of its members and the public.

AOTA Staff
Frederick P. Somers, *Executive Director*
Christopher M. Bluhm, *Chief Operating Officer*
Maureen Freda Peterson, *Chief Professional Affairs Officer*

Chris Davis, *Director, AOTA Press*
Sarah D. Hertfelder, *Continuing Education Program Manager*
Caroline Polk, *Project Manager*
Cynthia Stock, *Electronic Quill Publishing Services, Compositor*

Beth Ledford, *Director, Marketing*
Emily Zhang, *Technology Marketing Specialist*
Jennifer Folden, *Marketing Specialist*

The American Occupational Therapy Association, Inc.
4720 Montgomery Lane
Bethesda, MD 20814
Phone: 301-652-AOTA (2682)
TDD: 800-377-8555
Fax: 301-652-7711
www.aota.org
To order: 877-404-AOTA (2682)

Printed in the United States of America.

Library of Congress Control Number: 2010903788

ISBN-10: 1-56900-296-7
ISBN-13: 978-1-56900-296-4

Contents

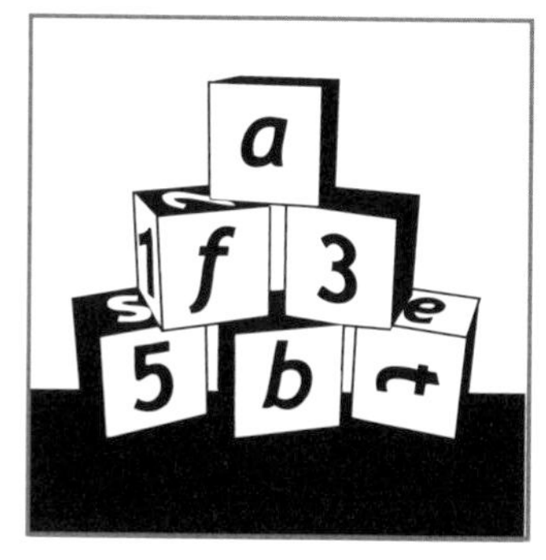

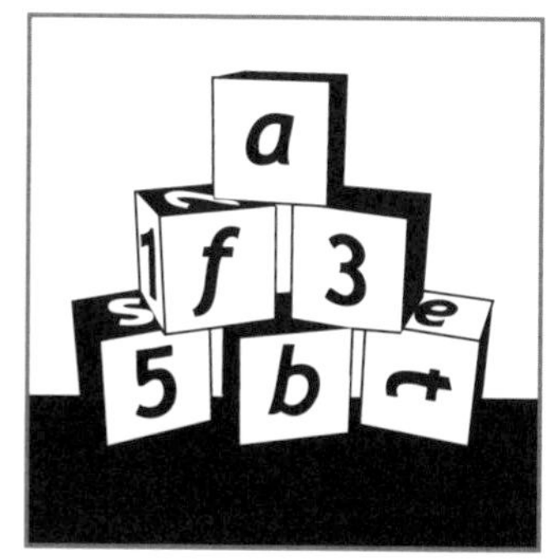

Dedication

In memory of my mother,
Mary Bernita "Betty" O'Donnell Chandler,
who, in her costume as the Red Queen
for a dress rehearsal of *Alice in Wonderland*
and wielding a cardboard sword, chased my
Brownie troop around our house shouting
"Off with their heads!" until they locked
themselves in the bathroom screaming
and I fell to the floor laughing.
She knew how to play . . .
and parent.

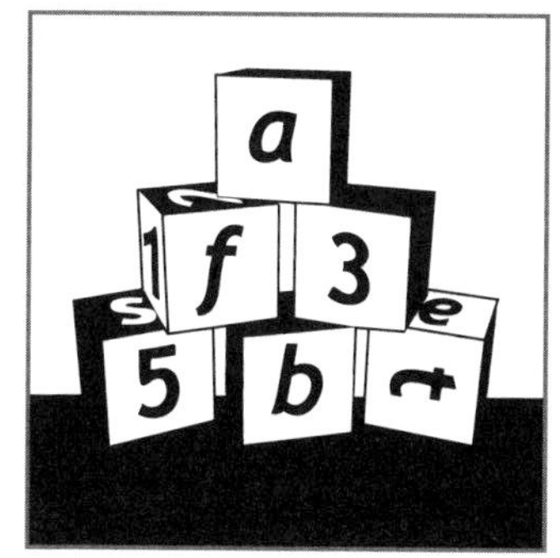

Acknowledgments

A work of this type is supported in many ways. Foremost are the authors, who agreed to go on this journey of writing a self-study. Other colleagues provided encouragement, guidance, resources, stories, and perspective. For their many and varied contributions, I thank my colleagues from my early years of practice, who continue to this day to be sources of practical wisdom and who welcomed me back to the Asheville, NC, therapeutic community as though I had never left: Rebecca Wallace, Janet Spletzer, Marian Reinsch, and Sarah S. Mims.

My colleagues at the Childrens' Developmental Services Agency in Asheville provide daily examples of dedication to young children and their families. I have learned from them.

Last, I thank my sons, Matthew Brady Allen, who never doubts that his mother can complete anything she starts as long as it does not involve motor coordination, and Zachariah Allen, who gave continual encouragement that this project would be completed and didn't seem to mind at all that I could not more closely monitor his senior year in high school.

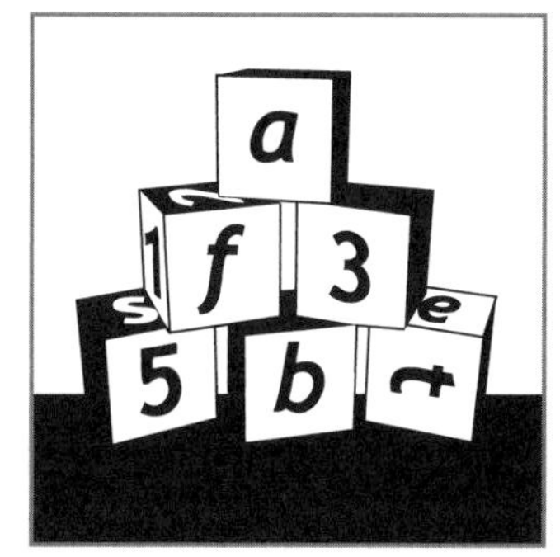

About the Editor

Barbara E. Chandler, PhD, OTR/L, FAOTA, has been an occupational therapist for 34 years. She received a bachelor's degree in American studies and sociology from the University of Tennessee and a master's degree in occupational therapy from Western Michigan University. She holds a doctorate in educational leadership.

Chandler is an occupational therapist with the Children's Developmental Services Agency, Asheville, North Carolina, the state early intervention program. She also provides consultative services through her private practice, Therapeutic Services and Design. She worked in the public schools and operated the private practice in western North Carolina for 12 years before serving as the first pediatric program manager of the American Occupational Therapy Association (AOTA) from 1988 to 1993. As assistant professor at Shenandoah University from 1993 to 1998 and associate professor at James Madison University from 1999 to 2006, she participated in the development of graduate-level occupational therapy programs.

Chandler writes the long-running "Classroom Clinic" in *ADVANCE for Occupational Therapy Practitioners* and has lectured and written extensively on occupational therapy services under the Individuals With Disabilities Education Act. She is the immediate past chairperson of the AOTA Early Intervention and School Special Interest Section.

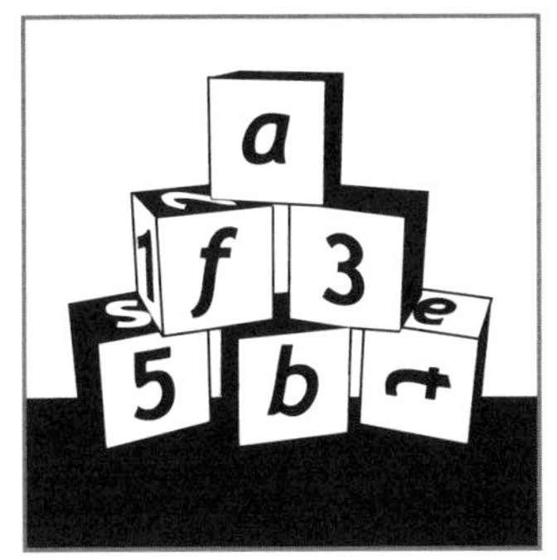

About the Authors

Frances A. Davis, MA, LPA, is senior research associate and developmental psychologist with the Family, Infant and Preschool Program in Morganton, North Carolina, a nationally recognized program for its innovative work with families and their young children. She received an MA in developmental psychology from the University of North Carolina at Greensboro and is a North Carolina–licensed psychological associate. Davis has 19 years of experience providing home-based early intervention supports to children and families. Her research activities focus on early intervention and early childhood practices that promote parent–child interactions important for the development of cognitive and social–emotional competencies in infants, toddlers, and preschoolers.

Gloria Frolek Clark, PhD, OTR/L, BCP, FAOTA, is a graduate of the University of North Dakota's occupational therapy program. She received her master's degree in early childhood special education from Iowa State University and received her doctorate from the Iowa State University Early Childhood Special Education Program.

Clark has focused on early intervention and school practice and policy. After working for more than 30 years as an early childhood/school occupational therapist and a state consultant for occupational therapy, she is employed by the Iowa Department of Education as an early childhood consultant. At the state and local levels, she has been involved in various research activities, including development of a statewide handwriting screening tool known as the IOWAN and a Web-based individualized family service plan outcome module.

Nationally, Clark presents on early intervention and school practice and methods of monitoring student performance. She has also served in various volunteer positions for the American Occupational Therapy Association (AOTA), including as a cofounder and first chairperson of AOTA's Early Intervention and School Special Interest Section (EISSIS), as a member of the Commission on Practice and of the

Pediatric Specialty Board, and as faculty for regional early intervention and school-based practice workshops. She has written several AOTA self-study chapters and an audioconference and has coauthored several AOTA official documents.

Joanne J. Foss, PhD, OTR/L, is the assistant dean of student affairs and a clinical assistant professor at the University of Florida College of Public Health and Health Professions. She is also the program director of the University of Florida's Master's in Occupational Therapy Program. Foss received her bachelor's degree in occupational therapy in 1975 from Colorado State University, her master's degree from Syracuse University, and her doctorate from the University of Florida. She teaches courses in applied lifespan human development and pediatric assessment and intervention.

Foss's research interests are in professional health education and pediatric assessment and intervention. She has served as an investigator, author, and editor of self-study programs to train occupational and physical therapists in early intervention services. She is specifically interested in neurobehavioral and neuromotor development in young children with disabilities.

Terry Giese, MBA, OT/L, FAOTA, is the lead therapist (occupational therapy, physical therapy) for Naperville Community Unit School District 203 in Illinois, where she also serves on the Early Childhood Diagnostic Team. She has been active in AOTA and Illinois Occupational Therapy Association leadership for more than 20 years and is the ex officio chairperson of the Naperville Mayor's Advisory Commission on Disabilities. For AOTA, Terry has served as the vice chair of the Nominating Committee, as Illinois representative to the Representative Assembly, and as an AOTA Representative Assembly Task Force leader. She authored the AOTA position paper on the role of occupational therapy in complementary and alternative medicine. Occupational therapy practice and presentations have taken her to Africa, Asia, Australia, Europe, and South America and across the United States and Puerto Rico.

Rebecca E. Argabrite Grove, MS, OTR/L, has a bachelor's degree in psychology from the University of Virginia and a master's degree in occupational therapy from Shenandoah University. She has worked with Loudoun County Public Schools in Virginia for 13 years as an occupational therapist, assistive technology (AT) practitioner and, most recently, elementary special education supervisor. She served two consecutive terms as president of the Virginia Occupational Therapy Association (VOTA) in addition to serving as the VOTA school system co-liaison and bylaws and ethics chair.

Argabrite Grove has served AOTA as vice chairperson of the Affiliated State Association Presidents and is the Virginia representative to AOTA's Representative Assembly and a member of the Bylaws, Policies, and Procedures Committee. She has conducted numerous presentations on occupational therapy and education-related topics at local, state, and national levels; has served as an adjunct professor and clinical lab supervisor for Shenandoah University; and has published on psychosocial practice, AT, and play. She is a recipient of the VOTA Award of Merit and the Shenandoah University Alumni Association Young Career Achievement Award.

Elise Holloway, MPH, OTR/L, is occupational therapy clinical specialist for Children's Services at Huntington Memorial Hospital in Pasadena, California. In addition, she is the occupational therapy consultant for the Early Start Program at Eastern Los Angeles Regional Center. She has worked in early childhood settings for more than 30 years.

Holloway has served on the standing committee for AOTA's Developmental Disabilities Special Interest Section and Sensory Integration Special Interest Section. She was a faculty member of AOTA's Family-Centered Care Trainings and coauthored AOTA's knowledge and skills paper on occupational therapy practice in the neonatal intensive care unit. She also cochaired the California Early Intervention Personnel Preparation Task Force, which defined best personnel practices for the state.

Holloway has published and lectured internationally on the topic of occupational therapy in early intervention; her expertise is in the Brazelton Neonatal Behavioral Assessment Scale, infant mental health, feeding, and sensory processing.

Anne L. Lucas, MS, OTR/L, is an early childhood technical assistance specialist at the National Early Childhood Technical Assistance Center at the University of North Carolina–Chapel Hill and the Western Regional Resource Center at the University of Oregon. She provides technical assistance to states and territories nationwide, focusing on Part C early intervention and preschool special education. In this capacity, she assists states with making systemic change and improving outcomes for young children with disabilities and their families. Her technical assistance focuses on helping states establish effective infrastructures; develop appropriate state policy; and implement evidence-based, family-centered practices in the context of everyday routines and activities.

Previously, Lucas was the state Part C coordinator in Virginia, the director of one of the nation's first early intervention programs, and a practicing occupational therapist in both early intervention and school-age services. As a practitioner, program administrator, state policymaker, and national technical assistance provider, she has consistently promoted occupational therapy as an essential and contributing profession for enhancing the lives of young children with disabilities and their families.

Judith Schoonover, MEd, OTR/L, ATP, earned a bachelor's degree in occupational therapy from Western Michigan University, a preliminary teaching credential from Chapman University, and a master's of education in integrating technology in schools from George Mason University. In addition to working as a school-based practitioner, Schoonover taught elementary school for more than 4 years. She is a RESNA-certified AT practitioner and a founding member of the Loudoun County (Virginia) Public Schools AT team.

Schoonover has been active in occupational therapy for more than 30 years, presenting nationally and authoring articles and chapters on topics related to school-based practice and AT. She has served as adjunct faculty for George Mason University and Shenandoah University. She is continuing education chairperson for VOTA, a past member of AOTA's EISSIS standing committee, and a member of AOTA's Transition Task Force. She represents AOTA on the National Joint Committee for the Communication Needs of Persons With Severe Disabilities.

Amy Russell Yun, MS, OTD, OTR/L, teaches in James Madison University's occupational therapy program. Her research interests are infant mental health and occupations of families with young children. She has worked as an occupational therapist within diverse settings, including early intervention, infant mental health, school-based therapy, clinic-based therapy, and transitional living. Yun has presented nationally and locally on topics related to family occupations and infant mental health.

Reviewers

Anne L. Lucas, MS, OTR/L
TA Specialist

- National Early Childhood Technical Assistance Center, Frank Porter Graham Child Development Center, University of North Carolina–Chapel Hill
- Western Regional Resource Center, Technical Assistance Consulting Services, University of Oregon, Eugene

Peggy McGrane, MA, OTR
Director, Early Childhood Intervention
ECI Keep Pace
Harris County Department of Education
Houston, TX

Tracy Miller, MHS, OT/L
Director
Rehabilitation Associates, PC
Virginia Beach, VA

Betsy A. Slavik, MA, OTR/L
Co-Owner, K.I.D.S. Therapy Associates
San Diego, CA

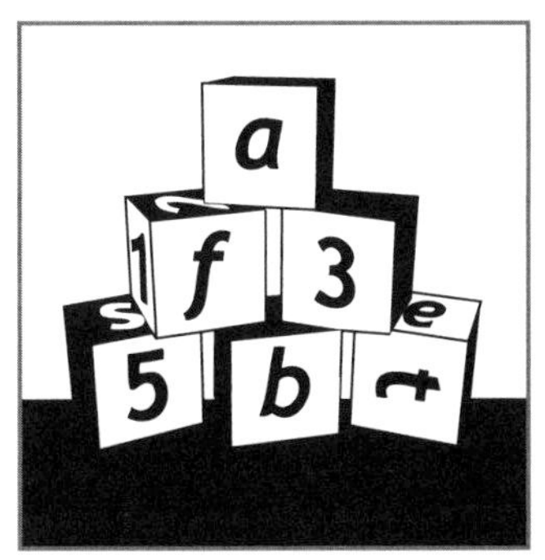

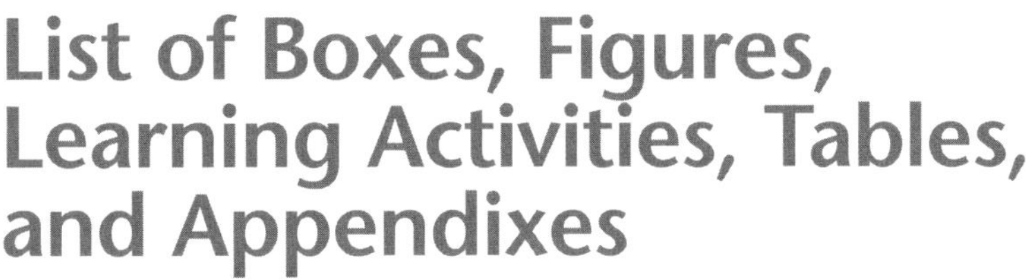

List of Boxes, Figures, Learning Activities, Tables, and Appendixes

Chapter 1

Chapter 2

Chapter 3

Chapter 4

Chapter 5

Chapter 6

Chapter 7

Chapter 8

Preface

Barbara E. Chandler, PhD, OTR/L, FAOTA

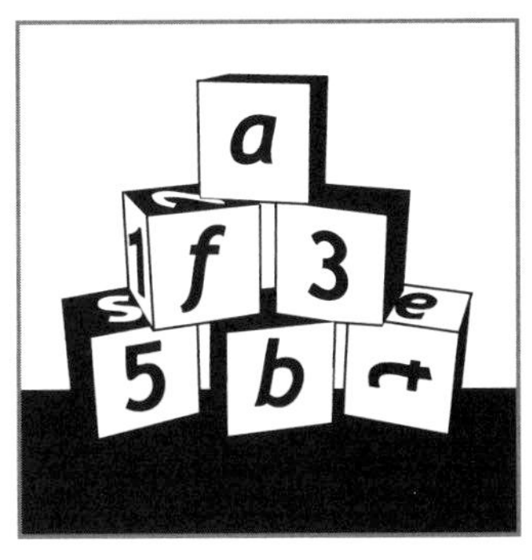

Welcome to *Early Childhood: Occupational Therapy Services for Children Birth to Five.* This publication has been designed as both an American Occupational Therapy Association (AOTA) Self-Paced Clinical Course (SPCC) and as an AOTA Press textbook to address occupational therapy practice in community-based programs for children from birth to age 5. SPCCs are a means for occupational therapists and occupational therapy assistants to develop perspective, knowledge, and skills to improve their ability to have a positive impact on the lives of the recipients of their services, including children, their families, teachers, and child care providers. Readers who successfully complete the SPCC exam can obtain continuing education credit for their efforts (continuing education materials and exam are in a separate packet). As a textbook, the content can be used in the classroom or on its own to provide information and serve as a resource.

Purpose and Objectives

The purpose of this volume is to provide an overview of the federal legislation and resulting programs and services in primarily community-based services for very young children and their families and of the role of occupational therapy within these programs. The following objectives for readers guided the selection of content for the eight chapters in this combination textbook and SPCC:

- Identify the legislative foundations of five primary community-based early childhood programs authorized by federal legislation.
- Delineate the various ways in which occupational engagement is supported by the interaction of the developmental processes.
- Identify the key principles of family-centered practices and how those principles are reflected in the services provided in the Infants and Toddlers With Disabilities Program, Head Start, and Early Head Start.

- Identify the similarities and differences in the ways in which multidisciplinary, interdisciplinary, and trandisciplinary teams are composed and work.
- Recognize the anticipated outcomes for children enrolled in the Infants and Toddlers With Disabilities Program and in Preschool Services under Part B of the Individuals With Disabilities Education Improvement Act of 2004 (IDEA).
- Delineate the use of the term *natural environments* in the implementation of the Infants and Toddlers With Disabilities Program and the profession of occupational therapy.
- Identify the uses and benefits of routines in occupational therapy with very young children and their families.
- Differentiate between play as means and play as occupation.
- Identify how assistive technology is used in early childhood programs.

Background

The content was developed with input from occupational therapists practicing in early childhood and is designed to articulate occupational therapy's perspective on, role in, and contributions to these programs. In addition, this work is informed by leading federal, state, and nongovernmental entities that are shaping current and future community-based early childhood programs. These entities include the lead agency in each state for the Infant and Toddlers With Disabilities Program, federal and state departments of education or public instruction, the Administration for Children and Families, the Maternal and Child Health Bureau, the Family Support Network, and many others.

Occupational therapy brings the perspective of occupational engagement to early childhood practice. Experiences in early childhood, beginning prenatally, resonate throughout a child's life and affect all aspects of development, both positively and negatively. How those experiences are addressed from a family-centered perspective lays the foundation and has profound implications for the child's quality of life. It is imperative that occupational therapists rise to the challenges of working in community-based early childhood programs, whose philosophies, purposes, and practices in many ways mirror long-standing beliefs and perspectives of occupational therapy. Too often, however, occupational therapy is not recognized by professional colleagues in early childhood as bringing broad-based, holistic, strengths-based, and functional perspectives and practices to early childhood community-based programs, and professionals in other fields present those practices as brand new.

This publication will assist in bridging that gap by helping occupational therapists more fully understand community-based early childhood programs and more completely articulate and practice the domain of occupational therapy. This text may also be used in preservice occupational therapy education programs to teach the structure and interaction of community-based early childhood programs and occupational therapy's role in and contributions to positive outcomes for children and families.

Overview of Chapters

This volume has an introduction and eight chapters, which are conceptually divided into three sections. The first section provides foundation information about early childhood and the community-based programs that serve young children. The introduction provides a brief historical overview of public efforts to address the needs of young children, emphasizing that legislation and programs evolve out of an interactive process of need and advocacy. Chapter 1, "Structure and Interaction of Service Provision Systems," describes the community-based early childhood programs in which occupational therapists typically practice: the Infants and Toddlers With Disabilities Program and Preschool Services, both created under IDEA; Head Start and Early Head Start; Smart Start; and child care programs under the Child Care and Development Block Grant. The commonalities and differences in these programs are discussed with emphasis on the different, yet related, purposes that they serve.

Chapter 2, "Infant, Toddler, and Young Child Development," provides a unique perspective on development as it contributes to occupational engagement. The most prevalent risk factors for interference in normal development are discussed, with implications for how those risk factors are expressed in the child's ability to engage in occupations appropriate to his or her age and the parents' ability to foster development.

Chapter 3, "Family-Centered Practice: It's All About Relationships," stresses the vital roles of parents and families in the lives of young children and how the early childhood programs are designed to strengthen the capacity of families to meet their child's needs. It closes with the eloquent voice of a parent describing her experiences raising her son with special needs.

The second section contains information about the personnel, team functioning, and evaluation requirements and processes used in early childhood programs. Chapter 4, "Models and Process of Service Provision in Early Childhood," describes types of teams working in these programs and the commonalities and differences between types of teams and how and why a type of team is used in a particular program depending on programmatic goals. The ways of interactions among these professionals, parents, and other personnel are discussed.

Chapter 5, "Evaluation, Assessment, and Outcomes in Early Childhood," describes requirements for and types of evaluation processes, assessment tools, and desired child and family programmatic outcomes. Rationales for the various types of evaluation processes in early childhood are discussed. The chapter also presents information about reporting requirements of child and family programmatic outcomes and indicators of program performance

The third section of this publication stresses the interactions of the person and the environment in the process of occupational engagement and using that knowledge in multiple ways to bring about positive changes for young children and their families. Chapter 6, "Working Where Life Is Lived: Promoting and Using the Rhythms of Daily Life," describes using and strengthening the routines, objects, and patterns of interactions found in natural environments to foster child development. The sense of place—philosophically, theoretically, and practically—is emphasized as the locus of occupational engagement. The domain of occupational therapy, as articulated in the second edition of the *Occupational Therapy Practice Framework: Domain and Process* (AOTA, 2008), is used to illustrate the process of working in natural environments (primarily the home) of young children and their families. The chapter includes information on evidence-based practice in the early childhood field.

Chapter 7, "Play in Early Childhood," coauthored by an occupational therapist and a developmental psychologist, discusses play as the primary occupation of childhood and the primary way of learning in young children. Play within the home, child care environments, and preschool; play materials; and positive play environments are discussed.

The book closes with a discussion of assistive technology. Chapter 8, "Assistive Technology and Young Children: Laying a Foundation for the Future," discusses both conceptually and practically the myriad ways in which assistive technology provides ways for people to learn and do. The chapter describes the critical role that assistive technology can play in the lives of young children by providing ways to explore and interact with people and objects in their environment. This exploration and interaction, which is vital to all later development, is described with multiple, practical examples.

Each chapter provides cases to illustrate important concepts. In addition, one case continues from chapter to chapter to illustrate the changes that have occurred in early childhood programs and services for children with disabilities over the past 60 years and the importance of advocacy in fostering those changes.

Use of the Term *Occupational Therapist*

The text refers specifically to *occupational therapists* rather than to *occupational therapy practitioners*. This choice is for ease of reading, because the occupational therapist has the primary responsibility for evaluation in the occupational therapy process; it in no way negates or diminishes the contribution of occupational therapy assistants in the evaluation and service delivery process, as outlined in the *Guidelines for Supervision, Roles, and Responsibilities During the Delivery of Occupational Therapy Services* (AOTA, 2009). The occupational therapy assistant delivers occupational therapy services under the supervision of and in partnership with the occupational therapist in accordance with state regulations, the AOTA *Standards of Practice for Occupational Therapy* (AOTA, 2005c), the *Occupational Therapy Code of Ethics (2005)* (AOTA, 2005a), the *Standards for Continuing Competence* (AOTA, 2005b), and the *Scope of Practice* (AOTA, 2004). The course is directed toward occupational therapy assistants and occupational therapists as well as occupational therapy students.

As much as possible, the terms *evaluation* and *assessment* are used in a manner consistent with the second edition of the *Framework;* however, some federal legislation, federal programs, or other discipline- or service-specific programs use the terms differently. Readers are advised to clarify the use of these terms when reading information about early childhood services from other sources.

Readers are now invited to read and reflect on the material in this volume as it applies to their current practice and future pursuits. The field of occupational therapy has significant potential to contribute to the growing understanding of the importance of the early years to a person's entire life. It is hoped that occupational therapists who use this text will be leaders in facilitating that goal.

If you want to make a difference, start at the beginning.

References

American Occupational Therapy Association. (2004). Scope of practice. *American Journal of Occupational Therapy, 58,* 673–677.

American Occupational Therapy Association. (2005a). Occupational therapy code of ethics (2005). *American Journal of Occupational Therapy, 59,* 639–642.

American Occupational Therapy Association. (2005b). Standards for continuing competence. *American Journal of Occupational Therapy, 59,* 661–662.

American Occupational Therapy Association. (2005c). Standards of practice for occupational therapy. *American Journal of Occupational Therapy, 59,* 663–665.

American Occupational Therapy Association. (2008). Occupational therapy practice framework: Domain and process (2nd ed.). *American Journal of Occupational Therapy, 62,* 625–683.

American Occupational Therapy Association. (2009). Guidelines for supervision, roles, and responsibilities during the delivery of occupational therapy services. *American Journal of Occupational Therapy, 63,* 797–803.

Individuals With Disabilities Education Improvement Act of 2004, Pub. L. 108–446, 20 U.S.C. § 1400 *et seq.*

Introduction

Barbara E. Chandler, PhD, OTR/L, FAOTA

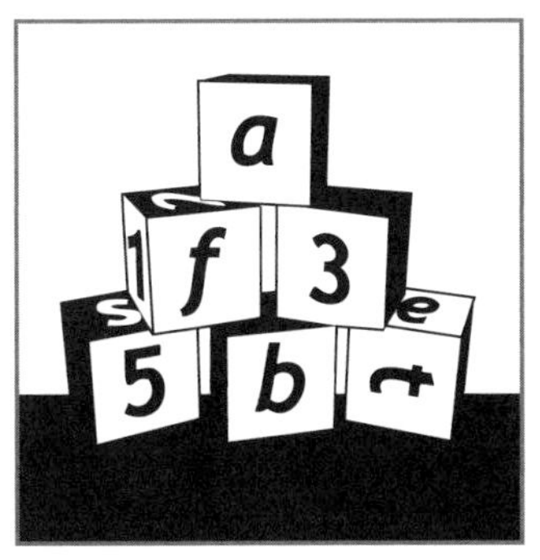

The childhood shows the man/As morning shows the day. . . .

—John Milton (1671/1823, p. 47)

When the framers of the U.S. Constitution, the Committee of Stile and Arrangement, wrote the Constitution in 1787, they began with a Preamble to state the reason for the document. It is important to remember and ponder these reasons as we discuss where we are 223 years later. The framers listed six reasons for the formation of the United States of America: "to form a more perfect Union, establish Justice, insure domestic Tranquility, provide for the common defense, promote the general Welfare, and secure the Blessings of Liberty to ourselves and our Posterity. . . ." Of the six reasons, promoting the general welfare is most closely tied to our discussions in this self-study. No matter how forward thinking these gentlemen may have been, it is a stretch of the imagination to think that they could have envisioned the early childhood programs we are about to discuss, much less occupational therapy's role in them.

What does the Constitution say about education? Nothing. Education is not mentioned. In 1787, education was predominantly a private affair, paid for by those who could afford it. By its omission, the responsibility for education belongs to each individual state as affirmed in the 10th Amendment. Ratified in 1791, the 10th Amendment states, "The powers not delegated to the United States by the Constitution, nor prohibited by it to the States, are reserved to the States respectively, or to the people."

Although the first public school in the United States was formed in the town of Dedham in the Massachusetts Bay Colony in 1634, until well into the 19th century, education was considered to be primarily the responsibility of the family. Over the next 140 years, various types of schools were formed with a variety of funding, including public funding through the Land Ordinance of 1785, which required that the 16th lot of each 6-square-mile township in the newly ceded territory west of the Appalachians be reserved for a public school. By 1870, all states provided free elementary education for children ages 6 and older.

Early childhood education was initially a private affair. The first public kindergarten in the United States opened in 1873 in St. Louis, Missouri. In 1876, Hull House in Chicago, Illinois, offered classes to teach women how to be kindergarten teachers. Kindergarten proliferated in cities, but it did not become universally offered by public schools until the 1990s.

The development of nursery schools for very young children began in the early years of the 20th century. During the Great Depression, the Works Progress Administration set up nursery schools to provide work for unemployed teachers. The nursery schools were replaced by child care centers funded by the Lanham Act in 1942 so that women who worked to support the war effort had available child care. At the end of the war, the nursery schools and child care centers closed, and 20 years passed before the federal government was again significantly involved in early childhood education.

Part of the Johnson administration's Great Society effort, Head Start was initially funded under the 1965 Elementary and Secondary Education Act (ESEA) as a cornerstone of the War on Poverty. Starting as a summer program, Head Start served 561,000 children. Fifteen of those children were in a classroom in downtown Atlanta, Georgia, taught by a 17-year-old rising high school senior—my sister. I, at 15, was her part-time assistant. The height of our technology was the flannel board (which actually was pretty nifty).

Untrained in teaching but full of good intentions, we were like many of the early "teachers." The need for a well-educated workforce to meet the complex needs of young children in poverty and the increasing number of child care facilities and nursery schools led to the development of preservice and in-service education programs to ensure the availability of competent, well-trained early childhood teachers. The dichotomy between whether the focus should be on development, on pedagogy, or on a mixture of the two and in what proportions remains unsettled.

Are early childhood programs developmental or educational? Or, because of the ages and needs of those who attend, are they both? And what of children who have some disability? Are they not part of "the people" whose "general welfare" should be promoted? As part of the Civil Rights movement, people with disabilities were being included in the initiatives that were changing how an entire nation lived, worked, and played.

The ESEA defined the role of the federal government in addressing inequality in educational opportunity on the basis of characteristics of the student (poverty). Drawing on this statutory basis (inequality), further legislation ensued. The ESEA delineated a comprehensive plan to address the differences in educational opportunity for poor children. The State Schools Act, authorized as the Elementary and Secondary Education Act Amendments of 1965, using this same basis (inequality), authorized grants to state-operated institutions and special schools in which children and youth with disabilities lived or were educated. This was the first federal grant program specifically targeted for children and youth with disabilities. Eventually, those funds became available to public school districts to assist them in integrating students with disabilities into regular and local public schools through Title VI (Aid to Handicapped Children) of the 1966 Amendments to the ESEA. This law also established the Bureau of Education for the Handicapped, which is now the Office of Special Education Programs, and what is now known as the National Council on Disability.

Services for young children with disabilities were addressed by demonstration projects (funded by the Handicapped Children's Early Education Assistance Act, passed in 1968), the purpose of which was to identify and model effective programs and practices to serve very young children (birth to age 5) with disabilities. Acknowledging the role that therapeutic services had long played with young children with disabilities, occupational therapy services were included in many of these demonstration and outreach projects (Reynolds & Fletcher-Janzen, 2001). Four years later, in 1972, children with disabilities were specifically identified as eligible for Head Start services through an amendment to the Economic Opportunity Act.

The most significant legislation in special education was passed in the late fall of 1975. The Education for All Handicapped Children Act (EHA) was the culmination of years of grassroots advocacy. At the time of its passage, it was the most heavily lobbied law in the history of Congress. Establishing aspects of public education now seen as a given, this law was revolutionary in its scope. "Free and appropriate public education" for all children with disabilities from ages 3 to 21 was mandated by Part B of the legislation. If a state did not provide education for children ages 3 to 5, however, it did not have to do so for children with disabilities in this age range, reflecting the emphasis on equality of services. Educational services in the least restrictive environment and as delineated in an individualized education program were also required.

The EHA went into effect in the fall of 1977. Although occupational therapists had worked in special education, their services were primarily provided in the specialized schools and institutional facilities in which the majority of children with disabilities had been educated or in which they lived. The passage of this law created thousands more jobs for occupational therapists. Occupational therapists, as well as physical therapists and, to a lesser extent, speech–language pathologists, who had always worked in public schools, met a critical need for educators unaccustomed to educating children with mental retardation, physical disabilities, and severe behavioral issues—not to mention feeding tubes, wheelchairs, and splints. Moving into the most public setting in many communities, occupational therapists were now visible on a daily basis to millions of people. Most teachers may not have known exactly what we could do or did, but they were glad we were there.

In 1986, 9 years after services to school-age children with disabilities were implemented, Congress amended the EHA. In recognition of greater understanding of the importance of early experiences on a child's life, Section 619 of the law mandated preschool services for students with disabilities, regardless of whether the state provided preschool for all children. In addition, a discretionary grant program (Part H in 1986, now Part C) was authorized to assist states in developing a "statewide, comprehensive, coordinated, multidisciplinary, interagency system that provides early intervention services for infants and toddlers with disabilities and their families" (20 U.S.C. § 1431(b)(1)).

This law, now known as the Individuals With Disabilities Education Improvement Act of 2004 (IDEA), reflects the continuing intersection of civil rights and special education and is a work in progress. Each reauthorization has strengthened the law and reflected current concerns, perspectives, advocacy, and knowledge. The most recent reauthorization more closely aligned IDEA with the ESEA, currently known as the No Child Left Behind Act of 2001.

Special education is increasingly viewed as a part of regular education and not a separate body of education. The early childhood programs—Part C and Section 619 of IDEA, Head Start, Early Head Start, and Smart Start—are all required to offer services in an integrated fashion, blending normal and customary services with supports, technology, enhancements, adaptations, modifications, and instruction in the natural environment in which children without disabilities live, are cared for, and are educated.

Head Start, Early Head Start, and Smart Start are designed for children whose needs do not necessarily relate to having a disability. The early childhood programs, especially Part C, have a primary emphasis on development and health, but the tension between development and education remains and is a topic of great concern as the push for academic accomplishment and "preacademic" experiences strengthens. The question of what constitutes appropriate experiences for young children is debated. Should programs foster development in all areas or focus on academics or preacademics? Is there an appropriate blend, and if so, what and how should such programs look, be organized, and staffed?

Occupational Therapy and Early Intervention

What are the roles of occupational therapists in this debate? We have a long history of working with children with disabilities, long before the laws discussed were in existence. What were our goals when working with children with disabilities? The goals focused on development and engagement in daily occupations, although we may have phrased the goals differently in the 1940s and 1950s. When development is fostered, education can occur. If formal education is attempted before the child is developmentally ready, the effort is wasted, and the outcome is not what was desired.

As we begin this study of occupational therapy in early childhood, focusing specifically on community-based programs, it is helpful to have a unifying perspective. Our profession provides us a unique and extremely important viewpoint of human development and behavior, but if unarticulated, it remains tacit and poorly understood by others. The seeming simplicity of that which is our focus—participation in daily life—belies the complexity that underlies what we do, how we do it, and why we do it. Our focus is the "magnificent mundane," carried out in our daily routines in our usual (natural) environments. We understand, perhaps better than any other profession, the complexity of what is required to foster development and participation in daily life. Our work with young children, their parents, and others must reflect this understanding and perspective.

The nation's perspective on people with disabilities was changed, in part, as it was framed in the view of equality and civil rights, leading to profound changes in legislation and practices. These changes resonated throughout society, slowly at first and then rapidly, bringing educators and others into work with young children with disabilities. These other professionals have changed how occupational therapists have practiced in early childhood and in some cases have limited practice and denied what is a rich history of home visiting, fostering parental competence related to their child's specific needs, embedding intervention into daily routines, and using play as an end and a means.

One of the most important perspectives that occupational therapists bring to early childhood practice is that of *resonation.* We look at children from a perspective of occupational engagement. What does it involve being able to do? From the ability to self-soothe at 2 weeks of age to the ability to wash hands and put on galoshes in preschool, what does it take to do a daily occupation? Like an inflated balloon that is squeezed in the hand and pops out between the fingers at the loosest point, a change or deviation in development or environment (human and nonhuman) resonates throughout the child's body and experience. How this resonation is expressed, experienced, and addressed has profound implications for the child's (and parent's) life, for the child's ability to engage in occupations that are meaningful and valuable, and for the child's quality of life.

This text is a journey of occupational therapy in early childhood. It is neither a complete clinical text nor all there is to be said about occupational therapy in early childhood in the early years of the 21st century. It is intended to provide an understanding of how federal legislation is driving practice. This legislation opens doors to occupational therapy practitioners or closes them. Legislation does not emerge from a vacuum. Remember that it was the advocacy of the American Occupational Therapy Association that ensured that occupational therapists were included in the Infants and Toddlers With Disabilities Program. As the early childhood programs grow and evolve, we are witnessing others use the language of occupational therapy and, often, our perspective and present it as though it were newly conceptualized. Occupational therapists are being told that they do not know infant and child development, daily routines, how to embed recommended activities into routines, how to work in natural environments, how to work with parents, and how to foster a child's ability to do what a child is expected to do at certain ages (Campbell, Chiarello, Wilcox, & Milbourne, 2009). This assumption is amazing because long before there were such programs, the practitioners who were then known collectively as *developmental therapists* (occupational therapists, physical therapists, and speech–language pathologists working with children with disabilities) were doing these very things.

Although other professions use the language of occupational therapy, they do not practice it in its rich fullness, and they do not fully understand occupational engagement in the manner that we do. This is not to say that these programs have not significantly enhanced the opportunities, resources, and supports available to all children, including those with disabilities. It is, however, to state that occupational therapy practitioners have much to offer children with disabilities and that we must clearly articulate and advocate for that which we bring to these programs. To do so, we must understand these programs, their conceptual basis and legislative structure, and the outcomes they foster. We must know who the fellow travelers are in these endeavors, how they perceive their roles and the programs, and how to work collaboratively with them. It is vitally important that we speak of development in terms of occupational engagement—how development allows the child to "do." We must understand the evaluation practices used in these programs and further our comfort level with the role of working as a member of a team in the evaluation process. We must be clear in articulating and demonstrating our longstanding expertise in working in natural environments and the profound depth of our understanding of the complexities of daily routines. We have always considered context as an integral part of occupational engagement, and we have always worked with families to help them build their capacity to help their children. We must be explicit about how we do so as a form of occupational engagement and the fulfillment of role. We can bring much-needed perspective to the role of play as an occupation in and of itself and as a means to further all aspects of development and self-esteem.

Probably the greatest area of change in early childhood practice is the greatly expanded use of assistive technology to support and enhance occupational engagement. From the days of the "made in the basement" laptop (which meant it fit "over the top of" the person's lap in the wheelchair) to the computerized toys readily available, occupational therapists have realized the value and used the means to provide what is now known collectively as *assistive technology.*

We cannot remain in the past or spend time lamenting that we used to do all this with our therapeutic colleagues in physical therapy and speech therapy and a few early childhood teachers. We can all do it better now because there are more supports, more funding, more fellow travelers, and greater knowledge that benefits all. We must adapt to the continuing changes that occur. We can and must articulate, demonstrate, and advocate for the unique and greatly needed services and perspective that we bring to early childhood services.

Our end is not only to educate the child but also to foster and provide what the child needs along the journey to participate fully through all the years of life.

How Very Far We Have Come

This book includes a case study that follows two children and their family for almost 60 years. The experiences of the family illustrate what many families experienced when raising a child with special needs. The case continues at the end of each chapter to assist readers in understanding the changes in attitudes, beliefs, knowledge, science, advocacy, legislation, and programs—and hope—that have occurred over this time frame. The stories of children and their families continue to unfold.

Lydia and Sam (1950)

Lydia and Sam were born during the Great Depression. They came of age during World War II, but luckily, the war ended before Sam was old enough to enlist. They married at 20 and worked in the textile mills. Lydia quit work when she became pregnant with twins. She grew a garden, canned and put up food for the winter, and started to sew for her babies. Twins ran in Sam's family, and they had a lot of advice about names and raising twins.

AnnaBelle and Daniel came 2 months early, in the winter of 1950, throwing the best laid plans awry. Annie was the larger of the babies; the doctors weren't sure that Danny was going to survive, because the cord had been around his neck, and he was blue at birth. He was stiff, had trouble feeding, and wasn't growing well. The doctors gave him oxygen because he had trouble breathing. Annie came home, but Danny had to stay in the hospital. The doctor recommended that Lydia and Sam put Danny in a state institution because he was "sure to be retarded and a cripple" and to go home and raise little Annie.

Their faith and their families would not let them do that. How were they going to raise a child like Danny? Were the doctors right? Could they care for him? Would he ever have anything but a baby's mind? When he was ready to leave the hospital, they brought Danny home.

Caring for two babies was exhausting, especially because Danny required feeding almost around the clock and threw up most of what he ate. Lydia was breastfeeding Annie and wanted to do so with Danny, but she could not stay awake all day and all night. A nurse from the health department came to help Lydia mix formulas that Danny could tolerate. When Sam's teenage sister, Maggie, graduated from high school, she came to live with them to help Lydia with the two babies.

They eventually settled into a routine. Lydia and Maggie took in sewing to make some money, and Sam worked double shifts when they were available and cut lumber on the weekends. They had medical bills to pay. When Danny was 8 months old, the pediatrician told them he was probably "some blind."

Questions

Consider what medical knowledge and procedures were available in 1950 for children who were born 2 months premature.

1. Why would the physician suggest that Sam and Lydia put Danny in a state institution?
2. Why was it common practice for a nurse to come from the health department when there was a new baby in the home?
3. What facilities were available at this time for residential care?
4. Why might Danny be blind?

References

Campbell, P., Chiarello, L., Wilcox, M., & Milbourne, S. (2009). Preparing therapists as effective practitioners in early intervention. *Infants and Young Children, 22*(1), 21–31.

Economic Opportunity Amendments of 1972, Pub. L. 92–424, 42 U.S.C. § 2701.

Education for All Handicapped Children Act of 1975, Pub. L. 94–142, 20 U.S.C. § 1400.

Education of the Handicapped Amendments of 1986, Pub. L. 99–457, 20 U.S.C. § 1400 *et seq.*

Elementary and Secondary Education Act of 1965, Pub. L. 89–10, 20 U.S.C. § 6301 *et seq.*

Elementary and Secondary Education Act Amendments of 1965, Pub. L. 89–313 (State Schools Act), 20 U.S.C. § 6301 *et seq.*

Elementary and Secondary Education Act Amendments of 1966, Pub. L. 89–750, 20 U.S.C. § 621 *et seq.*

Handicapped Children's Early Education Assistance Act of 1968, Pub. L. 90–538, 20 U.S.C. § 621 *et seq.*

Individuals With Disabilities Education Improvement Act of 2004, Pub. L. 108–446, 20 U.S.C. § 1400 *et seq.*

Lanham Act of 1942, Pub. L. 76–849.

Milton, J. (1823). *Paradise lost and paradise regained* (Book IV). Chiswick, England: C. Whittingham. (Original work published 1671)

No Child Left Behind Act of 2001, Pub. L. 107–110, 20 U.S C. § 6301 *et seq.*

Reynolds, C., & Fletcher-Janzen, E. (2001). *Concise encyclopedia of special education* (2nd ed.). Hoboken, NJ: Wiley.

CHAPTER 1

Structure and Interaction of Service Provision Systems

Barbara E. Chandler, PhD, OTR/L, FAOTA, and Anne L. Lucas, MS, OTR/L

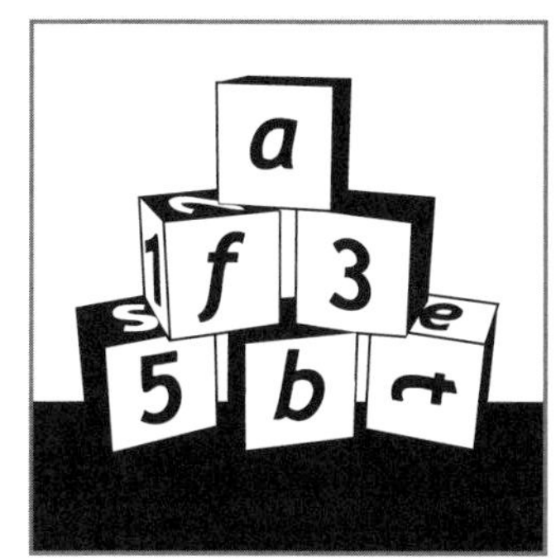

Learning Objectives

After reading this material and completing the examination, readers will be able to

- Identify the legislative foundations of early childhood programs for children with special needs in the United States;
- Delineate how the purpose and structure of a program drives the service provision process;
- Identify the basic mission and service components of the Individuals With Disabilities Education Improvement Act of 2004 (Infants and Toddlers With Disabilities Program and Preschool), Early Head Start, Head Start, and Smart Start;
- Identify the types of evidence used in early childhood developmental and educational services; and
- Identify the primary components of informed clinical opinion.

Historically, the care and education of *young children,* usually defined as birth to age 5, has been the responsibility of the family, primarily the mother. Formalized programs for young children have a relatively short history beginning in the late 19th and early 20th centuries. Formalized programs for children with special needs or disabilities have an even shorter history and have brought together health, developmental, and educational concerns. These programs have grown and evolved since their inception and now occupy a significant niche in the support systems that are available to children (and their families) with developmental issues or disabilities or who are at risk because of poverty or other factors. A thorough understanding of the purpose, structure, and function of such programs is necessary for occupational therapists to know how and why service provision is established and implemented as it is. It is also necessary to know how occupational therapy services contribute individually to and in collaboration with other services to ensure positive outcomes for children and their families who participate in these programs.

Head Start, Early Head Start, Smart Start, and the two early childhood programs of the Individuals With Disabilities Education Improvement Act of 2004 (IDEA 2004; discussed in detail in the next section) are the five most prominent federally funded programs. The involvement of occupational therapists varies in each program. Knowledge about all the programs is essential, however, because children and families transition from one program to another or may be involved in different programs at the same time, depending on need. The programs are intertwined in mission, philosophy, target population, and perspective. Although each program has its specific mission and funding, all share the belief that the early years are critically important and influence the rest of the child's life. A healthy, stimulating, and nurturing beginning is essential.

Programs and services do not emerge from a vacuum. They reflect current knowledge, a multitude of agendas, and the political will to authorize and fund them. In their final form, the programs and services are reflective of many competing interests reaching a compromise and a reconciliation of perspectives. Learning Activity 1.1 asks readers to consider the conceptual foundation of the federal early childhood programs.

Individuals With Disabilities Education Improvement Act of 2004

IDEA 2004 is the latest reauthorization of federal legislation addressing systemic efforts to foster the development of and educate infants, toddlers, children, and youth with disabilities. Each reauthorization has contained changes that strengthen and expand the scope and impact of the law. In 1986, in response to continued public advocacy and increasing evidence about the importance and influence of early

Learning Activity 1.1. Personal Reflection on the Conceptual Foundations of Early Childhood Programs

In 1988, as the American Occupational Therapy Association representative, I stood in a cavernous ballroom in a hotel in Washington, DC, and listened as C. Everett Koop, Surgeon General of the U.S. Public Health Service, dressed in a white officer's uniform, led more than 1,000 people in a chant. Although it had a cadence often heard at sports events, the chant was for a different cause. The event was the Surgeon General's Conference on Building Community-Based Service Systems for Children With Special Health Care Needs. In the call-and-response format of a preacher, he asked, "What do we want?" and the crowd responded, "Family-centered . . ." "Where do we want it?" "Community-based . . ." And how do we want it? "Coordinated care!" over and over and over again.

—*Barbara E. Chandler*

- Think about what the terms *family centered, community based,* and *coordinated care* mean individually and collectively.
- Alone or as part of a study group, identify literature in occupational therapy and other fields involved with early childhood that addresses how those concepts have been defined and implemented.
- Reflect on your own experiences with early childhood services as a professional or a parent.
- How did those conceptual foundations drive the programs and service provision?
- Do the programs deviate in any ways from the conceptual foundations? If so, how? What may have been or might currently be some reasons for this?

life experiences on all aspects of development, including learning and behavior, Congress made changes in the reauthorization of IDEA, through Part B of the act (20 U.S.C. § 1419), which added preschool to federally mandated services for children with disabilities, and Part H (now Part C), which established a discretionary grant program for early intervention services for children from birth to age 3, brought federally funded early childhood services to a large population of children with disabilities younger than age 5.

Infants and Toddlers With Disabilities Program: IDEA Part C

IDEA Part C, Infants and Toddlers With Disabilities (ITD), is a discretionary grant program that enables states and other government entities to apply for financial assistance in the development of a comprehensive, multidisciplinary, and statewide system of early intervention services for children with disabilities from birth to age 3. Part C has come to be known as *early intervention*. In the law, the term refers to the services that must be available through the ITD program.

All states, the District of Columbia, the Commonwealth of Puerto Rico, the Department of Defense, the Bureau of Indian Education, and four territories (American Samoa, Guam, the Northern Mariana Islands, and the U.S. Virgin Islands) participate in Part C. When participating in the program, states and other entities are required to make available appropriate services and supports to all eligible children and their families in accordance with an individualized family service plan (IFSP).

Whenever Congress initiates legislation to address specific needs, it provides the reasons for the legislation. Part C is based on the following five "urgent and substantial needs":

> FINDINGS AND POLICY.
>
> (a) FINDINGS.—Congress finds that there is an urgent and substantial need—
>
> (1) to enhance the development of infants and toddlers with disabilities, to minimize their potential for developmental delay, and to recognize the significant brain development that occurs during a child's first 3 years of life;
> (2) to reduce the educational costs to our society, including our Nation's schools, by minimizing the need for special education and related services after infants and toddlers with disabilities reach school age;
> (3) to maximize the potential for individuals with disabilities to live independently in society;
> (4) to enhance the capacity of families to meet the special needs of their infants and toddlers with disabilities; and
> (5) to enhance the capacity of State and local agencies and service providers to identify, evaluate, and meet the needs of all children, particularly minority, low-income, inner city, and rural children, and infants and toddlers in foster care. (20 U.S.C. § 1431)

These needs were translated into the purposes of the law. The purposes of the ITD program reflect the structure of the service provision system:

FINDINGS AND POLICY.

(b) Policy.—It is the policy of the United States to provide financial assistance to States—

(1) to develop and implement a statewide, comprehensive, coordinated, multidisciplinary, interagency system that provides early intervention services for infants and toddlers with disabilities and their families;
(2) to facilitate the coordination of payment for early intervention services from Federal, State, local, and private sources (including public and private insurance coverage);
(3) to enhance State capacity to provide quality early intervention services and expand and improve existing early intervention services being provided to infants and toddlers with disabilities and their families; and
(4) to encourage States to expand opportunities for children under 3 years of age who would be at risk of having substantial developmental delay if they did not receive early intervention services. (20 U.S.C. § 1431)

Remember this. . . .
A direct link exists between the need for the legislation and the purpose and manner in which early intervention is provided in each state.

A direct link exists between the need for the legislation and the purpose and manner in which early intervention is provided in each state. Federal regulations provide guidance on how laws are expected to be implemented by states. For IDEA Part C, the regulations that are in effect reflect IDEA 1997 (U.S. Department of Education, 1999). New Part C regulations were drafted to comply with IDEA 2004 (U.S. Department of Education, 2007); however, those regulations were withdrawn in January 2009 as a new administration came into office. As this book was going to press, final Part C regulations had not been issued. Until final regulations are issued, changes to Part C that were made in IDEA 2004 must be implemented by states while complying with the 1997 Part C regulations.

After Congress passes legislation, the implementing administrative branch of the federal government (in the case of IDEA, the US. Department of Education) issues draft regulations, accepts public comment, and eventually issues final regulations. The regulations provide specific guidance on how the law should be interpreted and the programs implemented. Learning Activity 1.2 asks you to compare the intent of the law with how is it operationalized.

The legislation dealing with the youngest of children was controversial and seen by some citizens as further and unnecessary intrusion into family life. Specific language in the law reflects this concern and allows states considerable latitude in how they establish and operate early intervention programs as long as they adhere to certain requirements. This latitude was also intended to allow states to design a system

Learning Activity 1.2. Does the Purpose Match the Product?

Review 34 C.F.R. §§ 303.1–303.5. Compare the language in the regulations with the "findings and policy" for the 2004 law (for the text of the regulations, see www.ed.gov/legislation/FedRegister/proprule/1998-2/041498d.pdf).

1. How do the regulations help to explain the law?
2. How are they the same? How are they different?

of service provision that reflected the specific needs of the state and to take advantage of and coordinate with existing programs and initiatives in the state. Congress allowed 5 years for states to plan and design a comprehensive coordinated system of early intervention services and begin full implementation of services. Most states met this deadline, but some states required more time and received a 2-year extension. Therefore, early intervention was not fully implemented until 1993, giving the program barely a 16-year history in its present form.

Since their inception, state early intervention programs have changed as a result of changes and clarification of the federal requirements, newly gained knowledge of evidence-based practices, and financial implications. Some states have changed lead agencies, whereas others have redesigned their system's infrastructure to improve accountability. Changes in practice and changes in eligibility have also occurred. For example, some states provided services to children "at risk for developmental delay" in their eligibility definition but, as a result of significant budget shortfalls, have now restricted their eligibility definition to limit eligibility to children meeting the state definition of developmental delay.

Minimum Components of a Statewide System for the ITD Program

IDEA 2004 requires that states implement 16 minimum components to ensure that a coordinated, comprehensive, multidisciplinary, interagency system of services is in place to provide appropriate early intervention services to all eligible infants and toddlers with disabilities and their families:

1. Rigorous definition of development delay
2. Early intervention services based on scientifically based research
3. Timely, comprehensive, multidisciplinary evaluation
4. Individualized family service plan
5. Comprehensive child find system
6. Public awareness program
7. Central directory
8. Comprehensive system of personnel development
9. Personnel qualifications
10. Lead agency supervision and monitoring of programs by a state
11. Policy for contracting or arranging for service providers
12. Timely reimbursement of funds/system of payments
13. Procedural safeguards
14. Data collection
15. State interagency coordinating council
16. Services provided in natural environments. (20 U.S.C. § 1433)

The law allows flexibility in how states implement and meet these 16 requirements. Therefore, it is important to understand that although each state must have these components, each state's early intervention system is unique. For example, each state must have a "rigorous definition of developmental delay," but the definitions vary from state to state. An excellent source for information about how each state has addressed the minimum components is the National Early Childhood Technical Assistance Center (NECTAC), a federally funded technical assistance center housed at the Frank Porter Graham Child Development Center of the University of North Carolina (www.nectac.org).

A review of the 16 required program components will assist occupational therapists in understanding the structure and function of the ITD (Part C) program in their state and how occupational therapy services contribute to the desired outcomes for infants, toddlers, and their families.

Component 1. Rigorous Definition of Developmental Delay

Each state is responsible for developing a rigorous definition of developmental delay. This definition determines who is eligible for early intervention services in the state. A child may qualify for early intervention in one state and not qualify in another. IDEA defines an *infant or toddler with a disability* as follows:

> (a) . . . an individual under three years of age who needs early intervention services because the individual
>
> (1) Is experiencing developmental delays, as measured by appropriate diagnostic instruments and procedures in one or more of the areas of cognitive development, physical development, communication development, social or emotional development and adaptive development; or
>
> (2) Has a diagnosed physical or mental condition that has a high probability of resulting in developmental delay. (20 U.S.C. § 1432(5)(a)(1)-(2))

Infants and toddlers at risk (both environmental and biological) may also be included in the state definition. At-risk populations may include children in extreme poverty, homeless children, or children whose parents have mental illness or mental retardation or are substance abusers. Most states do not include at-risk children. IDEA 2004 also allows states to continue to provide early intervention services to children, under certain conditions, older than age 3 until they enter kindergarten or an elementary school program (20 U.S.C. § 1435(c)). As this book was going to press, several states were in the process of adopting the Part C option.

Most states use quantifiable criteria to establish developmental delay (usually expressed as a percentage of delay) in one or more areas (such as 30% delay in one area or a 20% delay in three areas of development). *Delay* is often defined as a certain number of standard deviations (usually 1.5 or 2 standard deviations) below the mean on a norm-referenced test. All states must also use a qualitative measure, *informed clinical opinion* (also known as *clinical judgment*), which is based on professional judgment in combination with quantitative information to determine eligibility for the early intervention program

It is imperative that occupational therapists know the eligibility requirements for the early intervention program in the state in which they practice. Shackelford (2006) provided a discussion of eligibility standards and a table illustrating the eligibility requirements for each state.

Component 2. Early Intervention Services Based on Scientifically Based Research

Each state must have a policy in effect to ensure that appropriate early intervention services are made available to all eligible children and their families. The services must be based on scientifically based research to the extent feasible. It is expected that this research will guide and support effective practices to ensure positive

Learning Activity 1.3. What Is the Evidence?

Review the types of research referenced on the AOTA members-only *Evidence-Based Practice Resource Directory* Web site (www.aota.org/Educate/Research/EvidenceDirectory.aspx); the American Occupational Therapy Foundation's Evidence-Based Practice Resources site (www.aotf.org/html/evidence.html); and other databases, such as CanChild Centre for Childhood Disability Research (www.fhs.mcmaster.ca/canchild) and the Evidence-Based Practice Symposium of the University of Puget Sound (www.ups.edu/ot). Also review information at the the Orelena Hawks Puckett Institute's Web site (www.evidencebasedpractices.org) and ERIC Digests (www.ericfacility.net/ericdigests/index).

- How are the Web sites similar? How are they different?
- What levels of evidence are used? Why might they differ?
- What is the applicability of the research cited to your practice?
- How would you use this information?

educational results and outcomes for the children being served. Because the field of early intervention, in its current legislated form, is relatively young, the research base for this type of integrated service provision is continuing to evolve.

Occupational therapists are familiar with evidence-based practice. It is used to inform and guide our assessments and interventions. The American Occupational Therapy Association's (AOTA's) *Evidence-Based Practice (EBP) Resource Directory* (www.aota.org/Educate/Research/EvidenceDirectory.aspx) is an online service that links AOTA members to Web sites related to the evidence-based practice of occupational therapy. The challenge for all personnel providing early intervention services is to integrate evidence-based practices from their own discipline with the small, but growing, evidence in early childhood. Bringing together what we know and what we should do in working with young children with disabilities and their families is in its infancy in terms of evidence. Intuitively, many practitioners from various fields are in agreement.

The standards for evidence in medicine (which are based on epidemiology) are frequently based on the results of meta-analysis and randomized controlled studies, whereas the emerging evidence in the early childhood field is more often based on the synthesis of research and opinions of published experts. More information on evidence in early childhood services can be obtained from the Orelena Hawks Puckett Institute's Center for Evidence-Based Practices (CEBP; www.evidencebasedpractices.org).

The CEBP focuses on the preparation of reports and materials regarding effective early intervention, early childhood education, parent and family support, and family-centered and related practices. CEBP staff synthesize research findings, analyze databases, conduct research studies, develop evidence-based practice guides, and implement strategies to promote the adoption and use of practices informed by research findings. The integration of research and practice is guided by conceptual and methodological frameworks that emphasize the identification of practice characteristics that are associated with positive consequences and outcomes (Orelena Hawks Puckett Institute, 2009).

A helpful resource is *Evidence-Based Practice in the Early Childhood Field* (Buysse & Wesley, 2006), which discusses the evolving evidence in early childhood practices and the different perspectives on what constitutes evidence in the early childhood field, focusing on education. Learning Activity 1.3 provides an opportunity to explore some sources of evidence to guide practice in early childhood. Pay particular attention to what constitutes evidence at the different sites.

Component 3. Timely, Comprehensive, Multidisciplinary Evaluation

States must ensure a timely, comprehensive, and multidisciplinary evaluation of each infant or toddler with a disability. This evaluation must be completed within 45 days from the date of referral. The service coordinator, who is assigned for each child and family as soon as possible after referral, is responsible for coordinating the scheduling of evaluations.

Multidisciplinary means that two distinct professions or disciplines must conduct the evaluation. Ideally, one of the evaluators should practice in the area of referral need. For example, if speech concerns are the reason for referral, logically, a speech–language pathologist or someone with expertise in communication would be one of the disciplines involved in the initial evaluation and eligibility determination. This practice, however, is not required. The initial evaluation is designed to determine eligibility for the state early intervention program and to identify what services are needed. Additional evaluation may be required to further determine specific needs after the child is determined to be eligible.

The initial evaluation must focus on the following developmental areas: physical (including vision and hearing), cognition, communication, socioemotional development, and adaptive development. "When evaluating infants or toddlers, the occupational therapist considers their strengths and needs with respect to these areas of development and their ability to participate in the environment at home, school, day care and community" (AOTA, 2004, p. 683). As part of the multidisciplinary team, it is the responsibility of the occupational therapist to be sure that the tools used in the course of evaluation (e.g., diagnostic assessment instruments) are appropriate for determining eligibility in accordance with each state's requirements. A single screening instrument would not have the depth of content or specificity to determine eligibility. (See Chapter 5 for an in-depth discussion of the evaluation process and types of assessments.)

A "family-directed identification of the needs of each family of such an infant or toddler, to assist appropriately in the development of the infant or toddler" (20 U.S.C. § 1435(a)(3)) must also be conducted. Some states include this identification as part of the initial evaluation, and other states design it as part of the initial "get to know you and explain our program" visit done by the service coordinator. This process should identify the family's resources, priorities, and concerns and the supports and services necessary to enhance the family's capacity to meet the developmental needs of the child. The identification process should also yield information about what's working and what's challenging in the everyday routines and activities of the child and family. This information is used to assist in identifying appropriate IFSP outcomes and strategies for both the child and the family. Many resources regarding this process can be accessed at NECTAC (2008a, 2008b, 2009c).

"Occupational therapists have the knowledge and skills to conduct this assessment and may do so within the scope of practice and procedures of their state" (Clark, 2008, p. CE-3). As one of the basic tenets of the profession, addressing functional participation in daily routines has been a focus of occupational therapy practice since the inception of the profession, almost 100 years ago. Better than anyone else on the early intervention team, occupational therapists understand the complexity and value of routines to promote health, development, and functioning.

A required practice in determining Part C eligibility (34 C.F.R. § 303.322(c)(2)), and one supported by research (Bagnato, Smith-Jones, Matesa, & McKeating-Esterle, 2006), is the use of informed clinical opinion: "Available evidence suggests that clinical judgment or informed clinical opinion holds promise as a potentially effective strategy for use in early intervention for eligibility determination with the proper use of identified practice characteristics" (p. 6). Informed clinical opinion uses qualitative and quantitative information gathered from interviews with families, teachers, or caregivers; evaluation of the child at play; observations; and physical examinations, as well as record review and consensus among the members of the multidisciplinary evaluation team. This type of opinion has long been a part of occupational therapy practice and is an integral part of the clinical reasoning process through which decisions are made. More information about informed clinical opinion as defined by IDEA Part C can be found by reviewing Shackelford (2002).

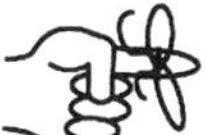

Remember this. . . . **Informed clinical opinion is often referred to as *clinical judgment* (and based on clinical reasoning) in occupational therapy and other professions that practice in medicine, health, and developmental care as well as in education.**

Informed clinical opinion is often referred to as *clinical judgment* (and based on clinical reasoning) in occupational therapy and other professions that practice in medicine, health, and developmental care as well as in education. Learning Activity 1.4 is designed to assist you in using informed clinical opinion and clinical judgment based on clinical reasoning more effectively.

Component 4. Individualized Family Service Plan

An IFSP is required to be developed for children who are determined to be eligible for Part C. The IFSP is developed by a team, which includes the parent, during an initial IFSP meeting. The meeting to develop the IFSP must be held within 45 days of referral. The IFSP is a commitment of appropriate supports and services that each eligible child and family are entitled to receive. The IFSP must contain the following elements:

- A statement of the infant or toddler's present level of development (in the five areas assessed for eligibility) based on objective criteria
- A statement of the families resources, priorities or concerns

Learning Activity 1.4. Using Informed Clinical Opinion

1. Review the issue of *NECTAC Notes* on informed clinical opinion (Shackelford, 2002; www.nectac.org/~pdfs/pubs/nnotes10.pdf).
2. Determine whether the evaluation teams in which you participate are using informed clinical opinion, as required.
   - If so, how does the use of informed clinical opinion occur?
   - If not, think about some strategies you might use to help your evaluation teams better use informed clinical opinion.
   - How does clinical reasoning contribute to informed clinical opinion?

- A statement of measurable results or outcomes for the child and family and the criteria, procedures and timelines used to determine the degree to which progress toward those outcomes is being made and whether modifications or revisions of outcomes or services are necessary
- A statement of early intervention services based on peer-reviewed research
- A statement of natural environments in which services will be provided
- The projected dates for initiation of services and the anticipated length, duration and frequency of services
- Identification of the service coordinator
- The steps to support the transition to preschool or other appropriate services. (20 U.S.C. § 1436(d)(1)-(8))

Both the law and the current regulations specifically state who must participate in the development of the IFSP. The IFSP cannot be developed solely by the service coordinator and the parent. At least one professional who participated in the multidisciplinary evaluation must be part of the team that develops the IFSP. As appropriate, service providers who will be providing services to the child and family must also participate. Just as the individualized education program (IEP) meeting for preschool and school-age children requires decision making, so too does the IFSP meeting. It is important for occupational therapists to participate in these meetings when occupational therapy services are identified and, ideally, when the occupational therapist has participated in the initial eligibility evaluation

The development of the IFSP results or outcomes (usually referred to as *goals* in occupational therapy practice) is a collaborative process. IFSP outcomes must be measurable and functional. IFSP outcomes for the child must reflect the child's developmental needs and be based on the family's priorities. IFSP results or outcomes should also reflect what is challenging for the child and the family in completing and participating in everyday routines and activities. Moreover, the family may have outcomes as well that reflect the services and supports needed by the family to enhance its capacity to support the child's development (NECTAC, 2008a). Many resources related to developing IFSPs and IFSP outcomes are available (e.g., NECTAC, 2008b, 2009b) and can inform practice in early intervention. Examples of states' IFSP forms (NECTAC, 2009d) and tools for evaluating the quality of IFSPs (NECTAC, 2009b) are also available. (See also Handley-More & Chandler, 2007.)

Component 5. Comprehensive Child Find System

Child Find under Part C is consistent with the Child Find activities under IDEA Part B. The purposes of Child Find activities under Part C are to identify, locate, and evaluate all potentially eligible infants and toddlers. IDEA 2004 requires that states establish policies and procedures for the referral of children who have been identified in "a substantiated case of child abuse or neglect" or "identified as affected by illegal substance abuse, or withdrawal symptoms resulting from prenatal drug exposure" (20 U.S.C. § 1437(a)(6)(A)-(B)). This language coincides with provisions of the Child Abuse Prevention and Treatment Act (CAPTA), which was most recently reauthorized in 2003.

> CAPTA requires that states that receive CAPTA funds develop provisions and procedures for the referral of a child under the age of 3 who is involved in a substantiated case of abuse or neglect to Early Intervention Services funded under Part C of IDEA. (NECTAC, 2009a)

States are allowed to use a screening process to determine whether a referral to early intervention is needed, and this screening process is the responsibility of the primary referral source (e.g., hospitals, physicians, social service agencies; 34 C.F.R. § 303.321(d)(3)).

Component 6. Public Awareness Program

To inform citizens of the existence of the early intervention program and how to make a referral, as well as what the program offers, the lead state agency is charged with developing a public awareness program. This program includes preparing and disseminating materials to all primary referral sources, especially physicians and hospitals but also schools, libraries, social service agencies, child care settings, and other places in the community. The materials should include information for parents (especially parents of premature infants or infants with other physical risk factors associated with learning or developmental complications) about the availability of services under Part C as well under Part B (preschool special education; 20 U.S.C. § 1419). Procedures for the dissemination of information to parents by primary referral sources must also be established along with procedures for making referrals.

Occupational therapists may participate in Child Find and public awareness activities by assisting the state in the development and dissemination of these materials, presenting to various groups on early intervention services, and participating in the screening of infants and toddlers.

Component 7. Central Directory

The state must compile a directory of early intervention services and resources, including services, resources, and experts in the state and available research and demonstration projects. These directories reside in different agencies in different states. The Family Support Network of North Carolina's Web site (www.fsnnc.org/other CDRs/otherCDRs.aspx) provides a list of central directory information in each state.

Component 8. Comprehensive System of Personnel Development

Systems of service provision like the ITD program are dependent on having adequate numbers of appropriately trained professionals and paraprofessionals who refer to and implement the program. Each state's comprehensive system of personnel development (CSPD) must include strategies for "recruitment and retention" of service providers and the preparation and training of personnel to "coordinate transition services" for infants and toddlers with disabilities from Part C to Part B of the act (20 U.S.C. § 1435(a)(8)(A)(i)-(iii)). IDEA also specifies that states may include training of personnel to work in rural and inner-city areas and on specific developmental areas (e.g., social and emotional development). "Occupational therapy practitioners can work with their states to enhance recruitment and retention of occupational therapy personnel. They also can work with states to set up a plan for ongoing continuing education for practitioners" (Clark, 2008, p. CE–4). Institutions of higher education (referred to as *IHE* in much of the information provided by federal government sources) in each state can look to the CSPD for guidance on the competencies practitioners should possess and be sure that content is incorporated in preservice education.

Component 9. Personnel Qualifications

Each state must develop policies and procedures related to the qualifications of personnel who provide early intervention services within that state. The qualifications should be "consistent with any state-approved or recognized certification, licensing, registration, or other comparable requirements that apply to the area in which such personnel are providing early intervention. . . ." (20 U.S.C. § 1435(a)(9)). The law also states that

> nothing in this subchapter (including this paragraph) shall be construed to prohibit the use of paraprofessionals and assistants who are appropriately trained and supervised in accordance with State law, regulation, or written policy, to assist in the provision of early intervention services. . . .

In other words, IDEA provides flexibility for states in establishing or recognizing new early intervention "paraprofessionals" within the parameters established by each state to do so. Some states are able, within the authority of state law, to develop or create new types of recognized early intervention disciplines filled by professionals or paraprofessionals that go beyond the professions listed in 20 U.S.C. § 1432(4)(F).

> Some states are also establishing additional requirements with regard to occupational therapy practice in the early intervention system; and in some instances, the requirements may restrict the role of occupational therapy. Occupational therapy practitioners must work with their state lead agency, regulatory agency, and state association to ensure that these Part C requirements do not restrict occupational therapy practice within the state. (Clark, 2008, p. CE–4)

Because each state's personnel requirements are different, it is imperative to know the requirements in your state for practicing occupational therapy in early intervention services.

Component 10. Lead Agency Supervision and Monitoring of Programs by a State

Part of the flexibility written into the law is the provision related to the designation of a lead agency. Recognizing that each state had different configurations of programs and agencies working with young children (e.g., health, development, and social services), the law requires the governor of each state to designate a lead agency whose responsibility it is to administer the state's early intervention program for infants and toddlers with disabilities. Although the early intervention program is authorized by federal education legislation and is federally administered by the Office of Special Education Programs (OSEP) in the U.S. Department of Education, Part C lead agencies include state health agencies, human services agencies, education agencies, social service, and other state agencies. The lead agency is the "single line of responsibility" for the early intervention program in the state. This responsibility includes the following activities:

- The general administration and supervision of the program
- Monitoring of regional and local Part C programs and activities
- Enforcement of the law
- Provision of technical assistance
- Ensuring the correction of noncompliance. (34 C.F.R. § 303.501)

The lead agency is also responsible for coordinating efforts among multiple state agencies and programs, coordinating financial matters, and developing formal interagency agreements within the state and procedures to resolve disputes or disagreements among these agencies or between individuals receiving services and the providing agencies. Occupational therapists should know what the state's lead agency is as well as the other cooperating agencies. A list of lead agencies is available at www.nectac.org/partc/ptclead.asp.

Component 11. Policy for Contracting or Arranging for Service Providers

The state must have contracts in place or make other arrangements with service providers to provide early intervention services in the state. These contracts must require that all early intervention services meet state standards and be consistent with Part C requirements. The state's policy on contracting or arranging for services must specify the conditions that must be met by service providers and the process for providers to enter into these contracts or arrangements. Because many occupational therapists work as providers in early intervention, it is particularly important that providers understand the conditions for participation as a provider of early intervention services.

Component 12. Timely Reimbursement of Funds/System of Payment

Funding levels and funding sources for Part C services vary from state to state. All states participating in Part C receive federal funds to support the provision of early intervention services. These funds may be used to support the structural aspects of the early intervention system, including coordination among the various agencies and the provision of direct services (e.g., the initial eligibility evaluation, IFSP development, service coordination, IFSP services). States must have interagency agreements with various public funding sources (e.g., Title V of the Social Security Act of 1935 [Maternal and Child Health]; Medicaid; Part B of IDEA, Developmental Disabilities) to pay for early intervention services. All federal Part C funds are considered "payor of last resort," meaning that all other funding sources must be exhausted before Part C funds can be used for the provision of services. However, Part C funds can be used on an interim basis while awaiting payment from other legitimate sources.

Medicaid has become one of the primary methods of payment for early intervention services. Families may be expected to pay through their private insurance or on a sliding fee scale based on income. These practices vary from state to state, but more and more states are implementing some methods of family cost participation.

As in any practice setting, when accessing third-party reimbursement, occupational therapists must be aware of the various funding sources used and meet the reporting and billing requirements of each, including prior approval of services.

Component 13. Procedural Safeguards

IDEA lists eight procedural safeguards (or rights) required in the statewide system, including the right to

(1) timely resolution of complaints by parents
(2) confidentiality of personally identifiable information
(3) accept or decline any early identification services
(4) examine records relating to screening, eligibility, and the IFSP
(5) protect the rights of infants or toddlers if parents are unknown or cannot be found through the appointment of surrogate parent
(6) written prior notice of initiated changes or refusal to initiate changes in any part of the infant's or toddler's eligibility for or participation in the program
(7) an assurance that the notice fully informs parents in their native language of all procedures
(8) the right of parents to use mediation. (20 U.S.C. § 1439(a))

Occupational therapists must be aware of these rights and, when serving as a service coordinator, review and adhere to these rights with the family. It is also essential to be knowledgeable about the states' procedures that families must use when filing a complaint or requesting a due process hearing or mediation.

Component 14. Data Collection

Each state must have a process for collecting, using, and reporting data to the federal government, the state legislature, and the governor, as required. One of the new federal reporting requirements for Part C (and Part B) established by IDEA 2004 is the state performance plan (SPP). The SPP, which is submitted to the U.S. Department of Education, is a 6-year accountability plan for states and local programs that summarizes IDEA priorities into 14 federally established indicators. The indicators were determined by the U.S. Department of Education to most closely align with improving educational results for children and families. Each indicator includes a rigorous target established by either OSEP (e.g., compliance indicators = 100%) or the state (performance indicators = state-established target).

States also must submit an annual performance report (APR) that describes their performance in meeting each indicator's target and compares current performance with the previous year's performance. The APR and the SPP are required to be posted on each state lead agency's Web site. The state is also responsible for publicly reporting each local early intervention program's performance on several of the SPP indicators. The U.S. Department of Education responds to each state's SPP and APR in writing and makes determinations of each state's performance. Determination letters for each state are posted on the U.S. Department of Education's Web site (www.ed.gov/fund/data/report/idea/partcspap/index.html; see Table 1.1 for a list of the SPP indicators).

Table 1.1. Office of Special Education SPP Indicators for Part C

No.	Indicator	Description
C1	Timely services	Percentage of infants and toddlers with IFSPs who receive the early intervention services in a timely manner
C2	Natural environment	Percentage of infants and toddlers with IFSPs who primarily receive early intervention services in the home or in programs with typically developing children
C3	Early childhood outcomes	Percentage of infants and toddlers with IFSPs who demonstrate improved A. Positive socioemotional skills (including social relationships) B. Acquisition and use of knowledge and skills (including early language and communication) C. Use of appropriate behaviors to meet their needs
C4	Family-centered services survey	Percentage of families participating in Part C who report that early intervention services have helped families A. Know their rights B. Communicate effectively with their children C. Help their children develop and learn
C5	Child Find 0–1	Percentage of infants and toddlers birth to 1 year with IFSPs compared with A. Other states with similar eligibility definitions B. National data
C6	Child Find 0–3	Percentage of infants and toddlers birth to 3 years with IFSPs compared with A. Other states with similar eligibility definitions B. National data
C7	Timely evaluation and assessment	Percentage of eligible infants and toddlers with IFSPs for whom an evaluation and assessment and an initial IFSP meeting were conducted within the 45-day timeline from referral
C8	Transition C to B	Percentage of all children exiting Part C who received timeline transition planning to support the transition to preschool and other appropriate community services by their third birthday, including A. IFSPs with transition steps and services B. Notification to local education agency if child is potentially eligible for Part B C. Transition conference if child is potentially eligible
C9	General supervision	General supervision system (including monitoring, complaints, hearings, etc.) identifies and corrects noncompliance as soon as possible but in no case later than 1 year from identification
C10	Complaints resolved within 60-day timeline	Percentage of signed written complaints with reports issued that were resolved within the 60-day timeline or a timeline extended for exceptional circumstances with respect to a particular complaint
C11	Due process hearings	Percentage of fully adjudicated due process hearing requests that were fully adjudicated within the applicable timeline
C12	Hearing requests to resolution sessions resolved	Percentage of hearing requests that went to resolution sessions that were resolved through resolution session settlement agreements (applicable if Part B due process procedures are adopted)
C13	Mediations that resulted in agreements	Percentage of mediations held that resulted in mediation agreements
C14	Timely and accurate date	State-reported data (618 and SPP and APR) are timely and accurate

Note. IFSP = individualized family service plan; SPP = state performance plan; APR = annual performance report.

Source. U.S. Department of Education (2010b).

Two SPP indicators deserve special mention: early childhood outcomes (Indicator C3) and family-centered services survey (Indicator C4). States are required to collect data on early childhood outcomes to report on the percentage of infants and toddlers who demonstrate improved

- Positive socioemotional skills (including social relationships),
- Acquisition and use of knowledge and skills (including early language and communication), and
- Use of appropriate behaviors to meet infants' and toddlers' needs (Indicator C3).

Local early intervention programs must report each child's performance in these three areas at entrance (near initial IFSP meeting) and at exit (near transition). Some states also collect child outcome data annually at the time of the annual IFSP meeting. Most states use the Child Outcomes Summary Form (COSF; Early Childhood Outcomes Center, n.d.) to compile evaluation and assessment data from numerous sources (e.g., observation, formal testing, and parent report) on the child's functional skills. Other states use data only from standardized or curriculum-based assessments.

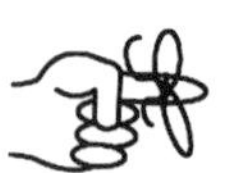

Remember this. . . .
A goal is what we work toward. An outcome is what the end result really is.

Occupational therapists working with IFSP teams must be aware of these requirements; as professionals who focus on function, they possess knowledge and skills related to these three outcomes areas. (See Chapter 5 for further discussion of outcomes and a recommended decision tree related to scoring the COSF.) The occupational therapist's input can inform the team on the scope of practice and expertise of occupational therapy and can help document the infant's or toddler's progress. The state is required to aggregate child outcome data and report on the state's overall performance on this indicator. More information on the purpose of child outcomes and the collection and use of child outcomes data can be obtained through review of resources provided by the Early Childhood Outcomes Center (www.fpg.unc.edu/~eco/index.cfm).

States must also report data in each APR on the percentage of families who report that early intervention services have helped their family

- Know their rights,
- Effectively communicate their children's needs, and
- Help their children develop and learn (Indicator C4).

States typically collect these data from families through a family survey. Each state is responsible for establishing its procedures for the dissemination of family surveys and the collection and analyses of family survey data. Just as the information on each child is aggregated for reporting child outcomes, so too are family outcome data.

Component 15. State Interagency Coordinating Council

To receive Part C grant funds, states must establish an interagency coordinating council (ICC) consisting of parents; service providers; state legislative personnel; personnel preparation institutions (e.g., universities); and representatives from the agencies responsible for early intervention services, preschool services, Medicaid, Head Start, child care, health insurance, office of coordination of education of homeless children and youth, foster care, mental health, and other representatives (e.g., Bureau of Indian Affairs). State agencies have different names in each state, and some agencies are responsible for several types of services. The governor is responsible for appointing the members and the chairperson of the council.

The ICC meets at least quarterly to advise and assist the lead agency in developing and implementing policies for the statewide system, achieving coordination and cooperation across agencies, and identifying necessary supports (e.g., fiscal, other) for the Part C system, including transition and other needs the state may have. The council's role in guiding the statewide system is crucial. In many states, local ICCs have been established to address specific needs in a geographical or jurisdictional area. Occupational therapists should consider serving on state and local ICCs, because they can provide strong positive direction for children and services in their state (Clark, 2008).

It is important to know and understand the functions of the lead agency in the state in which you practice. This information will help you identify and participate in opportunities to guide services and advocate for appropriate services and appropriate participation of occupational therapists in these programs. Learning Activity 1.5 will help you gain a better understanding of the work of the lead agency in your state.

Component 16. Services Provided in Natural Environments

States are required to develop policies and procedures to ensure that early intervention services are provided in natural environments to the maximum extent appropriate. The IFSP team is responsible for determining the natural environments in which early intervention services will be provided and developing a written justification if services will not be provided in natural settings.

The occupational therapy profession has always embraced the concept of natural environments. Consideration of a person's functioning in his or her living environment is an integral component of occupational therapy services in assisting the person in gaining or regaining daily occupations. A growing body of literature describes the provision of early intervention services in natural environments and its intent. Occupational therapists must be aware of this relatively new literature addressing natural learning opportunities, participatory learning (Dunst, Bruder, Trivette, Hamby, et al., 2001; Dunst, Bruder, Trivette, Raab, & McLean, 2001; Hanft & Pilkington, 2000), and teaming or coaching practices in early childhood (Hanft, Rush, & Shelden, 2004). This literature builds on the foundations of how children learn best and supports contextualized practice to assist family members and caregivers to enhance their child's learning and development through naturally occurring learning opportunities in everyday routines and activities. Contextualized

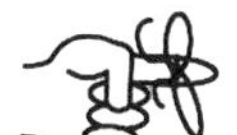

Remember this. . . .
Consideration of a person's functioning in his or her living environment is an integral component of occupational therapy services in assisting the person in gaining or regaining daily occupations.

Learning Activity 1.5. For a Coordinated System of Care

Identify the lead agency in your state for the Part C program.

- What other state agencies participate in your state interagency coordinating council (ICC)?
- Why were these agencies included? What role does each play in the funding and service provision process?
- Is there a local ICC in your area? What are the opportunities for participation? Remember, all politics is local.

practice takes advantage of the myriad opportunities available within the home or community setting for children to learn and use what they have learned. Occupation therapists are reminded that much can be learned from the rich history of home visiting in the health and social services field. In the natural environment, the distinction between expected support, embedded support, and enacted support is evident. In many ways, the provision of early intervention services is the current enactment of what Selma Fraiberg (1987) called "kitchen table therapy" in the early days of infant mental health. It is, indeed, providing services "where life is lived" (Chandler, 2009).

Further discussion of family centered care and working in the natural environments is provided in Chapters 3 and 6.

Transition From Infant–Toddler With Disabilities Program Services

As children "age out" of early intervention services, they often transition to preschool services. Although the transition from Part C to preschool special education and other community services is not a separate component of the law, its relevance to providing high-quality practices in early childhood and improving results for children and families requires special mention. States are responsible for ensuring a smooth transition for children receiving early intervention services to preschool or other appropriate services. Activities that the Part C program must carry out to support a smooth transition include the following:

1. Notifying the local education agency (LEA) in the area in which a child resides that the child will shortly reach the age of eligibility for preschool services under Part B of IDEA (This notification serves as referral to Part B services.)
2. For children potentially eligible for preschool special education services under Part B of IDEA, convening a transition conference (with parent approval) among the Part C program staff, the child's family, [and] LEA at least 90 days and up to 9 months prior to the child's third birthday
3. For children who may not be eligible for preschool special education services, with approval of the family, making reasonable efforts to convene a transition conference among the Part C program staff, the family, and providers of other appropriate community services that the child may receive at exit from Part C
4. Reviewing the child's program options from the child's third birthday through the remainder of the school year
5. Establishing a transition plan in collaboration with the LEA or providers of other appropriate community services. (20 U.S.C. § 1437(a)(9))

Occupational therapists need to be aware of their state's procedures related to transition from Part C to preschool special education services or other community programs, because each state has flexibility in determining how these requirements are implemented. For example,

- Some states begin conversations with families about transition when children enter services, whereas others wait until the child is about age 2.

- Some states combine the transition conference with an IFSP meeting or review, whereas other states have a transition conference separate from IFSP meeting or review.

Although service coordinators are responsible for facilitating the development of the transition plan and typically coordinate the transition process, some states permit service providers to initiate the transition referral to preschool special education or other community agencies.

The early intervention program has fundamentally altered the ways in which early intervention services are provided to our youngest citizens. In partnerships with families, health, developmental, and early learning experiences are coordinated with medical and social services so that infants and toddlers with (or, in some states, at risk for) disabilities experience coordinated care to minimize the effects of the disability or risk and, one hopes, to maximize developmental potential. Although early intervention continues to be a discretionary grant program in which states choose to participate, preschool services are required to be offered to children with disabilities under IDEA.

Preschool Grants Program: IDEA Part B

All states are now required by federal law to provide preschool special education services to children with disabilities from age 3 to age 5, regardless of whether they offer education to preschool children without disabilities. IDEA Part B says that states are eligible to receive federal funds:

> (a) In General.—The Secretary shall provide grants under this section to assist States to provide special education and related services, in accordance with this part—
>
> (1) to children with disabilities aged 3 through 5, inclusive; and
>
> (2) at the State's discretion, to 2-year-old children with disabilities who will turn 3 during the school year.
>
> (b) Eligibility.—A State shall be eligible for a grant under this section if such State—
>
> (1) is eligible under section 612 to receive a grant under this part; and
>
> (2) makes a free appropriate public education available to all children with disabilities, aged 3 through 5, residing in the State. (20 U.S.C. § 1419)

States may also reserve a percentage of funds

> (5) to provide early intervention services (which shall include an educational component that promotes school readiness and incorporates preliteracy, language, and numeracy skills) in accordance with Part C to children with disabilities who are eligible for services under this section and who previously received services under Part C until such children enter, or are eligible under state law to enter, kindergarten; or
>
> (6) at the state's discretion, to continue service coordination or case management for families who receive services under Part C. (20 U.S.C. § 1419 (f)(5)-(6))

These provisions reference the Part C Option (20 U.S.C. § 1435(c)) previously discussed and found in the law under Flexibility to Serve Children 3 Years of Age Until Entrance Into Elementary School. Although the intent is to have a seamless system of service provision that aids in transition from a family-oriented, home-based, developmental program to one that is educationally focused and provided in centers or schools, no state has yet implemented the Part C option. Because § 1419 is in Part B of IDEA, requirements for the provision of free appropriate public education (FAPE) also apply to preschool special education services.

Purpose of IDEA Part B

In accordance with IDEA 2004, the purposes of Part B are as follows:

> (A) To ensure that all children with disabilities have available to them a free appropriate public education that emphasizes special education and related services designed to meet their unique needs and prepare them for further education, employment, and independent living;
>
> (B) To ensure that the rights of children with disabilities and their parents are protected;
>
> (C) To assist States, localities, educational service agencies, and Federal agencies to provide for the education of all children with disabilities. (20 U.S.C. § 1400(d)(1))

The law also states that another purpose of Part B is "to assess, and ensure the effectiveness of, efforts to educate children with disabilities" (20 U.S.C. § 1400(d)(4)). For IDEA Part B, the regulations that are in effect reflect IDEA 2004 (U.S. Department of Education, 2006).

It is important that occupational therapists understand the purpose and implementing structure of each program authorized under IDEA. Learning Activity 1.6 provides an opportunity to compare and contrast the purposes and structure of the programs.

Child With a Disability

Children who are eligible to receive preschool special education services under Part B of IDEA must be determined to be a "child with a disability." The federal regulations implementing Part B define a child with a disability who may be eligible for

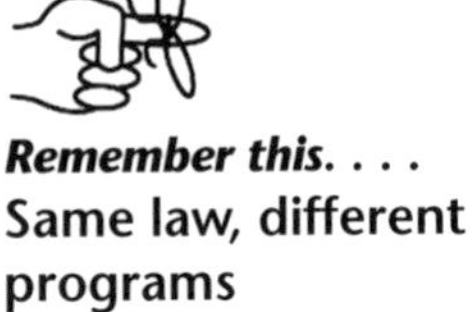

Remember this. . . .
Same law, different programs

Learning Activity 1.6. Same Law, Different Programs

Review the Findings and Policy section of the IDEA Infants and Toddlers With Disabilities Program (20 U.S.C. § 1431(b)(1)-(4)) and the Purpose of Part B (20 U.S.C. § 1400(d)(1)).

- After reviewing the purposes of Part C and Part B (which includes preschool), identify the differences in the purposes of these programs.
- What are the similarities?
- How do these differences affect how occupational therapy services are provided in these programs?

preschool services in one of two ways. An *eligible child* is defined as having been evaluated in accordance with Part B requirements and

> as having mental retardation, a hearing impairment (including deafness), a speech or language impairment, a visual impairment (including blindness), a serious emotional disturbance (referred to in this part as "emotional disturbance"), an orthopedic impairment, autism, traumatic brain injury, another health impairment, a specific learning disability, deafblindness, or multiple disabilities, and who, by reason thereof, needs special education and related services. (34 C.F.R. § 300.8(a)(1))

If a child has one of the disabilities but only needs a related service and not special education, the child is not considered a child with a disability unless the related service is considered special education rather than a related service under state standards. For example, in some states speech–language therapy is considered special education rather than a related service. A child may need occupational therapy as a related service to benefit from the speech–language therapy (which is considered special education). A child with a disability who does not need special education may participate in occupational therapy under what is known as a *504 plan,* which receives its name from Section 504 of the Rehabilitation Act of 1973. These services would focus on accommodations and modifications to allow the child to access the educational environment and would not include specialized instruction.

The second way in which a child may be deemed eligible for preschool services is through an evaluation process that determines the child is experiencing developmental delays as defined by the state. The evaluation criteria for the state definition of *developmental delay* may determine a child to have a disability and be eligible for special education and related services. The developmental delay must be measured by appropriate diagnostic instruments and procedures in one or more of the following areas: physical development, cognitive development, communication development, social or emotional development, or adaptive development (34 C.F.R. § 300.111(b)). Because IDEA allows each state to specify the definition of developmental delay and the age range, within the broader range of ages 3 to 9 years, a child may be eligible under this definition for preschool services in one state but not in another. Danaher (2007) provided a detailed discussion of the variability in states' definitions of developmental delay and eligibility requirements for preschool services.

Free Appropriate Public Education

Part B of IDEA defines *FAPE* as special education and related services that are provided at public expense, under public supervision and direction, and without charge and in accordance with an IEP (34 C.F.R. § 300.17). For children who have been receiving early intervention services, each state must ensure that FAPE is available to each eligible child beginning no later than the child's third birthday. As a result, an IEP (or IFSP, should any state exercise the Part C Option) must be in effect by that date. If a child's third birthday occurs during the summer, the child's IEP team must determine the date when services under the IEP or IFSP will begin (34 C.F.R. § 300.101(b)). Extended school year services must also be made available as necessary to ensure the provision of FAPE if determined by the IEP team (34 C.F.R. § 300.106) to be necessary. Although occupational therapy is a primary developmental service under Part C, it is defined as a related service in preschool special education, just as it is in school age services under Part B of IDEA. This distinction is extremely important. *Occupational therapy under Part C in the early intervention program should never be referred to as a* related service; *that term is only applicable under Part B of IDEA.*

Least Restrictive Environment (LRE)

Part B of IDEA requires that

> to the maximum extent appropriate, children with disabilities, including children in public or private institutions or other care facilities, are educated with children who are nondisabled; and . . . special classes, separate schooling, or other removal of children with disabilities from the regular educational environment occurs only if the nature or severity of the disability is such that education in regular classes with the use of supplementary aids and services cannot be achieved satisfactorily. (34 C.F.R. § 300.114(a)(2))

The proposed benefits of LRE are numerous for children with and without disabilities and their families, according to Wolery (1994). Wolery (1994) also reported that inclusion of young children with and without disabilities in the same class does not guarantee desirable outcomes. Desirable outcomes occur when the classroom is a high-quality environment and classroom staff have the necessary supports for individualizing instruction with children who have disabilities. More information about these two important conditions can be accessed on the NECTAC Web site (Wolery, n.d.). The same, of course, can be said for any classroom.

Because LRE requirements are similar to Part C's requirement to provide early intervention services in natural environments, many state preschool special education programs and Part C programs are working collaboratively to develop a continuum of community-based inclusive settings for children from birth through age 5. Occupational therapists can play a crucial role in ensuring the success of inclusion and LRE by supporting preschool teachers in adapting activities and environments to ensure that preschool children with disabilities are included and learning in regular education activities and environments.

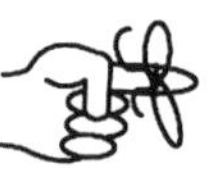

Remember this. . . .
Working in natural environments or where people must function on a daily basis is an integral part of community-based occupational therapy practice.

Working in natural environments or where people must function on a daily basis is an integral part of community-based occupational therapy practice. Even occupational therapy services in institutional settings, such as a rehabilitation center of a hospital, have the goal of enabling people participating in occupational therapy to function in their regular environment. Learning Activity 1.7 asks that you contemplate what it means to work in natural environments and LREs.

Evaluation and Eligibility Determination

For children referred to preschool special education services, local education agencies (LEAs) are required to conduct an initial evaluation to determine whether the child has a disability and to determine the educational needs of the child. The initial evaluation must be conducted within 60 days of receiving parental consent for the evaluation, unless the state has established a different time frame in which the evaluation must be conducted (34 CFR § 300.301). Reevaluations typically do not

Learning Activity 1.7. Least Restrictive Environments and Natural Environments

Preferably with a study group, read and then further explore through discussion how these terms are described and used in professional literature.

- What are the similarities between the LRE requirements for Part B and the natural environment requirements for Part C?
- What constitutes a high-quality classroom environment that is conducive for success with inclusive practices?
- Is the LRE always the "regular" environment? Why? Why not?

---

occur more than once a year but must occur at least once every 3 years (unless the parent and staff agree that the reevaluation is unnecessary). Reevaluations may occur more frequently if the child's educational or related services needs warrant reevaluation or if requested by the parent.

Occupational therapists participate in conducting evaluations and reevaluations of preschool children with disabilities or children suspected of having a disability on the basis of the educationally related needs of each child. Because each state establishes procedures for completion of evaluations, including assessment tools that are appropriate for use, occupational therapists must be aware of their state's protocols and the roles and responsibilities of the therapist in conducting evaluations. (See Chapter 5, which addresses considerations in choosing assessment instruments and evaluation procedures.)

Individualized Education Program

An *IEP* is defined as follows:

> a written statement for each child with a disability that is developed, reviewed, and revised in an [IEP] meeting (34 C.F.R. § 300.320(a)). The IEP must include—
>
> (1) A statement of the child's present levels of academic achievement and functional performance, including—
>
> (i) How the child's disability affects the child's involvement and progress in the general education curriculum (i.e., the same curriculum as for nondisabled children); or
>
> (ii) For preschool children, as appropriate, how the disability affects the child's participation in appropriate activities;
>
> (2)
>
> (i) A statement of measurable annual goals, including academic and functional goals designed to—
>
> (A) Meet the child's needs that result from the child's disability to enable the child to be involved in and make progress in the general education curriculum; and
>
> (B) Meet each of the child's other educational needs that result from the child's disability;
>
> (ii) For children with disabilities who take alternate assessments aligned to alternate achievement standards, a description of benchmarks or short-term objectives;

(3) A description of—

(i) How the child's progress toward meeting the annual goals described in paragraph (2) of this section will be measured; and

(ii) When periodic reports on the progress the child is making toward meeting the annual goals such as through the use of quarterly or other periodic reports (concurrent with the issuance of report cards) will be provided;

(4) A statement of the special education and related services and supplementary aids and services, based on peer-reviewed research to the extent practicable, to be provided to the child, or on behalf of the child, and a statement of the program modifications or supports for school personnel that will be provided to enable the child—

(i) To advance appropriately toward attaining the annual goals;

(ii) To be involved in and make progress in the general education curriculum in accordance with paragraph (a)(1) of this section, and to participate in extracurricular and other nonacademic activities; and

(iii) To be educated and participate with other children with disabilities and nondisabled children in the activities described in this section;

(5) An explanation of the extent, if any, to which the child will not participate with nondisabled children in the regular class and in the activities described in paragraph (a)(4) of this section;

(6)

(i) A statement of any individual appropriate accommodations that are necessary to measure the academic achievement and functional performance of the child on State and districtwide assessments consistent with section 612(a)(16) of the Act; and

(ii) If the IEP Team determines that the child must take an alternate assessment instead of a particular regular State or districtwide assessment of student achievement, a statement of why—

(A) The child cannot participate in the regular assessment; and

(B) The particular alternate assessment selected is appropriate for the child; and

(7) The projected date for the beginning of the services and modifications described in paragraph (a)(4) of this section, and the anticipated frequency, location, and duration of those services and modifications. (34 C.F.R. § 300.320(a)(1)-(7))

Similar to the requirements for the development of the IFSP under Part C of IDEA, the IEP must be developed by a team of professionals at an IEP meeting. The IEP meeting must be held within 30 days of determining that the child needs special education and related services. A model IEP form is available from the U.S. Department of Education (www.ed.gov/policy/speced/guid/idea/modelform-iep.doc).

Occupational therapists may be included as participants in the IEP meeting, depending on the needs of the child. Families are also important participants in the IEP meeting. In fact, LEAs are required to take steps to ensure that one or both of the

Learning Activity 1.8. What Is a Plan, and What Is a Program?

Review the model individualized education program (IEP) form at www.ed.gov/policy/speced/guid/idea/modelform-iep.doc and one state's individualized family service plan form (IFSP; available at www.nectac.org/topics/families/stateifsp.asp). Identify similarities and differences between the IEP and IFSP.

---

parents are present at each IEP team meeting or are afforded the opportunity to participate. OSEP has developed a model IEP form (U.S. Department of Education, n.d.) that complies with the federal content requirements for use and adaptation by states.

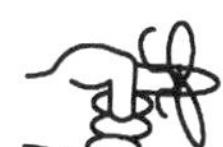

Remember this. . . .
Although both the IEP and the IFSP are individualized descriptions of services, the documents differ. One is a family plan, and the other is a program of services for an individual.

Although both the IEP and the IFSP are individualized descriptions of services, the documents differ. One is a family plan, and the other is a program of services for an individual. Learning Activity 1.8 asks you to compare and contrast the two documents.

Transition to Preschool or Other Services

States are responsible for ensuring that children participating in early intervention programs under Part C and that children who will participate in preschool special education services experience a smooth and effective transition. Each LEA is required to participate in the transition planning conference arranged by the local Part C agency and, at the request of the parent, invite the Part C service coordinator or other representatives to the initial IEP meeting to ensure a smooth transition. For children transitioning from Part C, the IEP team must consider an IEP that contains the IFSP content and is developed in accordance with IEP procedures. The IFSP may serve as the child's IEP if it is consistent with state policy and is agreed to by the LEA and the child's parents (parents must provide written consent). The LEA is also responsible for providing parents with a detailed explanation of the differences between an IFSP and an IEP (34 C.F.R. § 300.322(b)-(c)).

Procedural Safeguards

Like Part C, children with disabilities (including children ages 3 through 5 who are receiving preschool special education services) and their parents are guaranteed procedural safeguards (i.e., rights) with respect to the provision of FAPE under IDEA Part B. These include the following rights:

> (1) Examine all records related to the child; participate in meetings with respect to the identification, evaluation, educational placement, and provision of a FAPE; obtain an independent educational evaluation of the child
> (2) Have a surrogate parent assigned if the parents are unknown or cannot be found
> (3) Receive written prior notice in the native language of initiated changes or refusal to change the eligibility, placement or provision of FAPE
> (4) Access mediation
> (5) File a complaint
> (6) Inspect and review records
> (7) [Ensure] confidentiality of personally identifiable information. (20 U.S.C. § 1415)

Occupational therapists must be aware of these rights and knowledgeable about the states' procedures for filing complaints or requesting a due process hearing or mediation.

Monitoring and Enforcement

The state is required to monitor and enforce the implementation of Part B requirements and, as with Part C, report on its performance through an SPP and APR. The primary focus of monitoring is on improving education results and functional outcomes for all children with disabilities and ensuring that Part B requirements are met. The Part B SPP includes several reporting requirements specific to preschool services, child outcomes, LRE or inclusive settings, and transition from Part C to Part B preschool (Table 1.2).

For more information about the SPP and APR and early childhood outcomes, see the section "Component 14. Data Collection."

Summary

Occupational therapists working in preschool programs must adhere to all the requirements under Part B for providing occupational therapy services, including participation in the development of the IEP. The emphasis in preschool special education is on early education and preliteracy skills rather than on child development. One of the most important roles that occupational therapists can fill in preschool programs is to help keep the focus on appropriate expectations and activities for children ages 3 to 5. Our knowledge of all aspects of development is important as a basis for the recommendations that are made and the types of experiences that children have. Working collaboratively and cooperatively with teachers and others is vitally important in the design of classroom experiences and in how intervention is embedded in the daily experiences.

Table 1.2. Office of Special Education SPP Indicators for Part B Preschool Services

No.	Indicator	Description
B6	LRE	Percentage of preschool children with IEPs who received special education and related services in settings with typically developing peers (i.e., early childhood settings, home, and part-time early childhood/part-time early childhood special education settings)
B7	Early childhood outcomes	Percentage of preschool children with IEPs who demonstrated improved A. Positive socioemotional skills (including social relationships) B. Acquisition and use of knowledge and skills (including early language/communication and literacy) C. Use of appropriate behaviors to meet their needs
B12	IEP by age 3	Percentage of children referred by Part C before age 3 who are found eligible for Part B, and who have an IEP developed and implemented by their third birthdays.

Note. IEP = individualized education program; IFSP = individualized family service plan; LRE = least restrictive environment; SPP = state performance plan.

Source. U.S. Department of Education (2010a).

Head Start

Head Start is one of the most well-known and successful programs the federal government has initiated. Head Start was part of President Johnson's Great Society initiative, specifically, the War on Poverty. Citizens had been told that they could have both "guns and butter," meaning that the Vietnam war would not stop social progress on the home front. Head Start was controversial and initially not readily accepted. It has proven itself through its results and outcomes. The current Head Start Act, the Improving Head Start for School Readiness Act of 2007, was signed into law on December 12, 2007, and authorized Head Start through September 30, 2012, reflecting the 5-year cycle of most education and social service laws. The reauthorization contains significant revisions.

The Head Start program is administered by the Administration for Children and Families (ACF) of the U.S. Department of Health and Human Services (HHS) through the ACF's Office of Head Start. This program is housed in ACF because it administers programs that focus on children and families.

The purpose of Head Start is as follows:

> STATEMENT OF PURPOSE
>
> It is the purpose of this subchapter to promote the school readiness of low-income children by enhancing their cognitive, social, and emotional development—
>
> (1) in a learning environment that supports children's growth in language, literacy, mathematics, science, social and emotional functioning, creative arts, physical skills, and approaches to learning; and
>
> (2) through the provision to low-income children and their families of health, educational, nutritional, social, and other services that are determined, based on family needs assessments, to be necessary. (42 U.S.C. § 9831)

The ACF awards grants on application (i.e., formula grants) to "local public agencies, private non-profit and for-profit organizations, Indian Tribes and school systems for the purpose of operating Head Start programs at the community level" (ACF, 2009b). These grants are awarded directly by the ACF Regional Offices and the Office of Head Start's American Indian–Alaska Native and Migrant and Seasonal Program Branches. The grants provide funding for comprehensive child development services to economically disadvantaged (low-income) children and families, with a special focus on helping young (ages 3 and 4) preschoolers develop the early reading and math skills they need to be successful in school. Through the provision of health, nutritional, educational, social, and other services to enrolled children and families, Head Start programs promote school readiness by enhancing the development of enrolled children and the competence of parents to meet their child's needs. The services are offered on a normal growth and development continuum that promotes and uses physical, social, psychological, and cognitive activities.

By mandate, 10% of the population of children and families in all Head Start programs must be children with identified disabilities. During the 2005–2006 Head

Start Program year, 12.2% of the Head Start enrollment consisted of children with disabilities (mental retardation, health impairments, visual handicaps, hearing impairments, emotional disturbance, speech and language impairments, orthopedic handicaps, and learning disabilities), and nearly 48,000 children participated in home-based Head Start program services (ACF, 2009b).

Remember this. . . .
A significant aspect of Head Start programs, and most probably a key to their success, is the emphasis on the involvement of parents in the administration of local Head Start programs.

Formal family and community partnerships provide parents opportunities and support for their own growth so that they can identify their own strengths, needs, and interests and find their own solutions. A significant aspect of Head Start programs, and most probably a key to their success, is the emphasis on the involvement of parents in the administration of local Head Start programs. Parents are engaged in their child's learning and, through administrative responsibilities, are part of their community's efforts to help all children (ACF, n.d.-b). Head Start serves families within the context of the community. There is recognition that many other agencies and groups work with the same families, and efforts are embedded in Head Start services for cooperation and collaboration on behalf of children and families. For example, a child served under the preschool services of IDEA may receive that instruction in a Head Start program or a community child care center. In all Head Start programs, significant emphasis is placed on family involvement in the child's progress, program administration, and participation in support services designed to enhance the education, literacy, and eventual employment of the parents.

At all levels, Head Start programs follow a set of quality-based performance standards. Of particular interest to occupational therapists are the performance standards related to services for children with disabilities. Occupational therapists have a long history of working in Head Start centers and with Head Start teachers, initially through home health services and child development centers. Services provided specifically on behalf of a child with a disability are the most common form of involvement. However, occupational therapists work with Head Start teachers to help design the classroom environment to support the occupational functioning of all the children enrolled as well as specifically to identify any adaptations or modifications that may be necessary for children with disabilities. Particular support is provided in the establishment of routines and the transitions during the day that most children need to feel secure and thrive.

In some Head Start programs, occupational therapists are working with parents through the Family and Community Partnership as parents attend classes and participate in other activities to enhance their own education, improve literacy and, if needed, move toward employment.

Early Head Start

The 1994 reauthorization of the Head Start Act established the Early Head Start program for low-income families with infants and toddlers. The Early Head Start program is a child development program established in recognition of the mounting research evidence that the earliest years matter a great deal to children's growth and development. As part of Head Start, Early Head Start serves pregnant women and their husbands or partners and families with children from birth to age 3. Early Head Start promotes healthy prenatal outcomes, enhances the development of infants and toddlers, and promotes healthy family functioning.

The program offers two settings for infants and toddlers and their families: home based or center based. Both settings provide services at the child and family level; however, the setting(s) can differ according to the optimal combination for successful outcomes, state guidelines, and child or family needs. A combination of services can be provided in both environments.

Each Early Head Start program is responsible for determining its own eligibility criteria. Family income is a key factor in determining eligibility. The Federal Poverty Guidelines (HHS, 2009) are used to evaluate family income. Early Head Start programs may elect to target their services to a particular population to best meet the unique needs of families and children in their community (ACF, n.d.-a).

Early Head Start (community based) is based on nine foundations or principles, as follows:

1. *High quality:* A commitment to high quality means that programs will develop policies and practices founded in the knowledge, skills, and professional ethics embraced by the fields of child development, family development, and community building.
2. *Prevention and promotion:* The proactive promotion of healthy child development and family functioning begins before conception, and continues prenatally, at birth, and through the early years.
3. *Positive relationships and continuity:* Strong positive relationships that continue over time are key elements in a high-quality program.
4. *Parent involvement:* The Early Head Start initiative supports the highest level of parent involvement and partnership.
5. *Inclusion:* Programs will welcome and fully include children with disabilities.
6. *Culture:* The home culture and language of each family will be supported as an important aspect of early identity formation.
7. *Comprehensiveness, flexibility, responsiveness, and intensity:* Program services are grounded in the belief that all families can identify their own needs and strengths, set their own goals, and are capable of growth.
8. *Transitions:* Programs are responsible for facilitating a smooth transition from Early Head Start into Head Start or other high-quality programs and support services.
9. *Collaboration:* Collaboration with local community agencies and service providers will maximize the resources available to families with young children in a cost-efficient and comprehensive manner. (ACF, n.d.-a)

The framework of the Early Head Start program includes four cornerstones that reflect the needs of the target population:

1. *Child development:* Support the physical, social, emotional, cognitive, and language development of each child through
   - Early education services in a range of developmentally appropriate settings
   - Home visits, especially for families with newborns
   - Parent education and parent–child activities

- Comprehensive health and mental health services
- High-quality child care services provided directly or in collaboration with community child care providers.

2. *Family development:* Including adult literacy, safe housing, health and mental health services
3. *Community building:* Assessment of community resources for a comprehensive network of services and supports for pregnant women and families with young children
4. *Staff development:* Through ongoing training, supervision, and mentoring, staff will have the capacity to develop caring, supportive relationships with both children and families.

Early Head Start programs must coordinate with programs providing services in accordance with Part C of IDEA. Children with disabilities will be fully included in program activities (ACF, n.d.-b).

One way in which Early Head Start supports very young children and their families is through early childhood development and health services.

> Head Start's commitment to wellness embraces a comprehensive vision of health for children, families, and staff. The objective of Child Health and Development Services is to ensure that, through collaboration among families, staff, and health professionals, all child health and developmental concerns are identified, and children and families are linked to an ongoing source of continuous, accessible care to meet their basic health needs. (ACF, n.d.-a)

Occupational therapists work in Early Head Start in many of the same ways that they work in Head Start and early intervention. In collaboration with teachers and caregivers, they evaluate development, provide anticipatory guidance to teachers and parents, and help to design play and caregiving activities and environments that foster and promote development and a healthy lifestyle.

It is not unusual for children who are enrolled in the state early intervention program for developmental concerns to attend an Early Head Start center because their family is low income and the parents work and need child care. An occupational therapist would have many people to work with to help support the child in his or her development. Careful coordination is needed. In these circumstances, the role of the service coordinator from the early intervention program is invaluable. This person may be the occupational therapist or may be another professional or paraprofessional. Refer to Chapter 3 for discussion of the role of the service coordinator in early intervention.

Smart Start

As research revealed the importance of children's early experiences as highly influential on their entire life, Congress and state legislatures sought ways to improve and enhance the health and developmental and educational experiences of very young children. Coordinating efforts, rather than duplicating, was viewed as the most logical, politically expedient, and effective way to do so. *Smart Start* was a term used in some of these proposed initiatives.

In 1993, the North Carolina General Assembly authorized a public–private partnership, the Early Childhood Education and Development Initiatives, to enhance and upgrade child care services and facilities in selected locations in North Carolina so that the programs promoted child development in all areas and helped prepare children for public school. At that time, North Carolina's child care standards were among the worst in the nation. By 1998, however, every county in the state had received what became known as Smart Start funding, reflecting local partnerships and linkages, public and private, to address the needs of young children.

In 2001, federal legislation was passed that used North Carolina's Smart Start as the model for public–private partnerships for early childhood programs. The Early Learning Linkages Act of 2001 authorized for a short time a program of grants to fund services that would increase the availability, affordability, and coordination of services of programs in a community serving very young children. By 2003, 14 states were using Smart Start as their model for early childhood programs.

The original Smart Start was predicated on four basic perspectives:

1. Pre-K needs start at birth.
2. We should promote choice and diversity in pre-K preparation.
3. Standards matter.
4. Target the needy first and most.

These perspectives reflected years of program evaluation and societal trends. The federal response to Smart Start programs was to fold it into the 2001 reauthorization of the Elementary and Secondary Education Act, known as the No Child Left Behind Act (NCLB). NCLB focuses specific attention on services for children who are more likely to fall behind in reading. Recognizing that efforts to achieve preacademic skills must start before children enter kindergarten, an initiative called Good Start, Grow Smart was implemented in 2002. The goal of the initiative is to ensure that young children are equipped with the skills they will need to start school ready to learn.

> The Initiative focuses on strengthening Head Start; partnering with States to improve early learning; and providing parents, teachers, and caregivers with information on early learning to assist states to strengthen early learning for young children with an emphasis on literacy. (ACF, n.d.-b)

Smart Start (or Good Start, Grow Smart, depending on the state) requires that each community plan how best to meet the specific needs of their children and families. Therefore, each state and local community has expanded existing programs or designed and implemented new programs based on its unique needs. Although all funds are invested in early childhood education, by mandate the community must invest 70% in child care. Programs are usually a combination of child care subsidies and quality improvement activities. Funds are available for technical assistance, quality improvement, grants, teacher education and professional development, teacher salary, and family supplements to afford child care.

The agencies that administer Smart Start partnerships are required to establish Early Learning Guidelines for all children ages 3 to 5. These guidelines specify what children need to know, understand, and be able to do at certain ages. Many states have expanded these guidelines to younger children and have determined guidance (ACF, 2009c) for each developmental stage. Practitioners involved in Smart

Start–funded programs work within these guidelines when assessing and designing intervention programs for individual children (ACF, 2009c). Children with special health care needs or children with disabilities are involved in Smart Start program activities. In some communities, Smart Start centers offer preschool services under Part B of IDEA. It is imperative that every occupational therapist know the philosophy, funding mechanism, perspectives, and desired outcomes of any program in which they work with children and families.

Child Care and Universal Preschool[1]

All of a child's early experiences matter. They influence development and learning; can be positive or negative; and can have long-term consequences for the child, family, and society (American Academy of Pediatrics [AAP] Committee on Early Childhood, Adoption, and Dependent Care, 2005). For young children with disabilities and other special needs, the quality of early experiences can make the difference between full participation in their communities and at school with their typically developing peers and isolation from "normal" life experiences. Unfortunately, children with disabilities are among the least likely to have access to high-quality early education and child care (AAP Committee on Early Childhood, Adoption, and Dependent Care, 2005; Shonkoff & Phillips, 2000). This situation often results in negative experiences for children as well as for others who experience the delivery of inadequate early education and child care. High-quality early childhood education programs that are well versed in inclusion philosophies and practices can mitigate the impact of negative experiences for all children, particularly those with disabilities.

Policy, social, and economic changes over the past four decades have led to more women of child-bearing age in the workforce (Darlington & Rodger, 2006), resulting in more than 6 in 10 children being cared for regularly by someone other than their parents in some type of child care arrangement every week (National Association of Child Care Resource and Referral Agencies [NACCRRA], n.d.-a). In fact, children younger than age 5 whose mothers work spend, on average, 36 hours a week in child care (NACCRRA, n.d.-a). For this reason, Congress created the Child Care and Development Block Grant (CCDBG) in 1990 as section 5082 of the Omnibus Budget Reconciliation Act of 1990 (ACF, 2009a) and expanded it in 1996 as part of welfare reform. The CCDBG is the primary federal funding stream for child care in the United States and is administered by ACF. It provides formula block grants to states, which use the funds to subsidize child care for low-income working families, for Temporary Assistance to Needy Families recipients, and for families transitioning from welfare to work. In addition, a certain percentage of CCDBG funding is required to be spent on activities to improve the quality of child care (NACCRRA, n.d.-b).

Child care and universal preschool and prekindergarten programs present tremendous opportunities for occupational therapists. Occupational therapists can

[1]The material in the Child Care and Universal Preschool section is from "Inclusive Early Care and Education: An Opportunity for Occupational Therapy," by Leslie L. Jackson, 2009, *OT Practice, 14*(17), pp. 14–17. Copyright © 2009 by the American Occupational Therapy Association. Adapted with permission.

play an important role in increasing the capacity of these programs to meet the needs of children with varying abilities in their care, particularly for children with disabilities (Carrasco et al., 2007).

Occupational therapy is predicated on the notion that participation in meaningful activities (i.e., occupations) is vital to health and wellness (AOTA, 2008). Children are actively engaged in creating, negotiating, and interpreting their everyday worlds. The environment (i.e., context) and the people within it play an important role in this engagement and participation; it is an integral part of the action, not static or fixed (AOTA, 2008).

Early childhood program participation is associated with improvements in children's cognitive skills (Horton, 2007). Research on the brain has shown that the first years of life are crucial for intellectual, social, and general development (Horton, 2007). Other research on caregivers' effects on children during the early years has clearly shown that caregivers' education, training, and ability to provide a safe and stimulating environment affects children's cognitive and emotional development. One aspect of the environment is the level of support needed by a child, but this is particularly true for children with disabilities. Physical presence alone is no guarantee that children with disabilities will be successful in child care or other early childhood settings. Many of these children need supports to fit in. These supports help determine whether children with disabilities successfully participate and learn in the same settings as their typically developing peers (Easter Seals, 2008). Teachers, in partnership with parents, therapists, and other specialists, must design supportive strategies that facilitate and create learning opportunities within the context of activities and routines that focus on what children can do—not what they cannot do. Occupational therapists can help staff learn to target ways to support children's participation in activities and routines by framing what they need to learn within a context of engagement, identifying the skills needed to participate successfully, providing accommodations and adaptations and teaching–learning strategies to ensure children's success, and individualizing experiences for all children by matching learning opportunities with their strengths, developmental competencies, and needs (Campbell & Bruder, 2007; Odom et al., 1999). These characteristics hold true for programs serving children with and without disabilities.

Becoming an effective early childhood program for children with disabilities requires having skilled staff "who believe that their role and their skills will and can make a difference" (Schwartz & Brand, 2001, p. 289) for *all* children served by the program. Inadequate preparation and training of general childhood educators has been cited as perhaps the single most prominent barrier to inclusion (Buysse, Wesley, & Able-Boone, 2001; Buysse, Wesley, & Keyes, 1998; Easter Seals, 2008). Such educators are less likely to request or seek out training and education related to inclusion if they do not have a child with special needs in their classroom or such a child transitioning into their care (Campbell & Bruder, 2007). These same educators, however, often report that they are more comfortable and feel more confident in their ability to work with children with disabilities after they have participated in inclusion training. Occupational therapists can provide training for child care staff on how to meet the needs of children with a variety of disabilities and provide staff with strategies and educational activities to support children's developmental needs and encourage achievement of learning outcomes (Carrasco et al., 2007).

A major role for occupational therapists in early childhood settings is to advocate for supportive and developmentally appropriate child care and universal preschool and prekindergarten environments for children (Ziviani & Rodger, 2006). This role necessitates occupational therapists' collaboration with practitioners in other disciplines, which is key to successful inclusion (Bose & Hinojosa, 2008). The goal is to help programs enroll children with disabilities by increasing staff understanding of how to serve children with disabilities and their families more effectively and increasing staff competence in meeting the needs of all children in the program. Ultimately, this approach will also increase care options for families that provide access to high-quality early learning opportunities for their children and make it possible for parents of young children with disabilities to better care for their children. Moreover, parenting skills and home experiences improve when parents are supported and valued as equal partners in their child's education (AAP Committee on Early Childhood, Adoption, and Dependent Care, 2005).

Too few child care providers and universal preschool programs believe they are equipped to effectively meet the needs of young children with disabilities. Occupational therapists have an opportunity to support programs to provide high-quality, inclusive services that will enable all children to participate in nurturing environments that produce positive outcomes in all aspects of their development and learning. Additional benefits to occupational therapy include increased opportunities to develop new skills and share ideas and strategies, shared decision making, resources, and accountability for outcomes (Bose & Hinojosa, 2008).

Impact of Early Childhood Programs

Using Smart Start guidelines and Head Start Performance Guidelines, Head Start has developed an accountability system to assess student learning in language, early literacy, and premath skills. Research has shown a positive effect on children's academic attainment, emotional and behavioral outcomes, and health and safety, as well as on positive parenting and parental employment (ACF, n.d.-a).

To close the gap between the best research and current practices in early childhood education, HHS implemented a national training program providing information to parents, Head Start, and other early childhood personnel about techniques to promote prereading skills for Head Start students. All team members are included in these programs. Professional development activities that improve team collaboration and communication skills can foster successful achievement of outcomes in children.

We need to know the origins and organizations of these programs, but more important, we need to know how we can involve ourselves at the local level. Learning Activity 1.9 suggests ways in which you can gain greater understanding of the

Learning Activity 1.9. In Our Own Backyards

- With colleagues who may or may not work in early childhood programs, identify as many programs and services available in your local area that serve young children, with or without special needs, as you can.
- For each program, identify the purpose, sources of funding, administrative mechanism(s), and role of occupational therapy (real or potential).
- Identify the linking mechanisms among these programs.

programs that are available and in which occupational therapy services contribute to positive outcomes for young children and their families.

Other Models of Service Provision

Hospital

Most of us start our lives outside the womb in a hospital. It is our first place of care, even though we generally are there for only a day or two. Many babies, however, must stay at the hospital, often in the neonatal intensive care unit (NICU). With medicine pushing the viability of preterm infants to gestation of 24 weeks or younger, some babies will spend 3 or 4 months in the NICU—and some will be there even longer.

Many NICU graduates receive ongoing services in hospital-based "follow-up" clinics. These clinics work in collaboration with community-based services. The goal is to monitor development, obtain services if needed, and support the family as it cares for the child. Duplication of services and inconsistent or opposing recommendations should not occur. Hospital- and community-based practitioners should be in contact with each other so that costly resources are not wasted, and the child and family are not "lost in the paperwork." Simply because a child is enrolled in early intervention does not preclude the need for follow-up by the hospital-based team. However, if a child is receiving the same services in the community that would be provided by the hospital, it would be considered duplication of services unless the child had a specialized need (e.g., new orthotics) that would be more efficiently met in the hospital. Many referrals to state Part C programs come from the discharge planners and social workers at the hospital newborn services.

Once the child is home, a primary care provider (usually a pediatrician, but perhaps a family practice physician or family nurse–practitioner) provides well-baby care. These services are usually provided by private practices, but many children receive their well-baby care and periodic checkups through the local health department. Increasingly, these medical practices and health departments are monitoring development as well as growth and health using screening instruments such as the Ages and Stages Questionnaires (Squires & Bricker, 2009). If a delay or deviation in development is evident or suspected and the local Part C program has done outreach (through Child Find and public awareness), the child will be referred to the local early intervention program for an initial eligibility evaluation.

Provider Network

One required component of state early intervention programs is contracts or arrangements with service providers (e.g., therapists, educators, dieticians) to provide early intervention services. In many instances, these providers are located in private practices, sometimes as sole practitioners. A popular model in many states is the use of a private practice as a billing agent for contractual providers. Such practices handle the billing of the services (for a percentage of the fee collected), and the actual provider of the services is responsible for the rest of the service provision. For occupational therapists who work part time and want flexibility in their schedules, this arrangement may work well. However, it often limits the time available for any kind of meeting, phone call, or collaborative work because the therapist is only reimbursed for treatment time. The issue of distance in home-based services is critical because many early intervention programs have difficulty locating providers who will "drive out there" even if "out there" is 12 miles. Distance is a particular concern because one emphasis of the early intervention program is to serve children in rural areas.

Social Services

All early childhood program locations have close ties with local social services agencies. The children in these programs are among the most vulnerable and often have families that are the most stressed. Parenting is a demanding, 24-hour-a-day responsibility. Children with special health care needs and children with disabilities require constant care and attention—as, indeed, do all young children. Many communities have large numbers of people who are involved with illegal drugs; as a result, some children are born with prenatal exposure to opiates or other illegal drugs. Exposure to the ingredients of methamphetamine (e.g., by being in the house where the drug is made) has been shown to damage children's brains and other organs. Prenatal alcohol exposure is another risk affecting young children. Single mothers having limited or no support systems and those living in poverty increase children's risk for homelessness, inadequate diet, abuse, and other forms of neglect.

Understanding the structure of the local social and legal support system for young children is essential for any practitioner in early childhood. Because many early childhood services, especially in early intervention, involve home visiting, occupational therapists need to be familiar with their state's definitions of abuse and neglect of minor children and reporting requirements and processes. Being able to distinguish whether an unsafe home with a toddler in it is a situation of neglect or whether the child's teenage mother does not realize or know how to childproof the home, but could be shown and assisted to do so, is a skill that any home visitor should develop. One purpose of the early intervention program is to build family capacity to care for and promote a child's growth and development. Does one help the young mother rearrange the cabinets on a home visit (placing cleaning supplies at the top, pots and pans on the bottom) or problem solve, demonstrate, instruct, and check on the next visit? What is a reasonable timeline for the parent to make the home safe? The requirements for mandatory reporting of abuse or neglect should be periodically reviewed and discussed with colleagues from the courts and social services systems to be sure that all practitioners are aware of their initial and ongoing responsibilities. Of course, any actions and reasons for reporting a situation of child abuse or neglect should be documented.

It is likely that at some point while working in early childhood programs, you will find yourself with a subpoena in hand and a date on which you must appear in court as a witness. Before that happens, you should familiarize yourself with the types of courts in your area that deal with child abuse, neglect, and custody, which are the most likely reasons that you may be called on to testify. County social services departments periodically offer training sessions on social services involvement with young children, the guardian ad litem program, and other aspects of judicial proceedings dealing with young children.

Conclusion

Working in early childhood requires that you know the road that you are on; otherwise, the various programs, initiatives, services, mandates, and opportunities will seem like a blur. When you understand these entities and know their purpose, structure, focus, and mission, the paths become clearer and lead, one hopes, to a better life for parents and children. You must understand your part as an occupational therapist in these programs; your role is often that of a linking mechanism among programs. You should also comprehend and value what they mean to you as a citizen.

How Very Far We Have Come: Danny and Lydia (1950–1956)

Lydia and Sam switched pediatricians, which meant a drive to the next town, 10 miles away. With a new baby and the twins, they wanted a doctor who saw Danny's (and his siblings') strengths. Mark was born when Annie and Danny (as they had come to be called) were 2. Full term, Mark was a robust 8 pounds and grew quickly. Lydia and Sam realized again how very small and fragile the twins had been.

All three children were growing, though. Danny was still smaller than Annie, but he clearly could see, and he clearly could think! He watched his siblings and dragged or rolled himself to wherever Annie and, eventually, Mark was. The new pediatrician had referred Danny to the nearest Shriners Hospital, which was 3 hours away across the state line. The Shriners Hospital specialized in providing free medical care to children who had special needs. At Shriners, Danny was diagnosed with cerebral palsy (spastic diplegia) and fitted with braces to "keep his legs straight" so that he could eventually walk. He was also diagnosed with a "visual deficit," although the exact nature of it was unspecified at his age.

The trips to Shriners every 6 months were grueling because the roads were two lane, the waits were long, and the information was often provided quickly with little time to ask questions. Lydia understood that there were many children to be seen, and she certainly appreciated the care and the fact that it was free, but she often left frustrated, and she and Danny (and, sometimes, Mark and Annie) always arrived home exhausted. The doctors focused on what Danny couldn't do, not on what he could do. Again, she understood that that was their role and that their knowledge was something she didn't have. She wanted, however, for everyone to see Danny as a little boy with potential as she, Sam, and his pediatrician did.

Questions

1. How did the advocacy call for "family-centered, community-based, coordinated care" reflect the experiences of this family in seeking and obtaining care for Danny?
2. What is the difference between a deficit-based and a strength-based perspective in developmental care?
3. During this time, what resources were available to a family seeking care for a child with disabilities?

References

Administration for Children and Families. (2009a). *Child care and community block grants.* Retrieved November 22, 2009, from www.acf.hhs.gov/programs/ccb/ccdf/index.htm

Administration for Children and Families. (2009b). *Head Start Program fact sheet fiscal year 2008.* Retrieved November 22, 2009, from www.acf.hhs.gov/programs/ohs/about/index.html#factsheet

Administration for Children and Families. (2009c). *State early learning guidelines.* Retrieved November 21, 2009, from http://nccic.acf.hhs.gov/pubs/goodstart/elgwebsites.html

Administration for Children and Families. (n.d.-a). *Early Head Start Research and Evaluation Project, 1996–current.* Retrieved November 22, 2009, from www.acf.hhs.gov/programs/opre/ehs/ehs_resrch/index.html

Administration for Children and Families. (n.d.-b). *Program services.* Retrieved November 22, 2009, from www.acf.hhs.gov/programs/ohs/programs/index.html#fam

American Academy of Pediatrics Committee on Early Childhood, Adoption, and Dependent Care. (2005). Policy statement: Quality early education and child care from birth to kindergarten. *Pediatrics, 115,* 187–191.

American Occupational Therapy Association. (2004). Occupational therapy in early intervention and schools. *American Journal of Occupational Therapy, 58,* 681–685.

American Occupational Therapy Association. (2008). Occupational therapy practice framework: Domain and process (2nd ed.). *American Journal of Occupational Therapy, 62,* 625–683.

Bagnato, S., Smith-Jones, J., Matesa, M., & McKeating-Esterle, E. (2006). Research foundations for using clinical judgment (informed opinion) for early intervention eligibility determination. *Cornerstones, 2*(3), 1–14.

Bose, P., & Hinojosa, J. (2008). Reported experiences from occupational therapists interacting with teachers in inclusive early childhood classrooms. *American Journal of Occupational Therapy, 62,* 289–297.

Buysse, V., & Wesley, P. (2006). *Evidence-based practice in the early childhood field.* Washington, DC: Zero to Three.

Buysse, V., Wesley, P., & Able-Boone, H. (2001). Innovations in professional development: Creating communities of practice to support inclusion. In M. Guralnick (Ed.), *Early childhood inclusion: Focus on change* (pp. 179–200). Baltimore: Brookes.

Buysse, V., Wesley, P., & Keyes, L. (1998). Implementing early childhood inclusion: Barrier and support factors. *Early Childhood Research Quarterly, 13,* 169–184.

Campbell, P., & Bruder, M. B. (2007). *Including young children with disabilities in child care—What the research tells us.* Keynote presentations at the Easter Seals TMICC Train-the-Trainer Workshops, Chicago and Atlanta.

Carrasco, R. C., Skees-Hermes, S., Clark, G. F., Polichino, J. E., Ralabate, P., Thomas, L., et al. (2007). Occupational therapy service delivery to support child and family participation in context. In L. Jackson (Ed.), *Occupational therapy services for children and youth under IDEA* (3rd ed., pp. 89–127). Bethesda, MD: AOTA Press.

Carroll, L. (1872). *Through the looking glass.* London: MacMillan.

Chandler, B. (2009). Classroom clinic—Working where life is really lived. *ADVANCE for Occupational Therapy Practitioners, 25*(5), 8.

Child Abuse Prevention and Treatment Act (as amended by the Keeping Children and Families Safe Act of 2003), Pub. L. 108–36, 42 U.S.C. § 5106.

Clark, G. (2008). The Infants and Toddlers With Disabilities Program (Part C of IDEA). *OT Practice, 13*(1), CE-1–CE-8.

Danaher, J. (2007). *Eligibility policies and practices for young children under Part B of IDEA* (NECTAC Notes No. 24). Chapel Hill: University of North Carolina, FPG Child Development Institute, National Early Childhood Technical Assistance Center. Available at www.nectac.org/~pdfs/pubs/nnotes24.pdf

Darlington, Y., & Rodger, S. (2006). Families and children's occupational performance. In S. Rodger & J. Ziviani (Eds.), *Occupational therapy with children: Understanding children's occupations and enabling participation* (pp. 22–40). Malden, MA: Blackwell.

Dunst, C. J., Bruder, M. B., Trivette, C. M., Hamby, D., Raab, M., & McLean, M. (2001). Characteristics and consequences of everyday natural learning opportunities. *Topics in Early Childhood Special Education, 21,* 68–92.

Dunst, C. J., Bruder, M. B., Trivette, C. M., Raab, M., & McLean, M. (2001). Natural learning opportunities for infants, toddlers, and preschoolers. *Young Exceptional Children, 4(3),* 18–25.

Early Childhood Education and Development Initiatives of 1993, S. L. 93–321, 143B Gen. Stat. N.C. § 168.10 *et seq.*

Early Childhood Outcomes Center. (n.d.). *ECO resources: Child Outcomes Summary Form (COSF).* Retrieved January 14, 2010, from www.fpg.unc.edu/~eco/pages/outcomes.cfm

Early Learning Linkages Act of 2001, Pub. L. 106–554.

Easter Seals, Inc. (2008). *Training modules for Inclusive Child Care training curriculum.* Chicago: Author.

Fraiberg, S. (1987). The muse in the kitchen: A clinical case study. In L. Fraiberg (Ed.), *Selected writings of Selma Fraiberg* (pp. 65–99). Columbus: Ohio State University Press.

Handley-More, D., & Chandler, B. (2007). Occupational therapy decision making. In L. Jackson (Ed.), *Occupational therapy services for children and youth under IDEA* (3rd ed., pp. 89–127). Bethesda, MD: American Occupational Therapy Association.

Hanft, B., & Pilkington, K. (2000). Therapy in natural environments: The means or end goal for early intervention? *Infants and Young Children, 12*(4), 1–13.

Hanft, B. E., Rush, D. D., & Shelden, M. L. (2004). *Coaching families and colleagues in early childhood.* Baltimore: Brookes.

Horton, C. (2007). *Early care and education programs: What does research tell us about their effects on child development?* (Research brief). Chicago: Erikson Institute, Herr Research Center for Children and Social Policy. Retrieved March 12, 2009, from www.erikson.edu/hrc/publications/pubstopic.aspxwww.erikson.edu/hrc

Improving Head Start for School Readiness Act of 2007, Pub. L. 110–134, 42 U.S.C. § 9801 *et seq.*

Individuals With Disabilities Education Improvement Act of 2004, Pub. L. 108–446, 20 U.S.C. § 1400 *et seq.*

National Association of Child Care Resource and Referral Agencies. (n.d.-a). *Child care in America fact sheet.* Retrieved February 16, 2009, from www.naccrra.org/policy/docs/childcareinamericafactsheet.doc

National Association of Child Care Resource and Referral Agencies. (n.d.-b). *Reauthorization of the Child Care and Development Block Grant.* Retrieved February 16, 2009, from www.naccrra.org/policy/key_legislation/details.php?Area=ccdbg

National Early Childhood Technical Assistance Center. (2008a). *IFSP process: Planning and implementing family-centered services in natural environments.* Retrieved August 16, 2009, from www.nectac.org/topics/families/ifspprocess.asp

National Early Childhood Technical Assistance Center. (2008b). *Resources for writing good IFSP outcomes.* Retrieved August 16, 2009, from www.nectac.org/topics/families/famresources.asp

National Early Childhood Technical Assistance Center. (2009a). *CAPTA and IDEA laws.* Retrieved November 21, 2009, from www.nectac.org/topics/earlyid/capta.asp#capta

National Early Childhood Technical Assistance Center. (2009b). *Evaluating the quality of IFSPs.* Retrieved August 16, 2009, from www.nectac.org/topics/families/evalifsp.asp

National Early Childhood Technical Assistance Center. (2009c). *Family assessment: Gathering information from families and individualized family service plan outcomes.* Retrieved August 16, 2009, from www.nectac.org/topics/families/famresources.asp

National Early Childhood Technical Assistance Center. (2009d). *State examples of IFSP forms and guidance.* Retrieved August 16, 2009, from www.nectac.org/topics/families/stateifsp.asp

No Child Left Behind Act of 2001, Pub. L. 107–110, 115 Stat. 1425 (2002).

Odom, S. L., Peck, C. A., Hanson, M., Beckman, P. J., Kaiser, A. P., Lieber, J., et al. (1999). *Inclusion at the preschool level: An ecological systems analysis.* Retrieved May 13, 2008, from www.newhorizons.org/spneeds/inclusion/information/schwartz1.htm

Omnibus Budget Reconciliation Act of 1990, Pub. L. 101–508, as amended.

Orelena Hawks Puckett Institute. (2009). *Center for Evidence-Based Practices.* Retrieved August 16, 2009, from www.evidencebasedpractices.org.

Rehabilitation Act of 1973, Pub. L. 93–112, 29 U.S.C. § 701 *et seq.*

Schwartz, B., & Brand, M. E. (2001). Head Start and the inclusion of children with disabilities. In M. Guralnick (Ed.), *Early childhood inclusion: Focus on change* (pp. 277–292). Baltimore: Paul H. Brookes.

Shackelford, J. (2002). *Informed clinical opinion* (NECTAC Notes No. 10). Chapel Hill: University of North Carolina, FPG Child Development Institute, National Early Childhood Technical Assistance Center. Retrieved March 8, 2009, from www.nectac.org/~pdfs/pubs/nnotes10.pdf

Shackelford, J. (2006). *State and jurisdictional eligibility definitions for infants and toddlers with disabilities under IDEA* (NECTAC Notes No. 21). Chapel Hill: University of North Carolina, FPG Child Development Institute, National Early Childhood Technical Assistance Center. Retrieved March 8, 2009, from www.nectac.org/~pdfs/pubs/nnotes21.pdf

Shonkoff, J. P., & Phillips, D. A. (Eds.). (2000). *From neurons to neighborhoods: The science of early childhood development.* Washington, DC: National Academies Press.

Social Security Act of 1935, Pub. L. 74–271.

Squires, J., & Bricker, D. (2009). *Ages and Stages Questionnaires* (3rd ed.). Baltimore: Brookes.

U.S. Department of Education. (1999). Part II. Assistance to states for the education of children with disabilities and the early intervention program for infants and toddlers with disabilities; final regulations (64 FR 12406). 34 CFR §§ 300, 303.

U.S. Department of Education. (2006). Assistance to states for the education of children with disabilities and preschool grants for children with disabilities; final rule (71 FR 46540). 34 C.F.R. §§ 300, 301.

U.S. Department of Education. (2007).Title 34: Education. Part 303—Early Intervention Program for Infants and Toddlers With Disabilities; proposed rules (72 FR 26456).

U.S. Department of Education. (2010a). *Part B State Performance Plan (SPP) and Annual Performance Report (APR) Part B indicator measurement table.* Retrieved April 17, 2010, from www2.ed.gov/policy/speced/guid/idea/bapr/2010/b2-1820-0624bmeastable techedits10-29-09.pdf

U.S. Department of Education. (2010b). *Part C State Performance Plan (SPP) and Annual Performance Report (APR). Part C indicator measurement table.* Retrieved April 17, 2010, from www2.ed.gov/policy/speced/guid/idea/capr/2010/b2-1820-0578cmeatableexp113012.pdf

U.S. Department of Education. (n.d.). *Part B individualized education program model form.* Retrieved March 8, 2009, from www.ed.gov/policy/speced/guid/idea/modelform-iep.doc

U.S. Department of Health and Human Services. (2009, January 22). *Poverty guidelines, Research, and measurement.* Retrieved August 15, 2009, from http://aspe.hhs.gov/poverty/

Wolery, M. (1994). *Proposed benefits of preschool inclusion.* Chapel Hill: University of North Carolina, National Early Childhood Technical Assistance Center. Retrieved August 12, 2009, from www.nectac.org/inclusion/research/Benefits.asp

Wolery, M. (n.d.). *Conditions necessary for desirable outcomes in inclusive classrooms.* Chapel Hill: University of North Carolina, National Early Childhood Technical Assistance Center. Retrieved August 12, 2009, from www.nectac.org/inclusion/research/RS_conditions.asp

Ziviani, J., & Rodger, S. (2006). Environmental influences on children's participation. In S. Rodger & J. Ziviani (Eds.), *Occupational therapy with children: Understanding children's occupations and enabling participation* (pp. 41–66). Malden, MA: Blackwell.

CHAPTER 2

Infant, Toddler, and Young Child Development

Terry Giese, MBA, OT/L, FAOTA

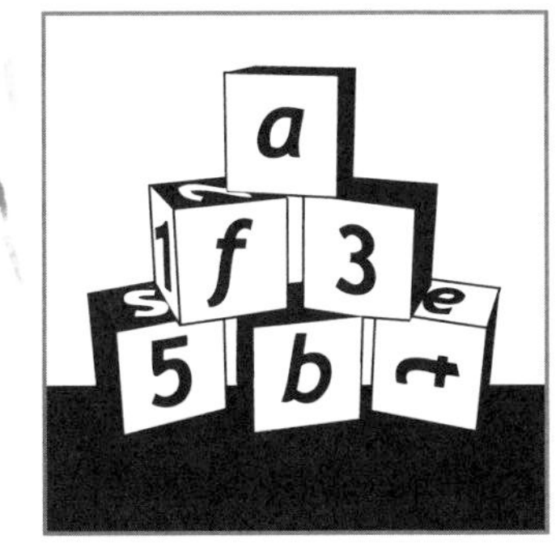

Learning Objectives

After reading this material and completing the examination, readers will be able to

- Delineate the concepts of occupational permanence and occupational equanimity as they relate to the development of the self;
- Differentiate the concepts of occupational development and occupational dissonance as defined in the Model of HOPE;
- Identify developmental consequences associated with engagement in impoverished maternal habits during the prenatal and perinatal periods;
- Delineate the behavioral characteristics associated with the easy, difficult, and slow-to-warm infant temperaments;
- Identify states of consciousness experienced by the full-term newborn;
- Delineate the primary contributions made by theorists Maslow, Erikson, Piaget, and Vygotsky to typical infant and young child development; and
- Identify motor sequelae that interrupt functional performance when typical development is interrupted by illness, injury, or environmental deprivation.

Holistic Perspective of Human Development

Occupational engagement is not only the outcome of the occupational therapy process; it is embedded in the developmental order of life. As infants, we are born into this world consciously whole and biologically immature. The newborn infant emerges to face a transitional challenge from the internal, protective, prenatal milieu to a rich, new, stimulating world outside the womb filled with novel sensory and social experiences. Human development occurs not as a singular trajectory of growth and maturation but as a dynamic, interactive process of occupational

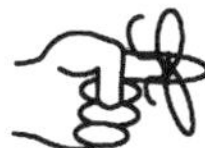

Remember this. . . .
Occupational engagement is not only the outcome of the occupational therapy process; it is embedded in the developmental order of life.

engagement with the human and nonhuman environment, spiraling in unique rhythms of exploration and discovery.

Meaningful occupations are incorporated into one's individual identity. As we participate in tasks associated with the roles that define us, we each develop a unique constellation of occupations that become integral to our sense of self. Priority occupations that take on longitudinal meaning are given *occupational permanence,* transcendental representation of purpose essential to one's self-concept. Occupational permanence contributes to a sense of stability that frees a person to choose new options for occupational engagement and to explore new contexts in which to participate. The meaning given to occupations by each individual determines an occupation's placement within the realm of occupational permanence.

The stability of occupational permanence is balanced by the flexibility of *occupational equanimity,* the extent and nature of engagement in occupational tasks that challenge a person toward occupational dysfunction or release. Just as any point of equilibrium is simultaneously in disequilibrium, the occupational being is in constant flux, flooded with opportunities for participation in a variety of novel and familiar tasks. Participation in these tasks is influenced not only by the person's physical capacities but also by the level of anticipated fulfillment associated with task participation or lack thereof. The dynamics of choice, satisfaction, and dissatisfaction influence the nature and extent of participation in occupations from one person and one moment to the next.

The scale of occupational equanimity undulates in waves of contentment or frustration from its individuated base of occupational permanence. At one end of the occupational equanimity continuum, *occupational development,* the successful learning of new tasks or skills, gives way to *occupational satisfaction,* the gratification and enjoyment of participation in functional activities. Extended occupational engagement with satisfaction may ultimately lead to *occupational release* as mastery of a chosen activity promotes giving of occupational skills by sharing them with others or giving up occupational skills because they are no longer necessary or valued.

The divergent wave of occupational equanimity starts with occupational dissonance, by which one is aware of a mismatch between the demands of the environment and one's affordances. "*Occupational dissonance* is a general sense of feeling incomplete or unresolved, disharmonious within the context of an otherwise satisfying life. It is a term that is more sensitive to picking up client needs within a wellness population" (Giese, quoted in Brachtesende, 2005, p. 13). Such a minor mismatch may be accepted or may motivate the person to seek greater competence in executing the task from which springs occupational dissonance. If dissonance is not accepted and does not fulfill occupational role demands, the person's perception of performance may move toward *occupational dissatisfaction,* whereby functioning yields frustration or discontent and, ultimately, to *occupational dysfunction.* The dynamics of occupational permanence and occupational equanimity comprise the Holistic Model of Occupational Permanence and Equanimity (Model of HOPE; Figure 2.1), presented here as an extension of the Holistic Theory of Human Development (Giese, 2002b).

The Holistic Theory of Human Development portrays human development as a lifelong process of individuation and transformation. On the most basic level,

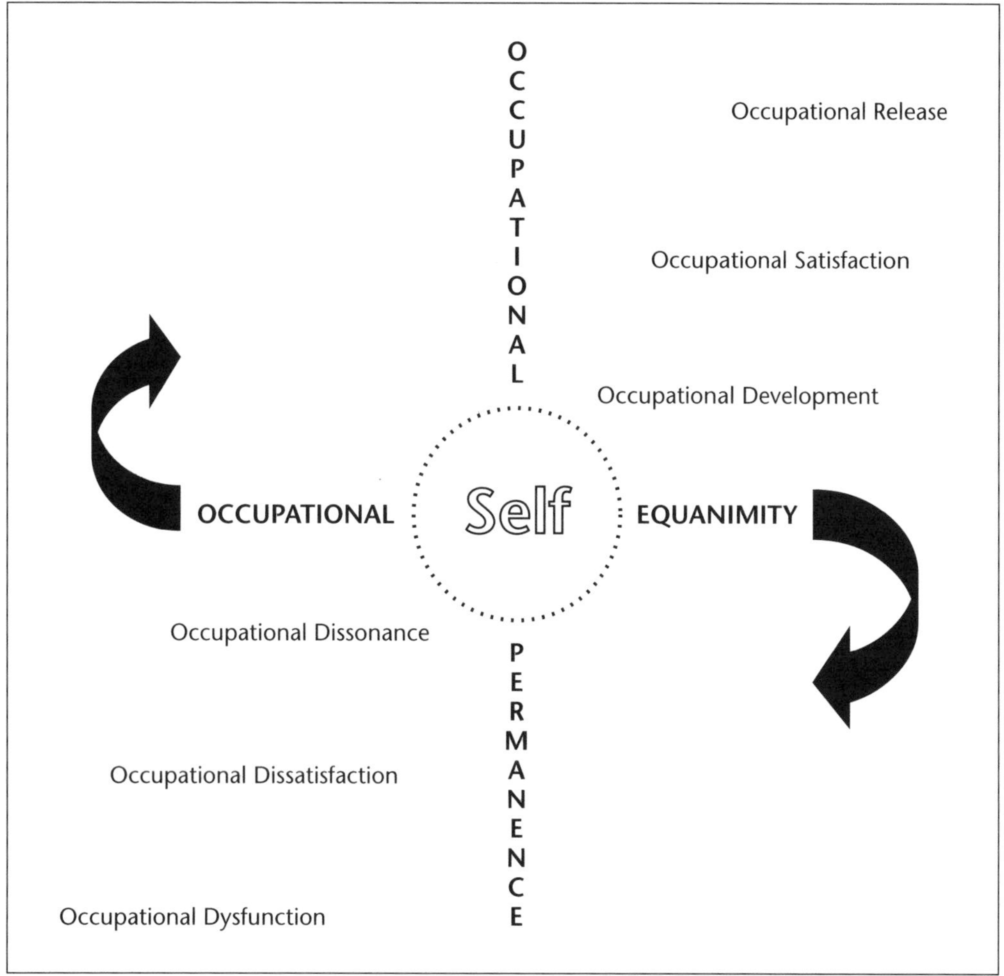

Figure 2.1. Holistic Model of Occupational Permanence and Equanimity (Giese, 2002b). Used with permission of the author.

• Individuation
• Transformation

individuation is the process whereby each person seeks to differentiate himself or herself from others, whereby the self is aligned with the soul, the true essence of each human being. *Transformation* describes the lifelong process of change that occurs by means of genetic expression of the physical body through biological processes, creative expression of the mind through emotional processing of perceptual interpretations, and spiritual expression of the soul through relationships with others. These attributes of human development reverberate along the axis of maturation as growth advances in predictable patterns and sequences (with individual variability in the timing and quality of performance outcomes relative to environmental pressures) and is simultaneously influenced by the social relationships that support the person. At the same time, each aspect of human development spirals toward progress or retreats from it as the locus of momentum shifts from the differentiating process of individuation to the exploratory process of transformation.

The holistic perspective (Figure 2.2) encourages us to look at the process of development with new eyes. With such vision, each person is seen as a deliberately whole creation from birth, even when born with a disability. Equal weight is given to the relationships that nurture the child and to the genetic characteristics with

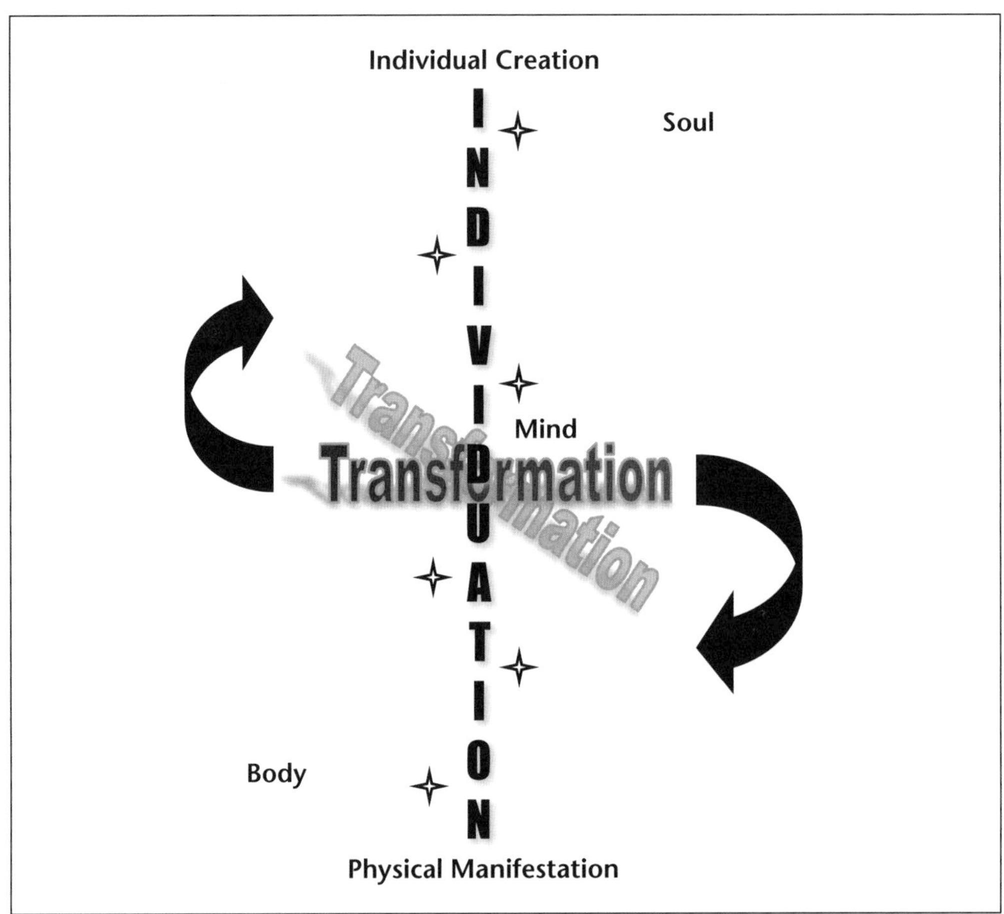

Figure 2.2. Holistic Theory of Human Development (Giese, 2002a). Used with permission of the author.

which each child is endowed. Transformational power rests within the way each person perceives the world. The way in which we think and feel about our individual experiences affects the choices we make and the encounters we initiate.

The developmental process begins at birth and, from a neurobiological perspective, even before. Human development is a complex dance of nature's genetic and environmental influences and of each caregiver's nurturing attention.

Community-Based Model of Practice

A thorough understanding of human development is paramount to proficient occupational therapy practice. During preservice training, occupational therapy students extensively study biological systems and processes across the lifespan as a foundation of professional knowledge. The medical model of training and practice was a hallmark of the occupational therapy profession during the biomedical or restoration era. Emphasis was placed on restoration of normal biological functioning, effectively marginalizing people who lived with long-term disabilities. The medical model focuses on dysfunction and vulnerability—deficiencies rather than strengths—so that problems can be addressed efficiently and effectively in a medical environment for correction, rehabilitation, or adaptation. In a medical setting, this model promotes precise diagnosis and treatment by the physician as the director of the medical team.

A medical team certainly has its strengths in addressing medical issues. Outside the acute care setting, however, current practice in early intervention and other early childhood programs is in a contextually referenced, community-based model of practice. The pace of development from birth through age 5 is a whirlwind of learning, adaptation, and change across all developmental domains. This transformation is both continual and contextual, because we are intrinsically programmed for growth and extrinsically flooded with opportunities for development. Such complex change creates solid foundations for future learning and success when handled positively. It can also create great vulnerability when family stresses become too great or caregiver resources are lacking. Public health policy supports the early identification and treatment of developmental concerns to facilitate future academic and social success and reduce the potential burden of care that may be borne by society as a whole. A community-based approach headed by the parents is needed to effectively address early intervention and early childhood needs.

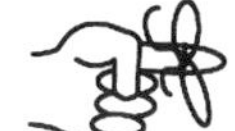

Remember this. . . .
This transformation is both continual and contextual, because we are intrinsically programmed for growth and extrinsically flooded with opportunities for development.

This chapter identifies the influence and interaction of socioenvironmental factors on growth and development from birth through age 5 and on future occupational engagement. Key challenges in social, cognitive, language and communication, motor, and adaptive domains are discussed, as are typical patterns and sequences of growth and development within each domain. The effects of occupational roles, occupational permanence and equanimity, and developmental processes on current and future occupational performance are viewed from a holistic perspective within a community-based model of treatment. The discussion begins, however, with anticipation and wonder and the changing occupational role dynamics that parents experience because typical development starts with the dreams of expectant parents for their unborn child.

Dreams of Parenthood: A New Occupational Role

The gentle kicks of an active fetus herald the arrival of new life. Each pregnancy journeys along its own path, varying from one mother to another and from one pregnancy to the next. After months of anticipation, the moment of birth is a time of great wonder and overwhelming emotion. Parents envisage the birth as a day of great joy, with dreams of 10 fingers and 10 toes, of smiling and laughing with their newborn child, of watching their child grow up to be healthy, happy, and successful. The moment of birth signals the initial fulfillment of—or interference with—those dreams.

Parents dream not only of what their child's life will be but also of what their own role as parents will entail. The occupations of parenthood include familiar activities of daily living (ADLs) that comprise performance patterns associated with adult life. Performance patterns may be habituated into automatic behaviors or may be consciously woven into the structure of daily life. Meals must be prepared or purchased. Work and recreation routines vie for attention. Restorative sleep cycles are incorporated into daily routines. Couples may already share these daily responsibilities as they care for themselves and each other. Single parents will have to manage not only ADLs but also the dynamics of choice or circumstance that result in raising a child alone.

Performance patterns may be health promoting, as when grooming and hygiene tasks become useful habits, or automatic behaviors. Performance patterns can damage health when impoverished habits, such as smoking or drug use, weaken the person. By adding an infant to any family, occupational responsibilities expand and grow to include new caregiving tasks. Some first-time parents may experience occupational dissonance with new skills such as breastfeeding or changing diapers. Others will have learned selected child-rearing skills as part of their role as older siblings in their families of origin or even as babysitters while growing up. What is common to all parents, regardless of their prior child-rearing experiences, is the profound change in occupational performance patterns that a new infant brings.

Parents must incorporate their new caregiving tasks into existing occupational roles. First-time parents must establish new function, whereas experienced parents must add new task demands to the parenting role they have already learned. Shared wisdom suggests that these demands multiply exponentially rather than incrementally with each new child in a family. The occupational tasks of this new role are learned through a dynamic interplay of occupational dissonance and occupational development. Where accurate anticipation and learning have occurred, occupational development will follow with individualized levels of challenge and success. Where individual capacities meet challenges that are greater than existing skills, or with unanticipated challenges, parents will be faced with occupational dissonance and the added stress of unmet needs.

The family constellation, with its changing tasks and routines, provides the contextual structure for the infant. It is into this dynamic environment that the newborn will be introduced. The dependent infant engages in occupational tasks of feeding, elimination, and sleeping as the newborn transitions to life outside the womb. With such dependent initial role function, the occupational profile  of the infant extends to caregivers as well. Because the family unit provides both dependent functional performance and contextual structure for the infant, the occupational profile of the infant extends to the parents. By carefully anticipating the changing occupational profile of new parents, plans for areas of anticipated occupational dissonance can be made to provide resources needed for learning and support.

Learning Activity 2.1 challenges readers to anticipate the changing occupational profile of new parents as they prepare for the birth of their first child. Performance skills related to child rearing and performance patterns of the couple illustrate the resources and stressors that may contribute to occupational development and occupational dissonance associated with new caregiving roles. The comparison of case study projections to the lived experience synthesizes wellness concepts into the changing occupational profile of new parents.

Preparation for Role Expansion: Environmental Influences

Healthy infant and young child development originates not only in expectations but also in preparation. Expectant parents modify many areas of occupation to prepare for the healthy arrival of their new child and for the changing role expectations

Learning Activity 2.1. Occupational Development and Occupational Dissonance: The Changing Occupational Profile

Kate and her husband, David, are expecting their first child. Kate is a 27-year-old tax attorney and an only child. Kate's parents believed that children should be allowed to enjoy childhood; she was expected to clean her room, make her bed, and set the table for dinner, and her few chores remained consistent as she grew older. Kate's college was paid for through a fund that her parents set up when she was born. Her leisure occupations throughout high school consisted of a variety of after-school clubs and activities. Kate entered paid employment the summer after her freshman year of college.

David, Kate's 26-year-old husband of 2 years, works in marketing and has two older sisters and one younger brother. His parents both worked outside the home while he was growing up. David had the same household chores as his wife, but he got his first job outside the home at age 15. Although David was the primary playmate for his younger brother during childhood, his older sisters helped with the caregiving tasks. David was not expected to feed or diaper his younger brother.

Kate and her husband are both health conscious. They walk together after dinner each evening and play tennis or golf on the weekends. David also plays on a local softball team in the spring and summer. The couple attends church frequently and plans to have their baby baptized. Both sets of grandparents and both of David's sisters live nearby. Kate and David are the first in the extended family to have a child.

Kate works full time and will stay home for 6 weeks before returning to full-time work after the baby is born. David works full time. David works near home in their suburban neighborhood, but Kate drives 40 miles each way to her law firm in a large urban area. The commute typically takes 60–90 min; parking and getting to her office on the 35th floor can take another 15–20 min. Kate recently said, "When the baby comes, I want to kind of incorporate it into our regular routine if we can." A typical daily routine for the couple is as follows:

Time	Kate	David
6:00 a.m.	Awaken—Hygiene and grooming Breakfast	Awaken—Work out
7:00 a.m.	Drive to work	Hygiene and grooming Breakfast
8:00 a.m.		Drive to work
9:00 a.m.	Work 9–5	Work 9–5
5:00 p.m.	Drive home	Drive home
6:00 p.m.		Prepare dinner
7:00 p.m.	Dinner; walk or tennis; softball spring and summer	
8:00 p.m.	Overtime work during quarterly tax seasons	Laundry, mail, cleaning tasks shared each day
9:00 p.m.		
10:00 p.m.	Down time and ready for bed	
11:00 p.m.	Sleep	

Part A

1. Is Kate in for a surprise or being unrealistic if she thinks she can just incorporate the baby into their regular routines?
2. What child-rearing skills did Kate and David learn in their families of origin?
3. How will the daily routine of each parent be affected by the birth of their child?
4. When during the year do you expect the levels of occupational dissonance to be greatest for this couple?
5. Who may be available to Kate and David as an additional resource for assisting with the occupational development of caregiving roles?
6. How will your answers to these questions change if the new baby is diagnosed with a developmental delay or is born prematurely?

Part B

1. Interview a new parent or set of new parents about the changes in routine they experienced with the birth of their first child.
2. Interview an experienced parent or set of experienced parents about the birth of their second child, and explore how that event differed from the first.

associated with child rearing. Occupational priorities may shift into or out of occupational permanence as activities are released in preparation for the role acquisition and expansion that child rearing brings.

The expectant mother experiences practical and protective alterations in ADLs throughout her pregnancy. Mild to moderate changes in individual hygiene, grooming activities, and functional mobility become practical realities as the mother's girth expands to accommodate the growing fetus. Individual energy expenditure may increase during the course of a pregnancy, affecting participation in normal daily routines and increasing the need for restorative sleep. Sleep patterns may also be altered by the activity of the fetus, which often intensifies at night. In complicated cases, medical orders for periods of bed rest may significantly affect routines and habits of the expectant mother as well as family occupations.

The expectant mother's attention to ADLs is especially important as it relates to the prenatal environment of the child. A child's fate is no longer thought to be predestined by genetics. The mapping of the human genome has catapulted the field of genetics to new heights of understanding. It is not just the presence of the genetic code but also the expression of it that alters human traits. The genetic record is expressed by the amount of proteins a gene produces and can be altered by epigenetic mechanisms such as genetic splicing, in which different proteins are created by the same gene. As a result of such genetic expression, identical twins may show different propensities for disease. Similar epigenetic change mechanisms may also be involved in altering proclivities for disease through individual differences in diet and lifestyle (Duke University Medical Center, 2009). As nature and nurture work in an integrated manner to affect human growth and development, rapid cell proliferation and growth during the prenatal period makes the fetus acutely susceptible to negative dietary and environmental influences. Scientific inquiry into the harmful effects of exposure to alcohol and tobacco, cocaine and other illicit drugs, nutrient deficiencies, and allergens has yielded various levels of evidence and concern (Jirikowic, Kartin, & Olson, 2008; Shonkoff & Phillips, 2000).

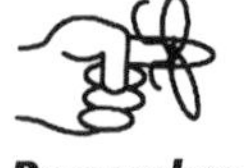

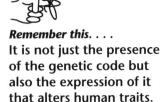

Remember this. . . .

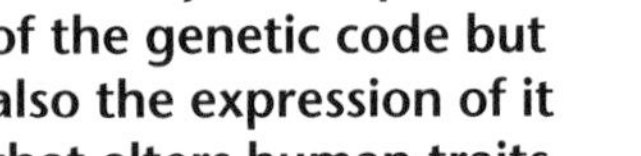

It is not just the presence of the genetic code but also the expression of it that alters human traits.

Infant Birth Weight

The conventional indicator of prenatal health has long been an infant's birth weight—the weight at birth compared with calculated gestational age. Although typical presentations vary widely among infants for both gestational duration and birth weight, the traditional indicator for a full-term infant is 37 to 41 weeks gestation with a birth weight of 2,500 g (5 lbs, 8 oz) or greater. Infants born at lesser weights with shorter gestations are identified as preterm infants, or babies of low birth weight (LBW). LBW babies have a higher incidence of neurobiological complications such as low oxygen levels at birth, poor body temperature regulation, difficulty feeding and gaining weight, bronchopulmonary distress, congenital malformations, chromosomal and metabolic abnormalities, intracranial hemorrhages, and neonatal diseases (Knobloch & Pasamanick, 1974). Prenatal exposure to environmental toxins, as well as low socioeconomic status, increases the risk of preterm birth (Prescott, 2006; University of Virginia [UVA] Health System, 2004). Ethnic health disparities are related to LBW in the United States; the incidence of LBW babies is twice as high in African-American births as it is in Caucasian births (UVA

Health System, 2004). Issues of LBW are of paramount importance for multiple-birth pregnancies: More than 50% of multiple births are LBW babies, compared with 6% of babies born as singletons (UVA Health System, 2004).

Very low birthweight (VLBW) babies—those weighing 1,500 g (3 lbs, 5 oz) or less—are surviving today at escalating rates. Technological, medical, and surgical advances in the past quarter century have dramatically increased the life-saving outcomes of infants of VLBW. These infants are at significantly greater risk than their full-term counterparts for neurological compromise and for developmental delay or disability within the first 3 years of life (Thompson et al., 2003). Researchers in Finland found that infants with VLBW with bronchopulmonary dysplasia use occupational therapy and physical therapy services more often than their counterparts of LBW only. LBW infants, however, also use occupational therapy services more often than children born at term. Parents in the Finnish study reported that the burden of care for infants with VLBW and bronchopulmonary dysplasia affected life for all family members long after the neonatal period of the new infant had passed (Korhonen, Koivisto, Ikonen, Laippala, & Tammela, 1999).

In the United States, researchers at Columbia University in New York, a cohort of the National Collaborative Perinatal Project, examined the relationship between early childhood respiratory disease and the risk of receiving treatment for mental health issues (Goodwin & Buka, 2008). More than 1,000 infants were followed from birth through adulthood. This cohort found that a higher respiratory rate in 4-month-old infants was associated with significantly greater risk of receiving treatment for anxiety by age 34. A diagnosis of respiratory disease at 1 year was also associated with increased risk of treatment for anxiety as an adult. It is easy to understand the relationship between difficulty breathing and anxiety; it is interesting that this anxiety may continue throughout life. Similar relationships were not found for increased risk for mood disorders.

Because LBW affects not only infant development and family occupations but also adult health issues, it is important to determine performance habit patterns that contribute to suboptimal maternal health and wellness and that are correlated with preterm births and LBW.

Fetal Alcohol Exposure

Fetal growth and development may be negatively affected by daily habits of both parents but particularly by the habits of the mother. Activities such as alcohol, tobacco, or drug use for recreation, emotional regulation, or calming responses to stress are impoverished habits that may harm the developing fetus. Excessive alcohol intake during pregnancy may result in fetal alcohol syndrome and resultant fetal alcohol spectrum disorder (FASD). Young children with FASD have been found to display poor social interaction and communication skills, variant gross and fine motor skills, delayed adaptive behavior, and sensory processing deficits (Franklin, Deitz, Jirikowic, & Astley, 2008; Jirikowic et al., 2008; Kalberg et al., 2006). These functional and component discrepancies interfere with a child's occupational performance in multiple environments and may persist throughout life, affecting school and work functions. Such challenges with self-regulation may further affect social skills well beyond childhood.

Fetal Drug Exposure

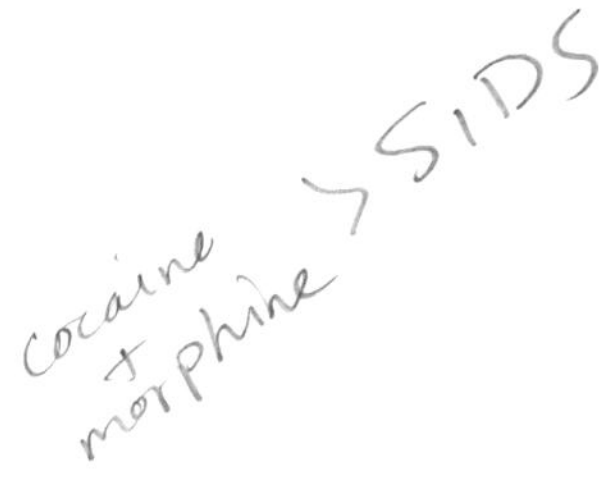

Fetal cocaine exposure yields medical risks associated with future developmental delays or deficits. Known pharmacologic and physiologic effects of cocaine include restlessness, depression, seizures, hypotension, and circulatory collapse. Potential complications of cocaine use during pregnancy include miscarriage, spontaneous abortion, or premature labor caused by increased contractions and hypertension (Morishima, Whittington, & Thadani, 1995). Olsen, Murphey, and Thadani (1995) identified that cocaine readily crosses the placenta and may be associated with sudden infant death syndrome (SIDS) in early infancy. The narcotic morphine, which depresses breathing, is even more strongly associated with SIDS when used by the expectant mother during pregnancy (Olsen et al., 1995).

Although pharmacologic and physiologic effects of prenatal cocaine exposure are widely known, later developmental delays appear to be related to more than cocaine exposure alone. In a study of 40 cocaine-exposed infants and 41 non-exposed infants of VLBW, Singer et al. (1994) found that cocaine-exposed infants had a higher incidence of mild intraventricular hemorrhage than their VLBW peers who had not been exposed to cocaine. The cocaine-exposed infants were also more likely to be placed in foster care or to be living with relatives because maternal occupational performance was often compromised by simultaneous addiction to alcohol, marijuana, and tobacco. Finally, at a mean corrected age of 8 months, these infants demonstrated cognitive and motor delays, even when statistics controlled for the effects of intraventricular hemorrhage and corrected chronological age (Singer et al., 1994). Such results suggest that the direct effect of cocaine exposure on infant development has not yet been definitively linked to only cocaine exposure itself.

A literature review by Tronick and Beeghly (1999) garnered variations in the developmental performance of cocaine-exposed infants when compared with their age-matched peers but revealed no direct relationship between prenatal cocaine exposure and delays in infant development. What the researchers did notice, however, was that among the cocaine exposure study populations there was a cumulative effect of multiple medical and social risk factors associated with long-term exposure to poverty. Risk factors included social isolation, child abuse and domestic violence, and maternal psychopathology and poor child-rearing practices. These findings suggest that long-term stress in an unsupportive environment can lead to the inclusion of a multitude of impoverished performance habit patterns into the daily lives of expectant mothers, thereby negatively affecting infant and young child development.

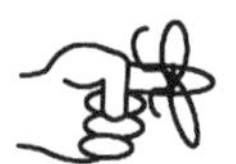

Remember this. . . .
These findings suggest that long-term stress in an unsupportive environment can lead to the inclusion of a multitude of impoverished performance habit patterns into the daily lives of expectant mothers, thereby negatively affecting infant and young child development.

Fetal Exposure to Smoke and Other Environmental Toxins

Smoking is an impoverished habit pattern that has a negative influence on early infant development through both active and passive exposure. Recent studies have confirmed the harmful developmental effect of prenatal maternal tobacco use on infants. At the Case Western Reserve University School of Medicine, more than 4,400 singleton pregnancies were studied at 10 to 19 weeks gestational age to determine the effects of maternal tobacco use on infant development. Small fetal size, early preterm birth, LBW, and poor fetal growth were all associated with maternal tobacco use during pregnancy (Mercer, Merlino, Milluzzi, & Moore, 2008). The Department of Health Services in Oakland, California, studied a similar number of pregnancies in 2000. This analysis found that when expectant mothers smoked more than 10 cigarettes per day, their infants faced neurodevelopmental risks similar to those reported by Mercer et al. (2008). Comparable incidences of LBW, small for gestational age (10th percentile for growth), and very early preterm birth (<35 weeks) were found (Windham, Hopkins, Fenster, & Swan, 2000). Maternal smoking during pregnancy has also been linked to impoverished self-regulation in infants and a greater need for handling in early infancy (Stroud et al., 2008).

The neurodevelopmental effects of early exposure to second-hand smoke and other environmental pollutants have also been studied. A literature review by Hermann, King, and Weitzman (2008) analyzed facts about the effects of prenatal tobacco and postnatal smoke exposure on child development. The review supported the correlation between tobacco exposure and adverse effects on infant behavioral and cognitive development. Challenging behaviors such as conduct disorders, attention deficit hyperactivity disorder, oppositional defiant behavior, and irritability have all been linked to prenatal and secondhand perinatal environmental smoke exposure (Hermann et al., 2008). The Columbia Center for Children's Environmental Health has estimated the cost of early intervention services related to environmental tobacco smoke exposure at $99 million per year for all New York City births; more than half of the estimated expense is borne by the Medicaid program (Miller et al., 2006). Clearly, the occupational performance habit patterns of parents can have a significant effect on early infant development, health, and occupational performance well beyond childhood.

Fetal Nutrition

Influential habit patterns include not only superfluous habits but also daily nutritional practices. Possible associations have been established between dietary habits that create suboptimal intrauterine conditions at critical periods of growth and findings of developmental disabilities, behavior problems, cognitive disabilities, speech–language impairment, learning disabilities, asthma, and adult-onset chronic health conditions such as Type 2 diabetes and schizophrenia (Kaiser, Kearney, Scott, DuClos, & Kurlfink, 2008; Opler & Susser, 2005; Opler et al., 2008; Prescott, 2006; Salvatore, Keymolen, Hauser, & Vandenplas, 2005; Yajnik & Dwshmukh, 2008). Even a strict vegetarian lifestyle has been shown, in some cases, to lead to severe Vitamin B12 deficiency, which may produce neurological symptoms in infants such as irritability, failure to thrive, apathy, feeding difficulties, and developmental regression (Dror & Allen, 2008). Proper nutrient intake with special attention to levels of folic acid, vitamin B12, iron, and calcium is widely accepted as playing an important role in creating an optimum intrauterine environment.

More controversial are other nonnutrient food additives, such as aspartame, a highly potent artificial sweetener contained in many foods and beverages to lower calorie content. Conflicting evidence exists about the long-term effects of aspartame ingestion as extrapolated to humans from toxicology studies on rodents. Although aspartame is regarded to be safe for human consumption with no direct effects on infant development, some studies have suggested negative health effects over the lifetime. Italian researchers have suggested that over the lifespan, the cumulative effects of aspartame ingestion may increase the rate of carcinogenic effects (Soffritti, Belpoggi, Esposti, Falcioni, & Bua, 2008; Soffritti, Belpoggi, Tibaldi, Esposti, & Lauriola, 2007). Similarly, rodent studies have advised that early aspartame ingestion may hasten the onset of cancer during adult life, particularly if intake begins through the expectant mother during pregnancy (Holder, 1989; McAnulty et al., 1989).

National Children's Study

Because of the far-reaching, widely diverse, and significant effects of genetic, nutritional, and environmental influences on health and development, a partnership of the U.S. Environmental Protection Agency and the U.S. Department of Health and Human Services, which includes the National Institutes of Health and the Centers for Disease Control and Prevention, has initiated the National Children's Study. This study, authorized by the Children's Health Act of 2000, is following the health and development of 100,000 children across the United States from before birth through age 21. The multisite project is examining the effects of environmental influences on health and development and is using a broad definition of *environment* to include natural and human-made environmental factors, biological and chemical factors, physical surroundings, social factors, behavioral influences and outcomes, genetics, cultural influences and differences, and geographic locations (National Children's Study, 2009). Results will be used to make recommendations to improve the health and well-being of children, develop prevention strategies, propose health and safety guidelines, and contribute to the possible development of new treatment for diseases and disabilities.

To date, the National Children's Study has focused on planning, pilot studies, research methodology, and recruitment of study partners and sites. Actual data collection began in January 2009 at a projected cost of nearly $200 million. Cohorts in Duplin County, North Carolina, and Queens, New York, will be the first to participate in the study work. These centers were chosen for their diversity. The North Carolina cohort represents a rural geographic area with a significant number of Hispanic residents, and Queens, New York, represents a racially and ethnically diverse urban area that is disproportionately affected by many of the health conditions the study will analyze. Although the study will span more than 20 years, results will be released as the study population reaches various developmental milestones. Global comparisons may eventually be included: The addition of a Japanese birth cohort study with 60,000 additional participants is under consideration (National Children's Study, 2009).

Daily Habit Patterns and the Fetal Environment

Remember this. . . .
Public policy that endorses community-based early intervention programs recognizes the need to address parental routines and habit patterns to facilitate healthy infant and young child development.

Just as the occupational profile of the infant encompasses the occupational performance history and routines of the parents, daily parental habit patterns shape the prenatal and perinatal environments of the developing child. The negative effects of impoverished parental habits on prenatal and perinatal environments has the potential to affect a child's health and well-being long into adult life. Public policy that endorses community-based early intervention programs recognizes the need to address parental routines and habit patterns to facilitate healthy infant and young child development. Performance patterns that have developed over time

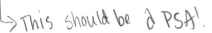

This should be a PSA!

to become automatic behaviors, however, may be difficult to change, even when motivation is high.

Prochaska, Norcross, and DiClemente (1994) studied successful change processes in people who have overcome habits of smoking, overeating, alcohol abuse, and the like; they identified six stages in the process of individual change.

1. The *precontemplation phase,* the initial phase of transformation, is highlighted by a person's inability or unwillingness to recognize and acknowledge the need for change. During this phase, clients may ignore change proposals because they feel overwhelmed by additional task demands or may feel hopeless about their ability to successfully adopt new habit patterns.
2. In the *contemplation phase,* people begin to weigh the pros and cons of adopting a personal change and eventually reach a tipping point where the advantages of making the change outweigh the perceived benefits of maintaining the current habit pattern.
3. The *preparation phase* marks readiness to initiate change; the person gathers resources and organizes routines and materials to facilitate the change process.
4. Social and physical supports may be assembled in preparation for the *action phase* of change, the hallmark of which is modification of behavior. Although this period of change is the most visible, each preceding phase prepares the groundwork for enduring transformation. Action without awareness and commitment easily dissolves.
5. During the *maintenance phase,* the person struggles to preserve new habits until they can become fully integrated into daily routines. The person fights to prevent lapses in commitment and performance and to overcome self-destructive behaviors as he or she adopts healthier habits. When lapses in the desired behavioral change occur, the person must find the resilience and social support to start again without abandoning the change process.
6. Finally, in the *termination stage* of change, the person no longer feels a sense of occupational dissonance or dissatisfaction as healthier habit patterns are effortlessly adopted into daily routines.

The maintenance and termination phases strengthen the durability of new habit patterns after the conversion has been initiated.

Learning Activity 2.2 invites the reader to apply the phases of the change process to personal experience. A progression of thoughtful contemplation is designed to enhance the reader's ability to empathize with others who are undergoing change.

Parent–Infant Relationships: Social–Emotional Development

Imagine yourself with nothing—no home, no clothes, no food—none of the basic necessities of life. Stripped of all your possessions, relationships are all that you have. Unable to provide for yourself, you are totally dependent on others.

Transfer now your imagination to the reality of the newborn. Infants enter this world with nothing but their genetic endowment and the kindness, love, and skills

Learning Activity 2.2. Personal Reflections on Changing Habits

Think about your own daily habits and their potential contribution to the physical environment of a developing child. Identify one impoverished habit or potentially damaging health routine that you have contemplated changing or have tried to change. You may have been successful in this process, or you may have fallen short of your goal. Answer the following questions with this daily routine or habit pattern in mind.

1. What happened in your daily life that made you aware of the need or desire to change this habit or daily routine?
2. What was the tipping point that made you believe it was time to change?
3. What preparations did you make to facilitate the change process? What resources did you garner? How did you reorganize your role expectations and daily occupations to support your intended change?
4. Briefly describe the actions you took to implement your change. What did you do that contributed to your success? What roadblocks did you encounter along the way?
5. How many false starts did you make? What did you do, or what supports did you receive to pull yourself back onto your plan of action? If you stopped and returned to your old ways, what was it that moved you to give up on the change?
6. If you were successful in your change quest, at what point did you realize that you had integrated this new habit into your daily routine?
7. Reflect on your journey toward integrating a new habit or routine into your daily life. Describe how these insights might help you to facilitate change in the daily habits and routines of parents to create a healthier environment for infant and young child development.

Learning Activity Discussion

Personal habits, particularly those of expectant mothers, have been shown to have a far-reaching impact on the development of infants across the lifespan. However, daily routines and habits may be deeply rooted, resistant to change, out of awareness, or even tied to one's identity with the stability of occupational permanence. By exploring your own journey toward changing routines and habits for healthier outcomes, you gain some insight into the difficulties your clients may encounter during the change process. Add to the desired change the major life adjustment of bringing a child into the world, and the dynamics of the change process are magnified. Personal routines and habits of both parents remain increasingly important after the child is born, because the social environment and cultural context of the home are equally important to the lifelong health of the child. Parent–infant relationships form the foundation for development across the lifespan. Such caregiving relationships are tangible assets to the infant. Relationships are the first real "things" that an infant experiences—for, in truth, infants enter this world with nothing.

Remember this. . . .
Each child's gifts are discovered gradually as life unfolds.

of others around them. The social context of an infant becomes more than a part of the external world; it permeates the activity demands of all that the infant does. Social relationships, as an extension of the infant and his or her occupational function, provide the foundation for all future development.

Although infants are dependent on others for occupational function and survival, every newborn brings a unique genetic capacity to life. Each child's gifts are discovered gradually as life unfolds. From physical aptitude to cognitive reasoning to individual skills and abilities, the genetic expression of traits unfurls as life progresses. At the beginning of life, however, one facet of development expresses itself immediately: Highly linked to genetics, the child's temperament surfaces as the novel environment greets the newborn. Life outside the womb is filled with sights, sounds, tastes, smells, and tactile experiences that are all new to the infant. No longer a constant recipient of nutrients through the placenta, even feelings of hunger and thirst are foreign to the newborn. The baby responds in its own way with its own disposition. This inherent nature of the child is known as *temperament,* the unique balance of emotional reactivity, sociability, and activity level that makes up the infant's responses to novelty and to distress. It is the infant's intrinsic approach to life—essentially, the emotional set point of the infant, the way in which each

how do they know?

* temperment

person is hard-wired to react to the world and to novel experiences. Temperament encompasses the unique behavioral pattern of how a person learns about, seeks from, and adapts to the environment and seems to share many features identified in Dunn's (2001) Model of Sensory Processing.

Temperament and Sensory Processing

Although Dunn (2001) specifically referred to earlier models of temperament when making comparisons to patterns of sensory processing, three types of temperament are now routinely identified in newborns: (1) the happy, or easy, child; (2) the fussy, or difficult, child; and (3) the moody, or slow-to-warm up, child (Box 2.1). Each type blends the three facets of temperament—emotionality, sociability, and activity levels—in different measure (Chess & Thomas, 1991).

Emotionality refers to the infant's susceptibility to emotional stimulation and response to distress. When upset, one infant might show fearful reactions and withdraw from the upsetting stimulus, whereas another infant might become angry and protest, typically with loud cries of discontent. These characteristics are similar to the emotional reactivity sometimes seen in response to sensory input. Occupational therapists may be challenged to determine whether an infant's emotionality is related to sensory input, communication frustration, or distress.

Sociability, or an infant's desire to be with others, is inferred by duration of eye gaze and turning toward others. When a sensory processing pattern of low registration of sensory input exists, more frequent and more intense sensory input is needed to produce an adaptive response. If the child and caregiver have different sensory processing patterns, especially if this difference is unrecognized, interactions may suffer as social signals are crossed.

Activity level is observed in the rhythm, intensity, and frequency of movements. In newborns, these movements typically indicate the presence of stress, periods of alert observation, or an infant's attempts to self-regulate emotions while learning to maintain longer periods of alertness throughout the day. Activity levels may also reflect an infant's unique sensory processing pattern. Some infants act in accordance with their sensory processing pattern, seeking the sensory input that their bodies need. Others seek to counteract their sensory stressors, decreasing active exploration or warming up slowly to new environments.

Temperament and Social Relationships

Although temperament appears to be principally programmed by genetics, it is further mediated by the social responses of adults in the child's environment. The sensitivity of the parent to the infant's emotional state and needs has been shown to have a significant impact on emotional bonding between the two. Healthy parent–infant relationships, especially during the first months of life, are critical to the health and well-being of the family unit. Occupational therapy professionals may provide support for positive parenting practices; the beneficial impact of occupational therapy in facilitating the parental role in child rearing has long been recognized as an important feature of occupational therapy practice with children (Allen & Hudd, 1987; Bazyk, 1989). A variety of supportive social structures increase maternal self-esteem and improve early parent–infant interactions. When caregivers are

Box 2.1. Three Types of Temperament Routinely Identified in Newborns

Happy: The happy, or easy, baby is one who is generally thought to be in a good mood and who tends to react mildly when hungry or experiencing discomfort. Easy infants effortlessly adapt to change and quickly establish regular routines. These babies are generally even tempered and independently find ways to calm themselves. They love to interact with others and to be involved in new experiences. Parents may respond favorably to the good nature of these infants or may spend less time interacting, erroneously thinking that the presence of the adult is not needed.

Fussy: The fussy, or difficult, infant experiences distress more frequently and intensely; he or she cries often, and becomes easily upset by new experiences. These infants are restless, distractible, and highly active. Crying is often loud and intense. These babies find it difficult to soothe themselves and may be difficult for parents to comfort. They are often very light sleepers. Difficult babies are apt to demand attention from their parents. Caregivers need to provide regular routines as well as calm and safe environments for these children. It is easy for parents of difficult children to become discouraged and to feel inadequate about their parenting skills. Therefore, it is important for parents to understand that self-regulation improves as the nervous system continues to develop and the baby grows.

Moody: The moody, or slow-to-warm up, baby is often known as a "shy" or "sensitive" child. These infants have a low activity level and a more negative mood. They are observant of the world around them, but they often become easily overstimulated. They demonstrate low adaptability and low intensity of movement. Slow-to-warm up infants often retreat from distress by looking or turning away. They take time to adapt to new experiences. As such, these babies require patience, a calm environment, and extra time to respond to new routines and activities. Caregivers may also need to recognize subtle signs of overstimulation in these infants and help them by removing them from the excessive stimuli.

Source. Chess & Thomas (1991).

stressed or perceive the infant as difficult or unlikable, they tend to respond and interact negatively with the infant. This interaction, in turn, negatively affects the bonding experience that is so important during the newborn's initial exposure to life, both for current occupational functioning and for future learning and mental health. (Chapter 3 provides further information about parent–child relationships.)

At the University of Chicago, Benjamin B. Lahey and colleagues (2008) followed nearly 1,900 children every 2 years from infancy through age 13 to study the effect of temperament and parenting style on the prevalence of conduct disorders later in life. Researchers visited the homes of study participants during the infants' first year of life to interview mothers about their child's temperament and to observe parent–infant interactions. Both parenting style and child's temperament were found to be good predictors of future behavioral problems, such as disobeying parents, acting out, lying, or bullying others. Babies with low fearfulness, whose mothers had provided meaningful stimulation during the first year of life, were less likely to develop conduct problems later during childhood. Similarly, infants with temperaments that were described as low in fussiness and high in predictability were also less likely to develop behavioral problems. Infants in the study who were rated by their mothers as having difficult temperaments in infancy were more likely to have maternally reported behavioral problems from ages 4 to 13. These findings suggest that parenting style, parent responsiveness, and infant temperament during the first year of life are predictors of future behavioral problems.

Remember this. . . .
"Caregiving is a co-occupation that involves active participation on the part of the caregiver and the recipient of care" (American Occupational Therapy Association, 2008, p. 629).

Such conclusions support the occupational therapy principle that occupations are often shared: "Caregiving is a co-occupation that involves active participation on the part of the caregiver and the recipient of care" (American Occupational

Therapy Association, 2008, p. 629). This dyadic process is a dance that is driven both by the parent's attunement to the infant's direct and indirect needs and the infant's expression of needs in predictable or unpredictable patterns and in pleasant or unpleasant ways.

The dyadic nature of the interplay between infant temperament and parenting styles has global support. Studies in Australia, Finland, the Netherlands, and Canada have found similar relationships between parental stress and children's mental health. An Australian study of 733 children, recruited from a socioeconomically and culturally diverse wellness sample, followed the children from ages 7 to 36 months. Multiple measures of parenting, child behavior, and contextual factors were surveyed over the course of the study. Results indicated that increased parenting stress and decreased positive parenting procedures contributed to negative behavior in toddlers (Bayer, Hiscock, Ukoumunne, Price, & Wake, 2008).

In Finland, researchers surveyed 214 couples about temperament and marital relationship, social support, and self-perceived efficacy in routine caregiving. Mothers who reported high self-esteem, adequate social support, and adaptive social strategies during early pregnancy also reported less parental stress during the toddler years. Conversely, pregnancy-related anxiety and depression, infant temperament, and low self-perceived competence in caregiving were associated with increased reports of parental stress by early childhood (Saisto, Salmelo-Aro, Nurmi, & Halmesmaki, 2008).

Researchers in the Netherlands looked at low socioeconomic status and its relationship to temperament during infancy. This study was broad in scope: More than 4,000 mothers were surveyed, providing a snapshot of the infant's temperament and behavior at age 6 months. Difficult infant temperament was associated with lower socioeconomic status on 83% of temperament dimensions. Family stress and compromised maternal psychological well-being were associated with increased infant distress, poorer recovery from distress, and shorter duration of social orienting (Jansen et al., 2008). As noted previously, infant temperament influences parental behavior as well.

Canadian researchers studied 987 mother–infant pairs annually from ages 5 months to 6 years. Through questionnaires and interviews, researchers learned that the presence of sleep disturbances in infants before 18 months of age was associated with maladaptive parental behaviors during toddler years. Even so, early sleep disturbances associated with a fussy or difficult temperament were found to be more predictive of sleeping difficulties from ages 50 months to 6 years than the maladaptive parental behaviors that developed in response to sleep difficulties during the toddler years (Simard, Nielsen, Tremblay, Boivin, & Montplaisir, 2008).

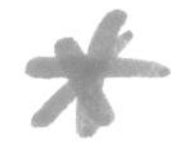

Humphry (1989) studied the influence of occupational therapists in early intervention and found that they can be relied on as a source of social support for parents. During this study, it was further noted that although parental stress and social support affect child-rearing occupations, a fussy or moody temperament in the infant had a negative effect on parenting as well. When occupational dissonance is created through differing infant temperament and parental sensitivity, it may lead to occupational dysfunction, particularly as it relates to the process of attachment and parent–infant bonding.

Attachment Theory

Ideas about the importance of parent–infant bonding are founded in attachment theory, which was developed and expanded on by psychologists John Bowlby (1977) and Mary Ainsworth (Ainsworth, Blehar, Waters, & Wall, 1978). Bowlby studied the effects of separation on the parent–child relationship and identified the early role of the parent as providing the ego and superego of the child. As the orienting center of the child's world, the caregiving parent permits the satisfaction of some impulses and denies others, acknowledging the duality of the parent–infant relationship. Bowlby posited that to grow up mentally healthy, the infant and young child should "experience a warm, intimate, and continuous relationship with his mother (or permanent mother substitute)" (Bowlby, 1951, as cited in Bowlby, 1988, p. 26). Building on Bowlby's early work, Ainsworth et al. (1978) observed parent–infant interactions. They found that infants who were *securely attached* cried little and comfortably explored the environment in the presence of their mothers, whereas infants who were *insecurely attached* cried often and did not explore the environment, even when held by their mothers. When attachment had not yet been established, infants did not display differentially referent behavior toward their mothers. Ainsworth et al. further documented that babies whose mothers were highly responsive to crying during infancy were later more reliant on facial expressions, gestures, and vocalizations for communication. The same pattern was true for tactile input. Babies whose mothers held them more during the first 3 months of life sought contact less often approaching 1 year, but the contact that did occur at 1 year was rated as more satisfying and affectionate.

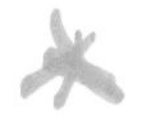

Parent–Infant Bonding

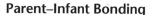

The role of the parent in fostering positive occupational outcomes in the child is related to patterns of responsiveness in parent–infant interactions. In Switzerland, Forcada-Guex, Pierrehumbert, Borghini, Moessinger, and Muller-Nix (2006) studied patterns of mother–infant play interaction in both term and preterm babies to determine their effect on developmental outcomes at 18 months of corrected age. Two patterns emerged as predictive of better outcomes in infant occupational performance: (1) a *cooperative pattern* with a sensitive mother and a cooperative–responsive infant and (2) a *controlling pattern* with a controlling mother and a compulsive–compliant infant. Other heterogeneous patterns were evident in 44% of the participants, but they did not readily correlate with outcomes. Of the full-term babies in the study population, 68% of the dyads were identified as cooperative pattern dyads, 12% were controlling pattern dyads, and 20% were other combinations. The study found that at 18 months of corrected age, preterm infants in cooperative dyads had similar occupational outcomes for sleep, eating, psychosomatic symptoms, and behavior and emotional problems as did their full-term counterparts. Preterm infants in controlling dyads had significantly more eating problems and behavioral symptoms than their full-term peers. Although overall developmental quotients were similar for both groups, controlling dyad patterns yielded significantly poorer personal–social development and hearing–speech development than did cooperative dyads. Thus, the cooperative pattern can be seen as having a protective function in infant development, whereas the controlling pattern appears to have a risk-precipitating function (Forcada-Guex et al., 2006).

The optimal time for facilitating parent–infant bonding and intervention effects was studied by Landry, Smith, Swank, and Guttentag (2008) for children of varying biological risk. This team examined interventions during infancy and toddlers and preschool-age children. Parent training in playing and learning strategies was provided at two intervention periods. Intervention during infancy fostered increased maternal warmth, whereas intervention during toddler and preschool age supported cognitive–behavioral outcomes in the youth. Across both age-related intervention periods, training was needed to increase the mother's sensitivity to a child's changing signals that contingent responsiveness or redirection was required (Landry et al., 2008).

Parent–infant bonding is critical as a foundation for emotional, cognitive, and social development and for learning adaptive behavior and social interactions (Brazelton & Cramer, 1990). Natural opportunities for bonding occur during routine ADLs. Feeding, diapering, bathing, dressing, and play activities are all cooperative functions between parent and child during a newborn's infancy. When a parent nurtures those functions through calm, supportive verbal modeling and physical support, infants develop a sense of emotional and physical security. This sense of calm amid the newborn's storm of novel internal and external stimuli helps the infant learn to regulate emotions and behavior in response to physiological needs. Especially during the first 4 months of life, parents and caregivers help the infant become skilled at maintaining the calm–alert state that is most effective for learning. Once infants learn to regulate their behavior and feelings, they begin to use their feelings to problem solve and act on the environment rather than only in response to it (Brazelton & Greenspan, 2000). As noted pediatrician Stanley I. Greenspan suggested, "We can say that the child first uses the expression of emotion as a probe to understand the world. It's through his first affective interchanges that his sense of causality is established" (Brazelton & Greenspan, 2000, p. 11). The sense of empowerment generated by initial understanding of causality is the next level of self-regulation that propels infants securely forward into the independence of childhood. The sense of self-esteem that develops not only through relationships in infancy but also in continuing relationships throughout the toddler years provides motivation for learning across the lifespan (Table 2.1).

Hierarchy of Needs

Abraham Maslow (1968) described a hierarchy of needs common to all human beings. Similar to the importance of bonding described in the literature, Maslow's hierarchy illustrates that basic needs must be met before children can focus on learning. Physiological needs are of the highest priority at the base of the hierarchy. Food, air, water, exercise, rest, bodily comfort, and health are the needs that the person is motivated to fill first. In infancy, caregivers help the infant meet those needs and learn to feel confident that they will be met. With increasing confidence, the infant develops a sense of security and stability that opens his or her heart to love and belonging. The infant feels included in the family unit and moves to meet ego needs through exploring and receiving positive feedback from the

Table 2.1. Newborn States of Consciousness

State	Quiet (Deep) Sleep	Active (Light/ REM) Sleep	Drowsy	Quiet Alert	Active Alert	Crying
Definition	Restorative	Greatest frequency of newborn sleep; usually precedes waking	Mild startles from time to time; may return to sleep or awaken further	Period of greatest attention to environment	Period of active body movement	Intense crying for minimum of 15 seconds
Sensory threshold	Very high	More responsive to hunger and handling	Delayed responses to sensory stimuli	Alert and responsive	Easily overstimulated	Has been crossed
Response to stimuli	Only very intense and disturbing stimuli will arouse	May remain in active sleep, return to quiet sleep, or arouse	May change to quiet alert, active alert, or crying	Will focus on any present stimuli	May change to quiet alert or crying	May self-soothe or need help to do so
Breathing pattern	Smooth and regular	Irregular	Irregular	Regular	Irregular	More irregular than other states
Body activity	Nearly still	Some	Smooth with variable activity level	Minimal	Variable level; startles; smooth motor activity	Increased motor activity; skin dark and ruddy
Eye movements	None	REM; fluttering of eyes beneath closed eyelids	Heavy-lidded, may open and close	Wide and bright	Open and glazed	Open or tightly closed
Facial movements	Occasional sucking movements	May smile and make fussy or brief crying sounds	Face appears still	Attentive	Face appears still	Grimaces
Impact on occupational performance	Wait for naturally occurring higher state of consciousness	Brief crying sounds normal; not indicative of need to nurse or feed	May arouse with visual, auditory, or suckling sensory input	Good time to feed infant; great time for socialization	Hunger, fatigue, noise, excessive handling may change to crying	Communicates response to unpleasant internal or external stimuli

Note. REM = rapid eye movement.

Sources. American Academy of Pediatrics (2010); March of Dimes (2003); Mesa Community College Psychology Department (1999).

environment. Self-actualization is reached incrementally as the child develops a sense of autonomy and achievement.

In toddler and preschool years, the same hierarchy of needs expresses itself in different ways. When a young child goes off to childcare or preschool without having had time for breakfast, the basic physiological needs of hunger and thirst may interfere with learning and behavior. The need for stability, provided by daily routines, does not get met when a household operates in chaos or when changing adult work schedules make it difficult to provide stable organization of routines. Unsupported by consistency, children may act out for attention in negative ways; they feel included in the social chaos, but do not realize the negative consequences of their behavior. Negative consequences lead to feelings of inadequacy, which can stifle learning. Such repeated behaviors become learned actions that habituate the child to poor performance, lack of self-esteem, and poor social skills.

Emotions and Learning

Erik Erikson (1982) also focused on the relationship of emotions and learning. His Eight Stages of Man theory identifies a sequence of emotional conflicts that need to be resolved for healthy development to occur. Successful resolution of conflict at one stage sets the foundation for higher level development. Erikson's first three stages encompass the period from birth through age 5.

The first stage of development focuses on the enhancement of trust versus mistrust in infancy. Recognizing the co-occupational nature of this time of life, Erikson (1982) posited that infants learn in this time to rely on others and to trust that others will meet their needs because they cannot meet them independently. When caregivers are sensitive and respond to infants' cries with calm, positive interactions, infants learn that they can depend on others for their physical survival and emotional security. When infants are met with angry adult interactions, they learn that their cries are inappropriate, regardless of their communicative intent. Social interactions are impeded, and the development of emotional bonds sets like a cracked foundation for future learning.

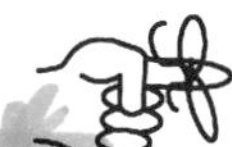

Remember this. . . .
When infants are met with angry adult interactions, they learn that their cries are inappropriate, regardless of their communicative intent. Social interactions are impeded, and the development of emotional bonds sets like a cracked foundation for future learning.

Erikson's (1982) second stage from ages 1 to 3 is characterized by the emotional conflict between autonomy versus shame and doubt. Autonomous or independent performance creates a sense of empowerment and self-respect. As infants explore the environment, the responses they receive can affect their emotional security about their ability to generate successful performance. If the environment is lacking in age-appropriate materials or if caregivers ignore or negatively respond to the infant's play and interactions, the child may feel ashamed about exploring and may learn to doubt his or her own abilities. When parental demands exceed the developmental capabilities of the child, frustration and shame create stress and further stifle performance. This situation creates a negative spiral that discourages learning and the development of self-confidence. Conversely, when infants are met with successful experiences and social interactions that match their own delight, they learn to be curious about the environment and feel confident to engage in new learning.

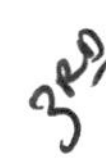

Finally, from ages 3 to 5, the child must resolve the conflict of initiative versus guilt. With initiative, a child feels positive about taking on new challenges and about initiating actions and interactions. A child with initiative is inventive and resourceful—perhaps creative and even mischievous. During this time, the emotional resources of parents and caregivers may be taxed as children make their own plans—plans that may conflict with existing rules, routines, or responsibilities. It is important to help children develop the ability to plan and make choices to feel confident about their ability to problem solve. As such, parents and caregivers need to provide age-appropriate choices such as which color shirt to wear or whether to don shorts or shirt first. Children need outlets for creative expression and the ability to get messy during creative play as their curiosity turns to the exploration of new materials in a variety of novel combinations.

When children are criticized for taking a stance, making a choice, or using materials with less than adult-level skill and precision, they blame themselves with self-reproach and take responsibility at a level that exceeds their physical and emotional capacities. Remembering that toddlers are only beginning to understand two-step related commands, adults need to modify their demands to match the developmental level of the child and set up the environment to support children's attempts at independence. Such sensitivity to children's emotional needs builds on the benefits of bonding that begin through co-occupational performance at birth.

Cognitive Development

For many years, researchers and child development specialists felt that babies entered this world as "blank slates"—as unthinking beings still growing without individual capacity for learning. Common wisdom held that because babies could not talk, they could not think. It was also thought until recently that very young babies did not experience pain. We now know that the human brain grows as a result of learning and experience and that learning new skills helps strengthen and retain neuronal synapses. Stress hormones can destroy brain cells and make learning more difficult. Emotional stability and physical safety and security play an important role in fostering receptivity to learning.

Perhaps the most influential developmental theorist was Jean Piaget (1936), who studied how infants and young children approached problem solving. He divided cognitive development into four stages (sensorimotor, preoperational, concrete operations, and formal operations) and showed that older children think differently from infants and young children. The first two stages are associated with infant and toddler development.

Piaget's (1936) sensorimotor stage spans from birth to age 2. During this time, babies learn through their experiences with the environment. Infants construct a cognitive representation of the world by building sensory experiences that tell about the environment and the child's relationship to it. This process starts with the reflexive movements of the infant. Because motor control is dominated by reflex activity at birth, the actions of the newborn result in unexpected sensory and motor experiences. In the process that Piaget labeled "primary circular reactions," the infant tries to re-create these experiences and thus learns about the human body and how it moves. By 6 months, as voluntary motor control increases, the infant begins to explore objects and to create similar accidental discoveries about the characteristics and capabilities of objects. At this time, the infant engages in "secondary circular reactions" by trying to re-create actions on objects that were originally discovered accidentally. Infants like to suck on fingers, kick mobiles with their feet, and play with their hands in their food. Eventually an infant learns that the finger he or she is sucking belongs to another person, that kicking a mobile causes it to swing, and that he or she can eat crackers independently by picking them up with the fingers. Thus, the infant begins to learn about the characteristics of objects in the external environment and about self as separate from the people and objects in the environment.

By the time a child is 1 year old, exploration is intentional and anticipatory. The infant develops a curiosity about the world that motivates new learning. Coupled with strong social bonding, the infant feels safe to move out into the world and try new things. By the time the child is age 2, an emerging sense of self frees the child to try ideas out with internal thought before trying them physically. An internal representation of objects has begun that allows mental manipulation of body parts and objects—the initial stages of motor planning. The child can now defer imitation—he or she can see something at one time and decide to imitate the action later. This is a time of *parallel play,* in which children play near each other but without significant interaction. During parallel play, children may notice what others are doing and can internalize that image to try observed play activities later on.

This phase leads to Piaget's (1936) preoperational stage of cognitive development, which lasts from age 2 through early childhood. During this stage, children see the world from their own point of view. Concrete and limited in their observations, they notice and respond to one characteristic at a time. Comparative attributes are based on what is directly observed, yielding errors in judgment without the benefit of logical reasoning. Social reasoning is based on the child's own experience of emotions; children during this phase do not yet understand perspectives that are different from their own.

Educational psychologist Lev Vygotsky (1986) brought a sociocultural perspective to cognitive theory. Vygotsky studied how children solved problems that were beyond their current level of development. His work suggested that a step-by-step change in a child's thought and behavior can be facilitated through social interaction and that such learning would vary widely from one culture to another. According to Vygotsky, cultural tools can be passed through the following types of learning:

- *Imitative learning,* which occurs when one child copies another
- *Instructed learning,* which is directed by the instructions of the adult and the use of these instructions to self-regulate learning
- *Collaborative learning,* which involves a group of peers who work together to learn a specific skill.

Vygotsky's (1986) sociocultural theory rests on four principles that provide the framework for learning.

1. *Children construct their own knowledge.* Preschoolers are often observed speaking to themselves as they work on a difficult task. This self-talk is a dialogue that guides them through the learning process, particularly as they are engaged in parallel play. Vygotsky (1986) posited that this externally voiced dialogue becomes quieter and eventually internal as knowledge is constructed over time.
2. *Learning cannot be separated from its social context.* Children can do more with the influence and assistance of others who are more skilled than they can do for themselves. They respond to the actions, suggestions, questions, and comments of others to facilitate their own learning. The term *zone of proximal development* refers to the difference between the actual developmental level of the child and the potential level of development determined through problem solving with an adult or more knowledgeable peer. The lower limit of the zone is marked by what the child can do independently; the upper limit is represented by what the child can do by watching and talking to others with greater knowledge and skills.
3. *Sociocultural learning can lead development.* This third principle of Vygotsky's (1986) theory leads to the possibility of great variability in rates of learning and development. With social learning, two people working together begin a task with different levels of understanding and arrive at a shared understanding as they work through the project. With the support of others, the child matches, categorizes, and organizes new

information with what is already known. This process of *scaffolding* builds a new cognitive structure on which future learning progresses. With careful attention to a child's task performance, others can facilitate learning through careful questioning and reflections on a child's performance.

4. *Language is an important part of social learning that furthers cognitive development.* Social interaction that is heavily laden with language also scaffolds one's internal dialogue, adding new elements of reasoning and logic from the experience of others to one's limited experience. Language is culturally based and therefore further contributes to the unique nature and cadence of learning that is mediated by cultural norms.

Language, Communication Development, and Social Skills

Communication comprises speech, language, and behavior. Language is closely related to cognitive development, because it is through language that we communicate learned information. *Language* is the symbolic representation of thought; it gives voice to ideas and meaning to relationships. After touch, it is the principal means throughout development for establishing and maintaining relationships with others. *Speech* is the element of communication concerned with the production of language, and speech development relies on oral–motor structure and function. It begins early in fetal development and increases in complexity after birth through play and feeding occupations.

The developmental period that precedes the infant's first word is the prespeech period. When the newborn arrives, all of his or her motor actions, including those of oral–motor structures, are guided by reflexive movements. The rooting reflex, for example, helps the child locate the source of food when the child's face is touched toward the region of the mouth. This reflex is present whenever the stimulus is presented, except for immediately after the child has been fed. The reflex persists until approximately age 3 months, at which time responses are differentiated for play and feeding in response to the same stimulus. The suck–swallow reflex is also present from birth to approximately 4 months. This reflex is an automatic, highly rhythmic pattern that allows the infant to close the lips around the nipple for feeding, suck repeatedly, and then swallow. It is closely coordinated with breathing patterns to allow successful ingestion of nutrients (Farber, 1982).

Additional reflexes serve both nutritive and oral–motor functions at various times throughout infancy. The gag reflex is a protective reflex that is present from birth throughout life, but it is more sensitive during infancy. The more experience the baby gains by mouthing objects and playing oral–motor games with others, the less sensitive the reflex becomes. The bite reflex, a repeated vertical chewing action, is present from 1 month and is integrated at approximately 6 to 8 months. Voluntary control gives rise to the more developmentally mature rotary chewing pattern used throughout adulthood. Although the infant is able to bring hands to mouth from birth, this movement comes under volitional control and becomes purposeful at approximately 5 to 7 months (Farber, 1982).

Infants' play with oral–motor sensations leads to language development. Initially random sounds emerge; later, the infant may attempt to reproduce the sounds, just as with other accidental motor actions. The discovery of single, repeated sounds leads to *ba-ba, ma-ma,* and *da-da,* to the delight of parents and friends. The occupation of feeding also contributes to oral–motor development. Lip closure attained during spoon feeding mimics the motor skills needed to produce closed consonant sounds like M and B. The introduction of different food consistencies promotes increasingly complex lip and tongue movements as well as increased coordination of respiration patterns later used for phonation. The child learns to integrate new breathing rhythms for drinking from a cup, because liquid must be drawn in before swallowing. Sipping, swallowing, and breathing are a new rhythmic pattern that must be mastered. Independent, consecutive swallowing is accomplished by approximately 1 year (Davis, 1978).

Before eating from a high chair, the infant is held in the caregiver's arms in a semireclined position. This position generates optimum natural opportunities for the reciprocal interactions that develop secure attachment and bonding. During feeding, the mother and infant gaze at each other, and the mother may engage in smiling, cooing, and vocal modeling to bond with the child. Infants respond to the speech of others with laughter, smiles, or other signs of pleasure at approximately 4 to 6 months. This communication interplay further contributes to bonding experiences and begins the development of social interaction skills. By 1 year, infants differentially respond to an adult's tone of voice and copy intonational patterns with jargon. The median age for an infant's first word is 11 months (Buch, Collins, & Gelber, 1978).

Once children begin to speak, language development proceeds exponentially. By 18 to 24 months, the child repeats syllables and uses two-word sequences. A vocabulary of 50 words at age 2 expands to more than 400 words within 1 year. During this time, the child is learning the meaning not only of individual words but also of words as they relate to each other. A hungry child quickly learns that "more cookie" may satiate a growling stomach, whereas "cookie" alone is simply declarative. By age 3, the child is using longer, more complex sentences and differentiating between their meanings.

Vocabulary development continues rapidly throughout preschool years. Children love to try new and bigger words. They enjoy the reactions from others as they communicate. Four-year-olds love to talk, to be spoken to, and to listen to books. They are beginning to understand increasing types of spatial concepts expressed through language. By age 5, children produce sentences with the same structure used by adults. Grammar is basically correct, and children begin to use language to read and write (Dodge, Colker, & Heroman, 2002).

Motor Skill Development

Until the higher centers of the central nervous system mature, the infant is dominated by automatic reflex movement. As the nervous system develops and matures, reflexes are integrated, and dominance gradually shifts to volitionally controlled motor function. Eventually, the infant is able to raise his or her body against gravity, maintain a stable posture against gravity, and move against gravity while maintaining dynamic equilibrium. Refined motor function leads to bilateral manipulation with coordinated fine motor capacities. Ever-imposed on motor execution is the process of motor planning or *praxis*. This sensorimotor sequence of registration, arousal, self-regulation, attention, focus, and motor execution increases in complexity as more complex motor capabilities are acquired (Farber, 1982).

Full discussion of typical motor development is far beyond the reaches of this synopsis. Occupational therapists study motor development in depth over multiple courses at preservice and postgraduate levels. What is important in this discussion of typical motor development is the impact on function when motor development is compromised, delayed, or disrupted.

Typical motor development may be compromised in several ways. Children born with cerebral palsy or spina bifida experience compromised motor function because of limitations of movement from paralysis or changes in muscle tone such as spasticity or athetosis. Children with trisomy 21 often have low muscle tone that interferes with motor control and execution. Low registration of sensory input in children with sensory processing disorders may compromise motor patterns and praxis. Delays in motor development are common for children born early or with LBW, because time spent hooked up to monitors in the neonatal intensive care unit (NICU) suspends opportunities for typical movement experiences associated with the newborn experience. Disruption of motor development is tragically seen in accidental or imposed trauma (e.g., abuse, physical violence). It has even been seen in care provided with the best of intentions, because of the overgeneralization of medical recommendations to have babies avoid the prone position during sleep to help prevent SIDS (American Academy of Pediatrics Task Force on Sudden Infant Death Syndrome, 2005).

When parents avoid the prone position altogether in an effort to avoid SIDS, infants lose the "tummy time" needed for optimal motor development.Typical motor development progresses in cephalocaudal and proximodistal directions. After this progression, the body's center of gravity moves from the head at birth to the pelvis at around 6 months. Within this sequence is the development of head control as the infant learns to raise and hold the head up against gravity. This motor skill is commonly developed and strengthened from the prone position, which also develops strength and stability around the shoulder girdle. When infants are not given time to play in this position, they lose opportunities for strengthening the shoulder girdle and developing head control. They also receive diminished vestibular stimulation and simultaneous visual stimulation that is stimulated by prone positioning. This paucity of sensory stimulation may lead to difficulties with coordinated visual function, which further impedes academic learning and may contribute to behavioral attending problems.

Motor function related to the cephalocaudal progression and the center of gravity can also be affected by seizure activity. A strong feature of tonic–clonic seizures is arching of the back during the active seizure. Repeated seizures may influence motor patterns to such an extent that the child's center of gravity may rest at the base of the rib cage rather than the pelvis. Even as typical developmental sequences emerge, the young child is affected by using the hands to support the body in seated and standing positions. Engaged in support, the hands are not free to manipulate objects, and fine motor development, bilateral coordination and, eventually, writing skills are disrupted.

Murray-Slutsky and Paris (2005) expanded on the cascading negative effect of a child's inability to tolerate movement or to move in typical ways. Interrupted movement patterns lead to decreased muscle strength in the motor groups needed to develop motor control. Poor motor control leads to diminished self-concept or knowledge about the body and its parts in relationship to the environment. Poor self-concept leads to decreased motor coordination, which can negatively affect the ability to organize and self-regulate emotional and behavioral responses. This problem may affect attending and, ultimately, visual–motor skills as the negative effect surges throughout multiple aspects of motor function (Murray-Slutsky & Paris, 2005). The term *resonation* is used to describe how a circumstance of one body part can affect or resonate throughout the entire body and affect multiple areas of development and, thus, learning.

Motor learning and motor function underlie occupational performance. They provide the physical capacities needed to provide adaptive responses to occupational task demands. Occupational roles may be fulfilled in various ways, but occupational tasks associated with childhood depend on motor functioning in some way to meet task demands. The occupational therapist brings clinical reasoning to naturalistic settings and sequences to critically observe, analyze, describe, and interpret human performance throughout early infant and young child development. The developmental progression of growth and occupational performance skills in infants and young children is summarized in Table 2.2. Changes in breathing, teething, and sleeping cycles over the first year demonstrate the amount of energy the infant exerts on these occupational tasks, above and beyond the motor skills often emphasized in early development.

Conclusion

Human development is a lifelong process of individuation and transformation, a dance of occupational permanence and equanimity. A thorough and integrated understanding of development as a reciprocal process between the individual and his or her environment (human and nonhuman) is essential to practice in early childhood, particularly in community-based settings, including the home. Working in community-based settings affords constant opportunities for occupational therapists and others to see and use this interaction to foster development and enhance the competence of the family and others to meet their child's needs. The Model of HOPE provides wellness language to support occupational therapy practice using a holistic view of human development. Programs such as Brazelton's Touchpoints (Brazelton Touchpoints Center, n.d.) help adults see the importance of early relationships on later development and to understand that a progression in one area of development might coincide with a regression in another and that the changes are part of the normal developmental process. Occupational therapists can facilitate greater understanding of the experiences of the young child and the importance of relationships to that experience. Using this information to frame your practice in community-based early childhood settings will allow you to see and participate in the beautifully orchestrated dance that is the development of a young child.

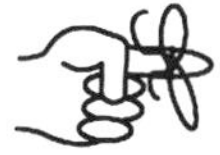

Remember this. . . .
Human development is a lifelong process of individuation and transformation, a dance of occupational permanence and equanimity.

Learning Activity 2.3 invites the reader to apply the material presented in this chapter to a case study. Comparisons of typical and atypical development within this single-case design challenge the learner to construct occupational performance expectations to facilitate development.

Table 2.2. Developmental Progression of Growth and Performance Skills

Age *(months)*	**Growth** *(Maturation of neurobiological systems)*	**Emotional Regulation** *(Identify, manage, and express emotions during activities and interactions)*	**Sensory–Perceptual** *(Locate, identify, respond to, and discriminate sensory stimuli)*	**Communication and Social** *(Understand, gesture, initiate, take turns, and interact)*	**Cognitive** *(Plan, prioritize, create, select, problem solve, manage tasks)*	**Motor and Praxis** *(Plan and execute skilled purposeful movements)*
Birth–1	• ≥2,500 g • Brain 25% adult • Body 5% adult • 85 breaths/min • Supine position	• 10–18 hr sleep • 2–3-hr cycle if breastfed • 3–5-hr cycle if bottle fed	• Eye gaze and tracking • Prefers high visual contrast	• Throaty sounds • Regards bell • Regards faces	• Reflexes are modified by experience	• Ocular control • Strong asymmetrical tonic neck reflex • Hands fisted
4	• Prone position • Voluntary sucking develops.	• 14–15 hr sleep • Differentiates delight from distress • 90% sleep through night	• Visual regard of rattle in hand • Plays with hands • Pureed foods added	• Coos • Laughs • Vocalizes • Imitates own sounds mirrored by others	• Primary circular reactions: repeats accidents to develop motor skill	• Head control • Prone play • Symmetrical postures • Hands open
7	• 60 breaths/min • Sitting position • Teething may begin.	• 14–15 hr sleep • Self-soothe after night waking • No more night feedings	• Plays with feet • Pats mirror • Transfers cube from hand to hand	• *Ba-ba, ma-ma, da-da* • Single-consonant sounds	• Secondary circular reactions: Repeats accidents with objects to develop skills	• Segmented rolling • Grasping and raking • Supported sitting
10	• Central and lateral incisors erupt.	• 14–15 hr sleep • Exhibits fear, disgust, anger	• Holds bottle, picks up pellet • Finger feeds solid foods • Begins cup	• One word • Imitates novel sounds	• Object constancy: Looks for objects that leave line of sight	• Sits alone • Creeps • Pulls to feet • Pokes
12	• 40 breaths/min • 4 front teeth on top and bottom present.	• 12–14 hr sleep, 11–12 hr at night • 2.5 hr during day, usually 2 naps • Expresses elation, affection	• Tower of 2 cubes • Releases cube in cup • Cooperates in dressing	• Two or more words • Imitates novel sounds • Recognizes objects by name	• Intention • Causality • Anticipation	• Stands • Cruises • Walks • Neat pincer grasp
18	• Cuspids and first molars erupt; locomotor period • Motor control for toileting emerges.	• 12–14 hr sleep • Usually 1 nap in afternoon for 1.5–2 hr	• Dumps pellet • Scribbles spontaneously • Tower of 3 cubes • Uses spoon • Assists with dressing	• Uses jargon • Recognizes pictures	• Curiosity • Classifies objects by shape, action, and function	• Walks without falling • Seats self
24	• Second molars erupt; often most painful • Bladder and bowel control continues to develop.	• 12–14 hr sleep • Attention span is <5 min.	• Tower of 6 cubes • Imitates circular stroke • Pulls on garments • Plays with dolls • Bottle free at 24–30 months • Drinks from cup without spilling	• 2-word phrases • 50–75-word vocabulary • Understands 1-step directions	• Internal representation: Practices trial and error in head before play • Deferred imitation • Uses multiple strategies • Understands pictorial object representations • Parallel play • Emerging sense of self	• Climbs • Runs well • Kicks ball

Table 2.2. Developmental Progression of Growth and Performance Skills (*cont.*)

Age *(months)*	**Growth** *(Maturation of neurobiological systems)*	**Emotional Regulation** *(Identify, manage, and express emotions during activities and interactions)*	**Sensory–Perceptual** *(Locate, identify, respond to, and discriminate sensory stimuli)*	**Communication and Social** *(Understand, gesture, initiate, take turns, and interact)*	**Cognitive** *(Plan, prioritize, create, select, problem solve, manage tasks)*	**Motor and Praxis** *(Plan and execute skilled purposeful movements)*
36	• All 20 primary teeth are present.	• 11–13 hr sleep • 11–12 hr at night, 1–3 hr during day • Sleep time 7–9 p.m. • Wake time 6–8 a.m. • Attention span is 5–10 min.	• Tower of 10 cubes • Imitates bridge of 3 cubes • Copies circle • Uses spoon well • Dons shoes • Plays group games led by adult	• 3–4 word sentences • 445-word vocabulary • First and last name • Takes turns • Understands *in, on, out, up, down* • 2-step related commands	• Symbolic thought • Fantasy play • Counts to 5 • Shapes, colors • Habituates to classes of objects vs. single objects • 2–3 picture sequence	• Stands on 1 foot • Jumps off bottom step • Static tripod grasp emerges
48	• Upper jaw widens to prepare for permanent teeth. • Toilet training is usually complete.	• 11–13 hr sleep • Attention span is 10–15 min.	• Imitates gate of 5 cubes • Copies cross • Cuts across thick, straight line • Washes and dries face • Manipulates large buttons	• 3–4 verbal exchanges on topic • Cooperative play, including simple board games • 3-step related commands • 2-step unrelated commands	• Analogies • Names 6–7 colors • Sorts by shape	• Broad jump
60	• 25%–40% of children age 36–60 months have nighttime growing pains.	• 11–13 hr sleep • Attention span is 15–20 min. • Accepts delayed reward	• Counts 10 objects • Copies triangle • Colors within lines • Blows/wipes nose without help • Dresses without assistance • Manipulates zipper	• Apologizes when breaks or damages property of others	• Names 8+ colors • 4-picture sequence • Counts to 10 • Tells weather conditions accurately	• Hops • Skips • Dynamic tripod grasp emerges

Source. American Dental Association (2009); Cassidy (2006); Furino et al. (1984a, 1984b); Scott (2004).

Learning Activity 2.3. Occupational Performance Expectations

Multiple client factors, parenting styles, environmental opportunities, cultural competencies, and contextual affordances affect occupational performance expectations. A client's medical history has the potential to indicate missed or altered opportunities for occupational development. Current levels of function may identify areas of occupational dissonance, dissatisfaction, or dysfunction. Review the team report below, then answer the questions that follow. Note that the report intentionally makes no conclusions or recommendations in order to facilitate the reader's participation in the learning activity.

MULTIDISCIPLINARY TEAM REPORT

Name: Jonah Smith Age: 2 years, 9 months

Reason for Referral

Jonah has a diagnosis of Down syndrome and has received early intervention services, including speech, occupational, and physical therapies, since age 6 months and early educational services through community-based teachers. Early intervention evaluations identified delays in all areas assessed. The purpose of this evaluation is for transition planning to preschool.

Medical History

Jonah was born full term with a birth weight of 7 lbs. He is his mother's second child. His family was aware that he probably had Down syndrome before he was born. Apgar scores were at 4, 4, and 6. He was diagnosed with a ventricular septal defect (VSD) at birth and spent 11 days in the neonatal intensive care unit for monitoring. The VSD was repaired when he was 3 months old. Jonah did very well postoperatively. He had a recent ear infection but has been generally healthy.

Social Developmental Summary

Jonah lives in a blended family. He sees two of his siblings every other weekend when they come to visit. Sibling relationships are reportedly good. Jonah's hobbies and interests include Elmo, songs, and TV/movies. Mrs. Smith is concerned about Jonah's general development and negative behaviors such as throwing items or clearing the table with a sweep of his arm when he does not want to complete a task.

Adaptive Behavior

Jonah relies on his parents for all his daily care needs. He assists with dressing by holding out his arms and legs when prompted, pushing up his sleeves when taken to the sink to wash his hands, and placing a toothbrush in his mouth and moving it around. Jonah was breastfed and transitioned to a bottle at 12 months. He feeds himself using his fingers and drinks from a spouted cup independently. He has no known food allergies and is not yet toilet trained. Although he adapts well to changes and transitions, Jonah does have some separation anxiety from his mother.

Behavioral Observations

Jonah was seen in his home with his mother and maternal grandparents present. He was eager to play with the evaluators and displayed a positive disposition throughout most of the evaluation. He smiled often and moved quickly from one task to another. Jonah used good eye contact and localized to environmental sounds.

Cognitive and Preacademic Skills

Cognitive skills (thinking, sequencing, problem-solving skills, basic concepts, and prereadiness abilities) were evaluated through observations of play, problem solving, imitative behaviors, and classification skills.

- *Play:* Jonah was noted to mouth and throw toys as well as push them off a surface, exemplifying exploratory play. Simple functional play was prompted whereby Jonah pushed balls down a sliding track.
- *Problem Solving:* Jonah used an emerging trial-and-error approach, repeating actions for their consequences. He was able to put a circle into a shape sorter and single-cell puzzle board. Jonah requested "more" by signing with prompts. Mrs. Smith stated that Jonah will push materials off the table using both hands when he does not want to participate.
- *Imitative Skills:* Jonah imitated a facilitator clapping and hugging a stuffed animal. He also imitated the use of a lever toy.
- *Preacademics:* Jonah was able to put a circle into a shape sorter and single-cell puzzle board. Mrs. Smith states that he points to his head, eyes, nose, and mouth on request, although he did not respond to these requests during the evaluation.

Communication

Mrs. Smith voices concern about Jonah's lack of verbal language and decreased communication skills with people unfamiliar to him because he primarily uses gestures and signs to communicate. The speech pathologist from Early Intervention has recently introduced a Go-Talk 9 augmentative device to aid in his expressive abilities. Mrs. Smith reports that Jonah uses the following signs: "all done," "more," "please," "cat," "dog," "horse," "bird," "thank you," and the sign "me" indicating "my turn."

- *Speech Production:* During this evaluation, Jonah spontaneously produced vowel sounds "uh" and "ah" without functional meaning. Minimal verbalizations or word approximations were otherwise heard during the evaluation. When prompted to imitate vowel sounds for "uh" and "ooooo" or to imitate oral–motor actions (such as "raspberries" with his lips), he did not respond. Jonah smiled when the examiner smiled at him and exhibited facial symmetry. Jonah's vocal quality and fluency were not assessed as a result of his limited verbal expression.

Learning Activity 2.3. Occupational Performance Expectations (*cont.*)

- *Expressive language* refers to the child's ability to communicate messages that convey meaning with others both familiar and unfamiliar to them. Jonah's expressive communication consisted primarily of gestures, facial expressions, and eye gaze.
- *Receptive language* refers to the child's ability to understand and process verbal information. Jonah did not demonstrate understanding of yes–no questions, identify specific objects, or follow simple 1-step directions during the evaluation. His attention to examiner-directed tasks was fleeting.
- *Pragmatic language* refers to a person's ability to successfully exchange communication using age-appropriate social skills such as eye contact, turn taking, initiating play or conversation, sustaining a conversation, and using age-appropriate body and verbal language. When Jonah's name was called by others, he inconsistently shifted his gaze toward the speaker. Jonah appropriately expressed happiness by smiling and laughing. He also expressed discontent by crying and looking for help from his mother.

Jonah displayed significant deficits in his expressive- and receptive-language skills, which were characterized by limited functional communication including making requests or choices. His articulation and speech sound production was minimal and consisted only of early developing vowel sounds. His pragmatic and social language was a relative strength but was significantly affected by his lack of expressive communication skills.

Foundational Motor Development

Jonah has low muscle tone throughout his trunk and extremities. He navigates the environment by bunny hopping and ring-sits with legs in full external rotation. Jonah has reportedly never used a reciprocal crawl. Jonah can pull to stand and cruise laterally for 6 ft. Jonah is able to use both hands functionally while in a seated position, but he leans forward at his hips and extends his back to maintain his balance. Parents report that they will be checking on the status of atlantoaxial stability at Jonah's 3-year physical.

Fine Motor Skills

The Peabody Developmental Motor Scales–2 (PDMS–2; Folio & Fewell, 2000) is a nationally standardized assessment used to assess motor development and plan interventions. It identifies sequential skills within the domain of fine motor development and measures interrelated motor abilities in children from birth to age 6. The two subtests that combine to determine a level of fine motor capabilities (Fine Motor Quotient) were administered.

Jonah received a raw score of 37 on the Grasping subtest, which equates to a standard score of 4 indicating performance well below average (Table 2.3). On the Visual–Motor Integration subtest, Jonah received a raw score of 75, which equates to a standard score of 4, also indicating performance well below average. These two subtests combine to yield a Fine Motor Quotient of 64 (average = 90–110 on PDMS–2 only).

Table 2.3. Jonah's Peabody Developmental Motor Scales–2 Scores

Subtest	Raw Score	Standard Score
Grasping	37	4 (well below average)
Visual–Motor Integration	75	4 (well below average)
Fine Motor Quotient		64 (well below average)

During play-based assessment, Jonah demonstrated visual–motor and grasping skills that indicated achievement of small gains within the same functional level reported in the occupational therapy evaluation from 1 year ago. Jonah occasionally uses an isolated index finger point and has a stable wrist for some visual–motor tasks and to wave goodbye. He does suck his thumb, however, and uses gravity-assisted wrist extension and forearm supination with his elbow flexed against his body. When eating finger foods, Jonah releases food by pushing off from the palm of his hand, even though he is able to use a more developmentally mature 3-jaw chuck grasp during play activities.

Sensory Processing

Jonah's mother expresses no concerns about sensory processing. Although Jonah doesn't enjoy getting his hands messy, he eats foods with a wide range of textures, accepts hand-over-hand assistance as needed, and reacts typically to a wide range of sensory inputs. As a result of decreased trunk stability, Jonah has had limited opportunity to develop functional balance reactions consistent with age-level expectations.

Questions

1. What markers in the medical history suggest missed or altered opportunities for occupational development?
2. What are the functional indicators of missed opportunities in Jonah's occupational performance?
3. Extrapolate from the team report areas of occupational dissonance, dissatisfaction, or dysfunction.
4. Using Table 2.2, identify Jonah's current levels of function and next steps in the expected developmental progression for each of the occupational performance areas.

How Very Far We Have Come: Annie Starts School (1956–1957)

Annie started school in the fall of 1956. In a new plaid dress Lydia sewed especially for the occasion, Annie excitedly got on the school bus and waved good-bye to her mother and two brothers. Mark was too young to go to school, but Danny, at 6, was not: State law specifically excluded him from attending public school because he had disabilities. The doctors at the Shriners Hospital had diagnosed Danny with cerebral palsy (spastic diplegia), a slight hearing loss in his left ear, and a visual impairment. Danny could see, but not well.

It did not seem fair to exclude Danny from school because he had disabilities. Certainly, school is where one goes to learn, figure out how to get along with other children and adults, and follow a structured routine, but it is also where one makes friends, some of whom you may know all your life. "We pay the same taxes that support the schools as everyone else; Danny ought to be able to attend," thought Lydia—and she was not shy about saying so.

At the library, which Lydia went to as often as she could to research how to help Danny, Lydia learned about an organization founded the year the twins were born: the National Association of Parents and Friends of Mentally Retarded Children. She didn't think Danny was retarded, but many of the children mentioned also had physical disabilities. There was a chapter in a town 28 miles away, where Maggie now lived. Sam didn't like Lydia driving alone that far at night, so they went together to the monthly meetings, leaving the children with Sam's sister Maggie and her husband, Jesse. The purpose of the association was to generate support and assistance for children and adults with mental retardation and their families. Most of the people they met had been given the same recommendation: institutionalization. And most were adamant that their children attend public school.

In 2 years, Mark would start school. Lydia swore that Danny would be attending then as well. She didn't know how long and how much effort change would take.

Questions

1. On what basis did most states exclude children with disabilities from attending public school?
2. What alternatives, if any, were provided for children with disabilities to attend school or to learn?
3. The National Association of Parents and Friends of Mentally Retarded Children still exists and advocates. How is it now known, and what role did it play in the passage of the Education for All Handicapped Children Act of 1975?

References

Ainsworth, M. D., Blehar, M.C., Waters, E., & Wall, S. (1978). *Patterns of attachment: Assessed in the strange situation and at home.* Hillsdale, NJ: Lawrence Erlbaum.

Allen, D. A., & Hudd, S. S. (1987). Are we professionalizing parents? Weighing the benefits and pitfalls. *Mental Retardation, 25,* 133–139.

American Academy of Pediatrics. (2010). *Ages and stages.* Retrieved January 5, 2010, from www.healthychildren.org/English/ages-stages/Pages/default.aspx

American Academy of Pediatrics Task Force on Sudden Infant Death Syndrome. (2005). The changing concept of sudden infant death syndrome: Diagnostic coding shifts, controversies regarding the sleeping environment, and new variables to consider in reducing risk. *Pediatrics, 116*(5), 1245–1255. Retrieved January 5, 2010, from http://aap-policy.aappublications.org/cgi/reprint/pediatrics;116/5/1245

American Dental Association. (2009). *Tooth eruption charts.* Retrieved January 28, 2009, from www.ada.org/public/topics/tooth-eruption.asp

American Occupational Therapy Association. (2008). Occupational therapy practice framework: Domain and process (2nd ed.). *American Journal of Occupational Therapy, 62,* 625–683.

Bayer, J. K., Hiscock, H., Ukoumunne, O. C., Price, A., & Wake, M. (2008). Early childhood aetiology of mental health problems: A longitudinal population-based study. *Journal of Child Psychology and Psychiatry, 49*(11), 1166–1174.

Bazyk, S. (1989). Changes in attitudes and beliefs regarding parent participation and home programs: An update. *American Journal of Occupational Therapy, 43,* 725–727.

Bowlby, J. (1977). The making and breaking of affectional bonds. *British Journal of Psychiatry, 130,* 201–210.

Bowlby, J. (1988). *John Bowlby: A secure base.* New York: Routledge Classics.

Brachtesende, A. (2005). Using complementary and alternative medicine in occupational therapy. *OT Practice, 10*(11). Retrieved January 5, 2010, from www.aota.org/Pubs/OTP/1997-2007/Features/2005/f-072705.aspx

Brazelton, T., & Cramer, B. (1990). *The earliest relationship: Parents, infants, and the drama of early attachment.* Cambridge, MA: Perseus.

Brazelton, T. B., & Greenspan, S. I. (2000). *The irreducible needs of children: What every child must have to grow, learn, and flourish.* Cambridge, MA: Perseus.

Brazelton Touchpoints Center. (n.d.). *Brazelton Touchpoints approach.* Retrieved July 20, 2009, from www.touchpoints.org/approach.html

Buch, L., Collins, S., & Gelber, S. (1978). Language. In F. P. Connor, G. G. Williamson, & J. M. Siepp (Eds.), *Program guide for infants and toddlers with neuromotor and other developmental disabilities* (pp. 209–217). New York: Teacher's College Press.

Cassidy, R. (2006, September 24). *The five stages of teething.* Retrieved January 28, 2009, from www.ezinearticles.com/?The-Five-Stages-Of-Teething&id=308739

Chess, S., & Thomas, A. (1991). Temperament and the concept of goodness of fit. In J. Strelau & A. Angleitner (Eds.), *Explorations in temperament: International perspectives on theory and measurement* (pp. 15–28). New York: Plenum Press.

Children's Health Act of 2000, Pub. L. 106–310, 42 U.S.C. § 201 *et seq.*

Davis, L. (1978). Pre-speech. In F. P. Connor, G. G. Williamson, & J. M. Siepp (Eds.), *Program guide for infants and toddlers with neuromotor and other developmental disabilities* (pp. 183–205). New York: Teacher's College Press.

Dodge, D. T., Colker, L. J., & Heroman, C. (2002). *The creative curriculum for preschool* (4th ed.). Washington, DC: Teaching Strategies.

Dror, D. K., & Allen, L. J. (2008). Effect of vitamin B12 deficiency on neurodevelopment in infants: Current knowledge and possible mechanism. *Nutritional Review, 66*(5), 250–255.

Duke University Medical Center. (2009, January 6). Gene expression and splicing vary widely from one tissue to the next. *Science Daily.* Retrieved August 16, 2009, from www.sciencedaily.com/releases/2008/12/081222221445.htm

Dunn, W. (2001). The sensation of everyday life: Empirical, theoretical, and pragmatic considerations (Eleanor Clarke Slagle Lecture). *American Journal of Occupational Therapy, 55,* 608–620.

Education for All Handicapped Children Act of 1975, Pub. L. 94–142, 20 U.S.C. § 1400 *et seq.*

Erikson, E. (1982). *The life cycle completed: A review.* New York: W. W. Norton.

Farber, S. D. (1982). *Neurorehabilitation: A multisensory approach.* Philadelphia: W. B. Saunders.

Folio, M. R., & Fewell, R. R. (2000). *Peabody Developmental Motor Scales (2nd ed.) examiner's manual.* Austin, TX: Pro-Ed.

Forcada-Guex, M., Pierrehumbert, B., Borghini, A., Moessinger, A., & Muller-Nix, C. (2006). Early dyadic patterns of mother–infant interactions and outcomes of prematurity at 18 months. *Pediatrics, 118*(1), e107–e114.

Franklin, L., Deitz, J., Jirikowic, T., & Astley, S. (2008). Children with fetal alcohol spectrum disorders: Problem behaviors and sensory processing. *American Journal of Occupational Therapy, 62,* 265–273.

Furuno, S., O'Reilly, K. A., Hosaka, C. M., Inatsuka, T. T., Zeisloft-Falbey, B., & Allman, T. (1984a). *HELP for Preschoolers Checklist: Ages: 3–6 Years.* Palo Alto, CA: Vort Corporation.

Furuno, S., O'Reilly, K. A., Hosaka, C. M., Inatsuka, T. T., Zeisloft-Falbey, B., & Allman, T. (1984b). *Revised HELP Checklist: Birth to Three Years.* Palo Alto, CA: Vort Corporation.

Giese, T. (2002a, June). *Kinetic educational approaches for developing therapeutic rapport: Giese's Holistic Theory of Human Development.* Paper presented at World Federation of Occupational Therapists Conference, Stockholm, Sweden.

Giese, T. (2002b, November). *Lifestyle patterns related to mind, body, and spirit: Giese's Holistic Theory of Human Development.* Paper presented at Illinois Occupational Therapy Association Annual Conference, Galena.

Goodwin, R. D., & Buka, S. L. (2008). Childhood respiratory disease and the risk of anxiety disorder and major depression in adulthood. *Archives of Pediatrics and Adolescent Medicine, 162*(8), 774–780.

Hermann, M., King, K., & Weitzman, M. (2008). Prenatal tobacco smoke and postnatal secondhand smoke exposure and child neurodevelopment. *Current Opinion in Pediatrics, 20*(2), 184–190.

Holder, M. D. (1989). Effects of perinatal exposure to aspartame on rat pups. *Neurotoxicology Teratology, 11*(1), 1–6.

Humphry, R. (1989). Early intervention and the influence of the occupational therapist on the parent–child relationship. *American Journal of Occupational Therapy, 43,* 738–742.

Jansen, P. W., Raat, H., Mackenbach, J. P., Jaddoe, V. W., Hofman, A., Verhulst, F. C., et al. (2008). Socioeconomic inequalities in infant temperament: The Generation R study. *Social Psychiatry and Psychiatric Epidemiology, 44*(2), 87–95.

Jirikowic, T., Kartin, D., & Olson, H. C. (2008). Children with fetal alcohol spectrum disorders: A descriptive profile of adaptive function. *Canadian Journal of Occupational Therapy, 75*(4), 238–248.

Kaiser, M. Y., Kearney, G., Scott, K. G., DuClos, C., & Kurlfink, J. (2008). Tracing childhood exposure to lead and developmental disabilities: Examining the relationship in a population-based sample. *Journal of Public Health Management and Practice, 14*(6), 577–580.

Kalberg, W. O., Provost, B., Tollison, S. J., Tabachnick, B. G., Robinson, L. K., Hoyme, H. E., et al. (2006). Comparison of motor delays in young children with fetal alcohol syndrome to those with prenatal alcohol exposure and with no prenatal alcohol exposure. *Alcoholism: Clinical and Experimental Research, 30*(12), 2037–2045. doi: 10.1111/j.1530-0277.2006.00250.x

Knobloch, H., & Pasamanick, B. (Ed.). (1974). *Gesell and Amatruda's developmental diagnosis: The evaluation and management of normal and abnormal neuropsychologic development in infancy and early childhood* (3rd ed.). Hagerstown, MD: Harper & Row.

Korhonen, P., Koivisto, A. M., Ikonen, S., Laippala, P., & Tammela, O. (1999). Very low birthweight, bronchopulmonary dysplasia and health in early childhood. *Acta Paediatrica, 88*(12), 1385–1391.

Lahey, B., Van Hull, C., Keenan, K., Rathouz, P., D'Onofrio, B., Rodgers, J., et al. (2008). Temperament and parenting during the first year of life predict future child conduct problems. *Journal of Abnormal Psychology, 36*(8), 1139–1158.

Landry, S., Smith, K., Swank, P., & Guttentag, C. (2008). A responsive parenting intervention: The optimal timing across early childhood for impacting maternal behaviors and child outcomes. *Developmental Psychology, 44*(5), 1335–1353.

March of Dimes. (2003). *Understanding the behavior of term infants.* White Plains, NY: Author. Retrieved February 22, 2009, from www.marchofdimes.com/nursing/modnmedia/othermedia/infantBehavior.pdf

Maslow, A. (1968). *Toward a psychology of being* (2nd ed.). New York: Van Nostrand Reinhold.

McAnulty, P., Collier, M., Enticott, J., Tesh, J., Meyhew, D., Comer, C., et al. (1989). Absence of developmental effects in CF–1 mice exposed to aspartame in utero. *Fundamental and Applied Toxicology, 13*(2), 296–302.

Mercer, B., Merlino, A., Milluzzi, C., & Moore, J. (2008). Small fetal size before 20 weeks' gestation: Associations with maternal tobacco use, early preterm birth, and low birthweight. *American Journal of Obstetrics and Gynecology, 198*(6), 673.

Mesa Community College Psychology Department. (1999, Spring). Infant states and temperament. *Developmental Psychology Student Newsletter.* Retrieved February 22, 2009, from www.mc.maricopa.edu/dept/d46/psy/dev/Spring99/infant/cogn.html

Miller, T., Rauh, V., Glied, S., Hattis, D., Rundle, A., Andrews, H., et al. (2006). The economic impact of early life environmental tobacco smoke exposure: Early intervention for developmental delay. *Environmental Health Perspectives, 114*(10), 1585–1588.

Morishima, H., Whittington, R., & Thadani, P. (Eds.). (1995). Species-, gender-, and pregnancy-related differences in the pharmacokinetics and pharmacodynamics of cocaine. In *Biological mechanisms and perinatal exposure to drugs*. (NIDA Research Monograph 158, pp. 9–14). Rockville, MD: U.S. Department of Health and Human Services, Public Health Service, National Institutes of Health. Retrieved August 16, 2009, from www.drugabuse.gov/pdf/monographs/158.pdf

Murray-Slutsky, C., & Paris, B. (2005). *Is it sensory or is it behavior? Behavior problem identification, assessment, and intervention*. San Antonio, TX: Psychological Corporation.

National Children's Study. (2009). *What is the National Children's Study?* Retrieved January 13, 2009, from www.nationalchildrensstudy.gov

Olsen, G., Murphey, L., & Thadani, P. (Eds.). (1995). Effects of morphine and cocaine on breathing control in neonatal animals: A minireview. In *Biological mechanisms and perinatal exposure to drugs*. (NIDA Research Monograph 158, p. 27). Rockville, MD: U.S. Department of Health and Human Services, Public Health Service, National Institutes of Health.

Opler, M., Buka, S., Groeger, J., McKeague, I., Wei, C., Factor-Litvak, P., et al. (2008). Prenatal exposure to lead, delta-aminolevulinic acid, and schizophrenia: Further evidence. *Environmental Health Perspectives, 116*(11), 1586–1590.

Opler, M., & Susser, E. S. (2005). Fetal environment and schizophrenia. *Environmental Health Perspectives, 113*(9), 1239–1242.

Piaget, J. (1936). *Origins of intelligence in the child*. London: Routledge & Kegan Paul.

Prescott, S. L. (2006). Maternal allergen exposure as a risk factor for childhood asthma. *Current Allergy and Asthma Reports, 6*(1), 75–80.

Prochaska, J., Norcross, J., & DiClemente, C. (1994). *Changing for good*. New York: Avon Books.

Saisto, T., Salmelo-Aro, K., Nurmi, J., & Halmesmaki, E. (2008). Longitudinal study on the predictors of parental stress in mothers and fathers of toddlers. *Journal of Psychosomatic Obstetrics and Gynaecology, 29*(3), 219–228. doi: 10.1080/01674820802000467

Salvatore, S., Keymolen, K., Hauser, B., & Vandenplas, Y. (2005). Intervention during pregnancy and allergic disease in the offspring. *Pediatric Allergy and Immunology, 16*(7), 558–566.

Scott, B. J. (2004). *Early developmental milestones: Checklists for observing and measuring a child's development; Pre-K–1st grade*. Greenville, SC: Super Duper Publications.

Shonkoff, J. P., & Phillips, D. A. (Eds.). (2000). *From neurons to neighborhoods: The science of early childhood development*. Washington, DC: National Academies Press.

Simard, V., Nielsen, T., Tremblay, R., Boivin, M., & Montplaisir, J. (2008). Longitudinal study of preschool sleep disturbance: The predictive role of maladaptive parental behaviors, early sleep problems, and child/mother psychological factors. *Archives of Pediatrics and Adolescent Medicine, 162*(4), 360–367.

Singer, L., Yamashita, T. S., Hawkins, S., Cairns, D., Baley, J., & Kliegman, R. (1994). Increased incidence of intraventricular hemorrhage and developmental delay in cocaine-exposed, very low birth weight infants. *Journal of Pediatrics, 124*(5, Pt. 1), 765–761.

Soffritti, M., Belpoggi, F., Esposti, D., Falcioni, L., & Bua, L. (2008). Consequences of exposure to carcinogens beginning during developmental life. *Basic Clinical Pharmacological Toxicology, 102*(2), 118–124.

Soffritti, M., Belpoggi, F., Tibaldi, E., Esposti, D., & Lauriola, M. (2007). Life-span exposure to low doses of aspartame beginning during prenatal life increases cancer effects in rats. *Environmental Health Perspectives, 115*(9), 1293–1297.

Stroud, L., Paster, R., Papandonatos, G., Niaura, R., Salisbury, A., Battle, C., et al. (2008). Maternal smoking during pregnancy and newborn neurobehavior: Effects at 10 to 27 days. *Journal of Pediatrics, 154*, 10–16.

Thompson, J., Carter, R., Edwards, A., Roth, J., Ariet, M., Ross, N., et al. (2003). A population-based study of the effects of birth weight on early developmental delay or disability in children. *American Journal of Perinatology, 20*(6), 321–332.

Tronick, E., & Beeghly, M. (1999). Prenatal cocaine exposure, child development, and the compromising effects of cumulative risk. *Clinical Perinatology, 26*(1), 151–171.

University of Virginia Health System. (2004). *High risk newborn*. Retrieved August 15, 2008, from www.healthsystem.virginia.edu/uvahealth/peds_hrnewborn/lbw.cfm

Vygotsky, L. (1986). *Thought and language*. Cambridge, MA: MIT Press.

Windham, G., Hopkins, G., Fenster, L., & Swan, S. (2000). Prenatal active or passive tobacco smoke exposure and the risk of preterm delivery or low birth weight. *Epidemiology, 11*(4), 427–433.

Yajnik, C., & Dwshmukh, U. (2008). Maternal nutrition, intrauterine programming, and consequential risks in the offspring. *Reviews in Endocrine and Metabolic Disorders, 9*(3), 203–211.

CHAPTER 3

Family-Centered Practice: It's All About Relationships

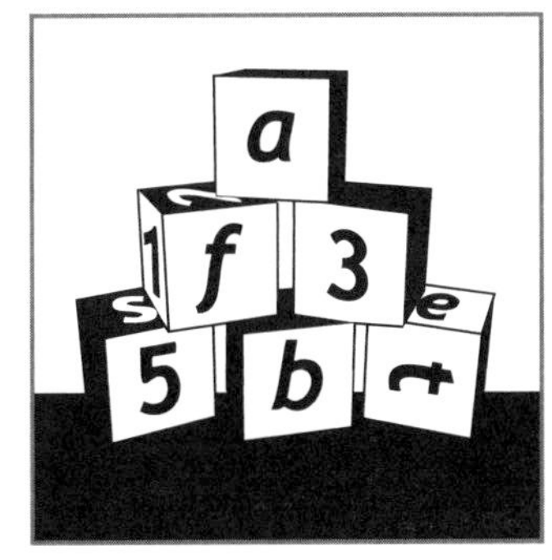

Elise Holloway, MPH, OTR/L, and
Barbara E. Chandler, PhD, OTR/L, FAOTA

Call it a clan, call it a network, call it a tribe, call it a family. Whatever you call it, whoever you are, you need one.

—Jane Howard (1978, p. 234)

Learning Objectives

After reading this material and completing the examination, readers will be able to

- Identify the seven principles of family-centered services,
- Identify and differentiate between the four most common types of service coordination in services under the Infants and Toddlers With Disabilities Program,
- Delineate the benefits and deficiencies of the primary provider model,
- Differentiate the coaching model in early intervention and the occupational therapy process,
- Identify current classifications of attachment and disorders of attachment,
- Identify different types of temperament and the implications of each type for interactions with parents and others,
- Delineate occupational therapy's role in infant mental health, and
- Recognize two examples of co-occupation of parent and child.

Jane Howard's statement on the importance of family speaks volumes: "You need one." This statement speaks to the primary, basic, foremost need of humans as we enter the world. We need someone to care—to care about us, to care for us. Without that, we are lost, adrift. In our society, we have set up safeguards so that the government will step in if the parent indicates unwillingness or inability to care for a very young child. If the parent abrogates that responsibility and does not realize it or see to it that someone else takes that responsibility, the experiences of the infant are profoundly compromised, perhaps to the point of death. Family: Yes, you need one.

Thankfully though, for most children, the family anticipates and welcomes the child and provides for its needs. Almost all parents have dreams about how they will nurture their child and how they will help their child thrive and become a happy, independent person. These dreams are rooted in their own experiences of having been parented, being an aunt or uncle, media portrayals, and observation of friends' relationships. In recent years, research and experience have shown that the relationship between infant and parent is the foundation for all other aspects of development. In orphanages in Romania, "without warm nurturing or appropriate social and intellectual interaction, children developed severe physical, intellectual, and social deficits" (Brazelton & Greenspan, 2000, p. xi). A child needs to be able to move or to pay attention or to communicate. The development of these abilities takes place within the context of the child's most important relationships with the family. Those relationships determine the child's experience of himself or herself as a separate person, able to act on his or her world, and able to engage in meaningful activities or occupations. We can never separate the child, the parent, and the child's developmental outcome.

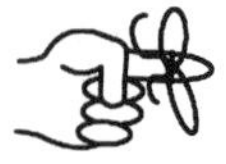

Remember this. . . .
We can never separate the child, the parent, and the child's developmental outcome.

All professionals in early childhood are working with families in new and extended ways. As occupational therapists working with very young children, we must work with families in comprehensive ways. To promote optimal participation in activities of daily living (ADLs) and family life for the young child, we must draw on our psychosocial origins and address how all experiences affect the parent–child relationship and family life. The daily parenting experience becomes a focus of therapy because the child is seen as an inextricable part of the family.

Child-centered issues, deficits, and needs are not the only focus of therapeutic intervention. They may have been the reason the family has come in contact with an occupational therapist, but enhanced parental competence to meet their child's needs is a goal of therapy. Occupational therapists must engage with parents and make the daily parenting experience a focus of therapeutic interaction.

What does it mean to practice family-centered care or engage in family-centered practices? What does it mean to help someone develop his or her role as a parent? Working with families is not new to human services providers, nor is the study and examination of how families structure themselves, their "work," and their daily routines. Families have always been a fertile field for study; anthropologists and sociologists have been engaged in these types of studies for many years. What is new is the interest that has recently (in the past 25 years) been paid to families of young children, particularly young children with special needs. Recognizing the increasing understanding of the importance of early relationships and nurturance and in response to family advocacy, the federal legislation (the Individuals With Disabilities Education Improvement Act of 2004 [IDEA 2004]) that defines services in early childhood requires that services for infants and toddlers be provided in the natural environment. One of the main purposes of those services is to support the natural nurturing relationships that occur in the daily dance between young children and their caregiver(s). Originally termed *family-centered care,* the phrase became *family-centered services* and is now usually phrased as *family-centered practices,* providing a subtle but important shift in thinking and acting.

Learning Activity 3.1 provides an opportunity to further examine the progression of these terms as reflective of social perspectives and advocacy. Remember the statutory language from Part C of IDEA 2004: "Congress finds there is an urgent and

Learning Activity 3.1. Defining *Family Centered*

Although the phrases *family-centered care, family-centered services,* and *family-centered practices* are similar, they connote subtle differences.

- Review literature in human services for the terms *family-centered care, services,* and *practices.*
- Discuss with an interdisciplinary group of colleagues the progression of these terms in the broad field of human services and their specific application in early childhood services.
- How are these termed applied or operationalized in early childhood services today?

---

substantial need. . . . to enhance the capacity of families to meet the special needs of their infants and toddlers with disabilities" (20 U.S.C. § 1431(a)(4)).

Key Principles of Family-Centered Practices

In the early childhood field, seven family-centered principles have been identified through research, professional wisdom, literature review, and consensus building, as follows (Pletcher & McBride, 2000, p. 2):

1. The overriding purpose of providing family-centered help is family empowerment, which in turn benefits the well-being and development of the child.
2. Mutual trust, respect, honesty, and open communication characterize the family–provider relationship.
3. Families are active participants in all aspects of services. They are the ultimate decision makers in the amount and type of assistance and the support they seek to use.
4. The ongoing work between families and providers is about identifying family concerns (priorities, hopes, needs, goals, or wishes), finding family strengths, and the services and supports that will provide necessary resources to meet those needs.
5. Efforts are made to build on and use families' informal community support systems before relying solely on professional, formal services.
6. Providers across all disciplines collaborate with families to provide resources that best match what the family needs.
7. Support and resources need to be flexible, individualized, and responsive to the changing needs of families.

The Office of Special Education Programs (OSEP) Workgroup on Principles and Practices in Natural Environments also developed seven key principles for working in the natural environment. They are similar to those above but provide more specificity through examples (National Early Childhood Technical Assistance Center [NECTAC], 2009a).

The principles of family-centered practices are reflected in the current language of the laws authorizing the programs serving young children and their families. The challenge is to honor and adhere to these principles in everyday practice.

Each family is a reflection of all the members of that family who have gone before. The culture, values, mores, beliefs, habits, attitudes, and perspective of each family are uniquely expressed on the basis of the family's history, experiences, and circumstances. Thus, each family should be treated with sensitivity to and respect for the culture and values of individual family members and each family's structure and function (i.e., the family's ecology). Without respect, no trust can exist. Some examples of being sensitive to individual family dynamics include acknowledging the decision maker(s) in the family, the temporal aspects of the family's day such as work schedules, the time spent commuting, and the child "handoffs" from one parent to another and their viewpoint(s) of help seeking and help accepting.

The focus on enhancing family strengths and the family's capacity to enhance their child's development is a critical aspect of family-centered practices. The term *family capacity* includes the ability to adapt to the changing needs of the family and includes ways that develop and strengthen the knowledge, skills, abilities, processes, and resources that the family needs to meet the needs of all members of the family individually and as a family unit (Philbin, 1996). Indeed, strengthening family capacity is one of the purposes of the early intervention programs under IDEA 2004 Part C, but it is also an inherent element of the Head Start and Early Head Start programs. Head Start and Early Head Start both include programmatic components to assist parents in developing their own skills in multiple ways to support their child's growth and development. These components include adult literacy, coordination with job training programs, instruction in preparing healthy meals, and similar individual capacity-building activities.

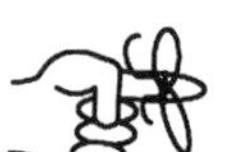

Remember this. . . .
Congress finds there is an urgent and substantial need . . . to enhance the capacity of families to meet the special needs of their infants and toddlers with disabilities. (IDEA 2004, 20 U.S.C. § 1431 (a)(4))

Family Competence and Confidence

Occupational therapists are familiar with practices that help build family capacity because they are critical considerations in the clinical reasoning process (Mattingly & Fleming, 1994), particularly in terms of conditional reasoning. Recognizing and assisting in the mobilization of formal and informal family and community supports is important for occupational therapists. Social support networks are critical to families, especially families of young children, whether or not the children have a disability or special health care need. These types of support may be crucial to helping the family deal with various situations or make positive changes.

Barrera (1986) distinguished between the terms *perceived support, embedded support,* and *enacted support*. The terms are used slightly differently in occupational therapy practice, however. *Perceived support* includes "logical" sources of support, such as close relatives and others living in the home. *Embedded support* arises from the specific circumstances or experiences of the person's life, such as a family support group for parents of children in the neonatal intensive care unit (NICU). *Enacted support* is support that is actually given, received, and perceived as a support to the family. These three types of support are obviously interconnected; however, the enacted support (i.e., that which really happened) is the most important support, particularly in times of stress or change.

Family-centered practice means that the family is an active participant in early intervention and early childhood programs. *Active* means that the family participates in all aspects of the service provision process as an equal to all providers. The family's perspective leads the way to what is most important to address. To that end, a hallmark of family-centered practices is the provision of information and links to resources to assist the family in making well-informed decisions. One of the most important roles of the service coordinator in early intervention (discussed in depth later in this chapter) is to provide information and assist the family in evaluating information because a family often has much to review, consider, and assimilate.

Families are not stagnant entities. They change day by day. The family's needs and priorities drive the service provision system in early intervention and are a heavy influence in Head Start and Early Head Start. As children age and as their condition changes or the family's circumstances change, the family's needs and priorities will change as well. Occupational therapists must be cognizant of and responsive to changing needs. Changing levels of competence result in changing needs as well and are interconnected with family capacity building.

Principles and Practices in Natural Environments

As the multidisciplinary field of early childhood continues to grow and develop, it has become increasingly important that all practitioners speak and understand the same language. To that end, consensus has been sought related to the most important terms and perspectives. When the early childhood field says that it uses family-centered practices in natural environments, what does it mean? (See Chapter 6 for in-depth information on natural environments and routines.) A multidisciplinary workgroup (arising from the OSEP-sponsored Communities of Practice on working in natural environments and including two occupational therapists) on principles and practices in natural environments developed a set of consensus statements (NECTAC, 2009b) that were based on legal requirements, research, and professional wisdom to help articulate what working with families in natural environments to support their child's or children's development means. The principles are the "foundations necessary to support the system of family-centered services and supports" in early childhood (NECTAC, 2008, p. 1):

1. Infants and toddlers learn best through everyday experiences and interactions with familiar people in familiar contexts.
2. All families, with the necessary supports and resources, can enhance their children's learning and development.
3. The primary role of a service provider in early intervention is to work with and support family members and caregivers in children's lives.
4. The early intervention process, from initial contacts through transition, must be dynamic and individualized to reflect the child's and family members' preferences, learning styles, and cultural beliefs.
5. IFSP [individualized family service plan] outcomes must be functional and based on children's and families' needs and family-identified priorities.
6. The family's priorities, needs, and interests are addressed most appropriately by a primary provider who represents and receives team and community support.
7. Interventions with young children and family members must be based on explicit principles, validated practices, best available research, and relevant laws and regulations.

These statements and the perspectives and practices they represent are familiar to occupational therapists. Two, though, bear further discussion. Principles 3 and 6 identify the service coordinator as the key to effective early intervention processes and speak of a primary provider who represents and receives team and community support. These principles suggest a somewhat different and, in many ways, conceptually new model of service provision and, in some ways, blend coordination of services and provision of services into one process.

Service Coordination

Initially, *service coordination* was thought of in terms of case or care management; indeed, the term is used in the implementing regulations. The regulations implementing IDEA identify specific responsibilities for service coordination (34 C.F.R. § 303.23(a)-(b)):

> Service coordination (case management).
>
> (a) General.
>
> (1) As used in this part, except in Sec. 303.12(d)(11), service coordination means the activities carried out by a service coordinator to assist and enable a child eligible under this part and the child's family to receive the rights, procedural safeguards, and services that are authorized to be provided under the State's early intervention program.
>
> (2) Each child eligible under this part and the child's family must be provided with one service coordinator who is responsible for (i) Coordinating all services across agency lines; and (ii) Serving as the single point of contact in helping parents to obtain the services and assistance they need. . . .
>
> (b) Specific service coordination activities. Service coordination activities include (1) Coordinating the performance of evaluations and assessments; (2) Facilitating and participating in the development, review, and evaluation of individualized family service plans; (3) Assisting families in identifying available service providers; (4) Coordinating and monitoring the delivery of available services; (5) Informing families of the availability of advocacy services; (6) Coordinating with medical and health providers; and (7) Facilitating the development of a transition plan to preschool services, if appropriate.

Under Part C, service coordination has evolved to encompass more than these specific responsibilities. As the informal, changing definition of service coordination and the role of the service coordinator have evolved, the effects of this transformation have reverberated throughout the early intervention systems. The relationship between the service coordinator and the family has grown in importance. States have considerable flexibility in how they define the role of the service coordinator and in how they structure the service provision process. A variety of service coordination practices are evident across the country (Markowitz, 2001). These practices fall into four broad types or models of service coordination: (1) dedicated service coordinator, (2) early interventionist and service coordinator, (3) interagency service coordination, and (4) interim or intake service coordination (Hurth, 1998).

How service coordination is defined and operationalized has a significant impact on how the entire early intervention system operates in a state. Learning Activity 3.2 provides an opportunity to compare the most common models of service coordination in early intervention.

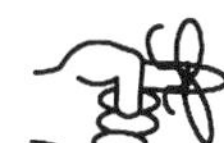

Remember this. . . .
How service coordination is defined and operationalized has a significant impact on how the entire early intervention system operates in a state.

Dedicated Service Coordinator

In the dedicated service coordinator model, the primary role of the dedicated service coordinator is to coordinate services to and for the family and child. This model is most closely akin to the case or care management model. People in this position are usually employed by the state early intervention program or a contracted agency. They do not serve as one of the evaluators for the multidisciplinary developmental assessment, although they would handle the coordination of the process. They continue past the initial eligibility process; coordinate the development of the IFSP; continue to coordinate, but not provide, all services; and serve as the primary early intervention contact for the family related to their child's needs. They would facilitate the transition to preschool or other services when the child turns 3.

Early Interventionist and Service Coordinator

In the early interventionist and service coordinator model, the coordinator carries out two distinct roles: (1) providing direct services to the child and family and (2) acting in the role of care manager and coordinating all services, including his or her own, for a select caseload of families. Responsibilities for both service provision and service coordination are shared among team members (trans-, inter-, or multidisciplinary). This model requires a great deal of ongoing communication so that the interventionist is not just knowledgeable of the services the child and family are receiving but also able to provide discipline-specific services in collaboration with others. This model is specifically mentioned in IDEA 2004.

Interagency Service Coordination

In interagency service coordination, the responsibility for service coordination falls to several different agencies, because several different agencies are involved with the

Learning Activity 3.2. Service Coordination Models

Review information from the Research and Training Center on Service Coordination at the University of Connecticut, which archives information and products from a 5-year federally funded project on service coordination (http://uconnucedd.org/projects/rtc/rtc.html), and the information on service coordination at the National Early Childhood Technical Assistance Center (www.nectac.org/topics/scoord/scoord.asp). Consider the information on different models of service coordination. With colleagues who have experience with service coordination in early childhood, identify the positive and negative aspects of each.

- Identify certain situations or certain types of family situations that would benefit from one type of service coordination over another. Why?
- What are the financial implications of each type of service coordination (consider interagency agreements)?
- What type of service coordination does your state use? How does this influence how occupational therapy is provided?

child and each coordinates its services with the services of other agencies. Ideally, the agency that has the closest tie to the child and family's needs would "coordinate the coordination." The benefit of this model is perceived to be better coordinated services for the individual family. The deficit of this model is that no one agency has the responsibility for service coordination, and the program may appear fragmented to potential clients. Some states use this model and do attempt to have the agency that is most related to the child and family's needs serve as that child's overall service coordinator.

Interim or Intake Service Coordination

The interim or intake service coordination model has a single point of entry into the early intervention program or system of early intervention services. In this model, the service coordinator is responsible for all the intake services, coordinates all activities during the first 45 days of evaluation and eligibility decisions, and is responsible for coordinating the IFSP. The service coordinator then continues as the ongoing service coordinator, or a new service coordinator is appointed to work with the child and family until they exit out of the program when the child is age 3 or the family decides it no longer wants or needs the service before the child is age 3.

Role of the Service Coordinator

No matter which model is used, the service coordinator is an extremely important person to the child and the family while they are enrolled in the early intervention program. The advocacy that led to the passage of Part C was fueled in many respects by families' frustration with fragmented services that they had to identify, chase down and, often, drive long distances to for their children with special health care needs. The mantra of "family-centered, community-based, coordinated care" emerged from these frustrations and led, in part, to the design of the Part C legislation.

Service coordination has been approached in many different ways in the different states. The competencies and knowledge base for service coordinators, at a minimum, includes knowledge of the federal and state laws that support early intervention and a knowledge about infants and toddlers who may need these services (34 C.F.R. § 303.23(d)):

> Service coordination (case management).
>
> . . . .
>
> (d) Qualifications of service coordinators. Service coordinators must be persons who, consistent with Sec. 303.344(g), have demonstrated knowledge and understanding about (1) Infants and toddlers who are eligible under this part; (2) Part C of the Act and the regulations in this part; and (3) The nature and scope of services available under the State's early intervention program, the system of payments for services in the State, and other pertinent information.

Occupational therapists may be able to provide service coordination, depending on the rules that the state has adopted for service coordination. Some states have developed training programs for service coordination, and no degree is required to be a service coordinator. Other states have developed stringent qualification standards for service coordination, often requiring a degree in early childhood or education.

The service coordinator is the face of the early intervention program to families and plays a pivotal role in how services are provided and integrated. The service coordinator may act as a gatekeeper for services. Because of the close nature of service coordination as it is implemented in early intervention, it is important to maintain professional distance while facilitating and advocating with the family. If problems exist or if desired outcomes are not achieved, the service coordinator can become the target for a family's animosity toward programs and services.

Primary Provider Model

One model of early intervention services that has emerged from practice, not legislation, is that of the primary provider or primary service provider. The *primary service provider* (PSP) is a member of the early intervention team who accepts information and guidance from all other members of the early intervention team. This transdisciplinary service delivery model requires role release and role expansion as well as extensive communication among all members of the team (including the parents). It challenges the entire concept of what early intervention is intended to be. The model is built on the premise that one person is able to receive and discuss information from a multitude of other professionals through regularly scheduled and attended team meetings, distill this information, and share it with parents to identify and expand the learning opportunities in the home or other natural environments and support achievement of the IFSP outcomes. The benefit of a family and child having to interact with one lead provider is stressed as most effective, because a rapport is established that leads to desired outcomes, is functional in its approach, and allows the primary provider to gain proficiency in varied areas of expertise.

Several states are in the process of implementing the primary provider model. Because each state is able to construct its system of early intervention services within the essential requirements of Part C, how the primary provider model is actually implemented varies. Much of the literature on the primary provider model stresses the purported differences between "traditional" intervention, which is portrayed as deficit focused, expert driven, practitioner dependent, decontextualized, provided in isolation and nonfunctional—a "dose of therapy" once a week with no thought given to working with the parents and family (Coaching in Early Childhood, 2010; McWilliams & Scott, 2001). It is not a description most occupational therapists would recognize. This approach sounds similar to that of the "multiskilled practitioner" that was proposed for medical care in the 1990s. Although cost containment is usually not mentioned when discussing this model, it cannot be ignored as a reason for its promotion.

Although an overload of services has never been the intention of early intervention, an ounce of caution is recommended when considering the primary provider model. This model may be inappropriate for some infants and toddlers. One fundamental intent of early intervention is to provide *individualized services* to meet the specific needs of the child and family in relation to the child's needs. Teams must be careful that what is actually occurring is not diminished by how it is provided. The actual logistics of implementing such a model, which calls for extensive and lengthy communication, does not lend itself readily to the realities of professional practices, the specific needs of infants and toddlers and their families, the necessity

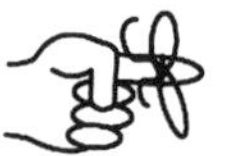

Remember this. . . .
Intervention is not just "doing"; it is also the critical thinking processes that professionals have learned through years of training and experience.

of responding during intervention, and reimbursement for services. The possibility of dilution and diminishment of quality of services and the potential for legal scope-of-practice issues are vast. Intervention is not just "doing"; it is also the critical thinking processes that professionals have learned through years of training and experience. To potentially reduce these individualized services to implementation of activities must not be done without careful research, especially on the outcomes using this model.

Using natural learning opportunities, focusing on daily routines, and working in the natural environment have been an integral part of occupational therapy practice. For many years, occupational therapy was looked down upon and seen as simple. "Those occupational therapists just teach folks to do the regular everyday stuff. Anybody can do that, big deal." Well, it is a big deal, but it was never simple. Occupational therapy is a complex and powerful process, simple only in its appearance. There is now an incredible amount of increased attention on and more widespread acceptance of this perspective; how to best implement it is still open to question. In the past, when we said, "Occupational therapy: We put the FUN in functional," people laughed. Now, they listen.

Facilitating Family Capacity: Coaching

One of the skills required of the primary provider—or of any provider in early childhood services—is the ability to share knowledge in such a way that the family is able to take that knowledge and use it all day, every day, until it becomes ingrained in the patterns of daily life. For most of what is fostered through intervention with young children, this approach is far more effective than the "dosing" of widely spaced interventions. Daily life is where skills are learned, practiced and, frankly, needed. This premise also underlies home care services for elderly people, visiting nurse visits for newborns and those who are chronically ill, and supportive living arrangements.

Clinical reasoning, with its primary emphasis on reflection in action (Mattingly & Fleming, 1994), building on the strengths of individual recipients of services, and considering all contextual factors, provides guidance for working with caregivers and others to build capacity to meet the needs of care recipients. In early intervention, this approach has been reconceptualized, called *coaching,* and directed specifically toward enhancing a family's capacity to meet the child's needs. It is termed a *learner-focused* intervention. "Coaching in early childhood is an interactive process of observation, reflection, and action in which a coach promotes, directly or indirectly, a learner's ability to support a child's participation in family and community contexts." (Hanft, Rush, & Shelden, 2004, p. 4). *Coaching* has also been defined as

> an adult learning strategy in which the coach promotes the learner's ability to reflect on his or her actions as a means to determine the effectiveness of an action or practice and develop a plan for refinement and use of the action in immediate and future situations. (Rush, 2003, cited in Rush & Shelden, 2005, p. 3)

Occupational therapists will see components of the clinical reasoning process in coaching. The processes are kindred, but they are not the same. In early childhood, coaching is focused on developing the competencies of the adult learner (usually the parent) so that the parent may increase the child's "learning opportunities and participation in daily life, knowing when the strategies are successful, and making necessary changes in current situations, as well as generalizing ideas and solutions to different circumstances and settings" (Hanft et al., 2004, p. 12). It is part of a process of capacity building of the family to meet the child's needs—not one day, but every day.

Rush et al. (2003) proposed coaching as a model for building relationships and promoting parent competence and participation (i.e., capacity building). When an occupational therapist is acting using coaching, the interactions between occupational therapists and families occur in the context of real-life situations and include joint planning and the analysis of existing activities to determine which actions should continue or be modified to obtain the intended outcomes for the family. In addition, occupational therapists provide informative feedback and opportunities for observation to expand parents' understanding about evidence-based practices that support children's learning and development (Rush et al., 2003).

Example of Coaching Intervention

The parents of two young children were having problems completing all tasks necessary to get the oldest to the bus stop on time while caring for the toddler. During a home visit by the occupational therapist, the mother mentioned the stress this issue was causing everyone in the family, and the therapist worked with the parents to establish a calmer and more efficient morning routine (J. J. Foss, personal communication, March 2009). During conversations, the parents identified problems, listed the steps needed to accomplish the tasks, and assigned responsibilities for each one. Over the next week of practice, the routines and tasks were revised, and the process was fine tuned. Reflecting on the process, the team of parents and professional found that some tasks (e.g., clothing selection and backpack packing) could be completed best the night before, and others (e.g., waking and feeding the younger child) were assigned to one parent while the other supervised the older child's breakfast and walked her to the bus stop. Both parents reported that this "tag team" approach was satisfying and gave them a sense of working together. They also commented that with less stress, morning tantrums and outbursts were minimized, and that a variation of this routine was working well for other visits outside the home, such as visits to relatives or shopping. Table 3.1 summarizes the intervention from the coaching and occupational therapy perspectives.

Working in a natural environment side by side with the parent or other caregivers is a familiar aspect of practice for many occupational therapists. This perspective in practice models appears to enhance developmental outcomes and empower families to function more effectively (Bruder & Dunst, 1999–2000; Pilkington, 2006). Occupational therapists receive education and training in clinical reasoning, observation techniques, task analysis, and therapeutic use of self, and these basic skills of occupational therapy practice are being recognized and used in early childhood programs across the nation. Readers are encouraged to investigate further coaching as practiced in early childhood and reflect on the similarities and differences from the therapeutic process as implemented through sound clinical reasoning.

Table 3.1. Comparison of Terminology to Describe the Same Process

Parents' Concern	Coaching	Occupational Therapy
Problem: Mornings are hectic and stressful for all.	Parents and children are stressed by daily demands.	Lack of routine for morning activities of daily living creates stress (area of occupation).
Goal: Calmer and more efficient morning routine	Calmer and more efficient morning routine	Establish routine that meets environmental press (eat, dress, bus stop) (activity demands and performance patterns)
Process: Identify problem, list steps to accomplish task, and assign responsibility	List steps; identify who will do what	Activity analysis; client factors, activity demands, performance skills and patterns, context (temporal)
Practice new procedures; reflect on implementation and refine based on experience	Practice, revise on the basis of aspects not anticipated and since learned	Occupational-based intervention: create, promote
Outcomes: Routine for morning: • Met bus on time • Expectations clear • Parents worked together • Behavior issues reduced • Generalized behavior to other "get ready" situations	More satisfying and effective daily morning routine for entire family; aspects generalized to other situations	Establishment of daily routine that meets contextual demands, reduces stress, and is applicable to other situations (generalization of behavior to similar environmental demands)

The Primary Relationship

Inherent in the discussion of service provision models, service coordination, and coaching is the theme of relationships: relationships between families and service coordinators, relationships among members of transdisciplinary teams, relationships between providers and families and, most important, relationships between parents and children. If the intent of early childhood programs is to foster development, the importance of the primary relationship(s) in a young child's life cannot be overemphasized. How those relationships develop and unfold is crucial: "Physician and psychoanalyst D. W. Winnicott strongly influenced the study of the infant's early emotional development by suggesting that the infant cannot be studied in a vacuum" (Holloway, 1998, p. 168). "A baby cannot exist alone, but is essentially part of a relationship" (Winnicott, 1964, p. 10). "The mother's 'good-enough' holding of the infant in both a physical and psychological sense helps to establish the foundation for the infant's sense of self" (Holloway, 1998, p. 169).

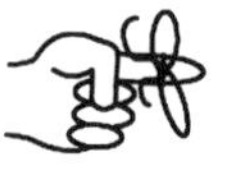

Remember this. . . .
"A baby cannot exist alone, but is essentially part of a relationship" (Winnicott, 1964, p. 10).

Although all occupational therapists have education and training in psychosocial aspects of functioning, content on infant and young child development typically does not emphasize early emotional development. Social skills may be included, but those skills are not synonymous with emotional milestones and emotion regulation. A growing body of research has demonstrated the importance of an infant's emotional development as the foundation for all other aspects of development (Shonkoff & Phillips, 2000). Essentially, the infant develops within the context of his or her earliest relationships with his or her family (or his or her most important consistent caregivers). It then follows that to facilitate a child's development, the therapist must understand and support the child's emotional development by means of relationship-based intervention with both the parent and the child participating. A *relationship-based* intervention is one in which there is an appreciation for the notion that child development, including neurological function, only progresses within the context of interpersonal experiences or relationships (Lillas & Turnbull, 2009). Early intervention's focus, therefore, must always include the interaction and ongoing relations between parent and child, child and therapist, and parent and therapist while determining therapeutic activities, because these relationships are the context for maturation and learning. The parent's role in therapeutic activity is determined by the child's emotional readiness to feel close, be dependent, begin to feel separate and, then, increasingly become independent. "The simultaneous engagement of parent and child within related occupations is referred to as *co-occupations* [italics added]" (Zemke & Clark, 1996, p. 213).

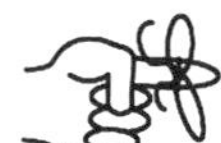

Remember this. . . .
"The simultaneous engagement of parent and child within related occupations is referred to as co-occupations" (Zemke & Clark, 1996, p. 213).

> These co-occupations forge the relationship between the infant and caregiver in a process of continued development of skills and behavior. This "dance" is a type of social reciprocity. This relationship has long-lasting effects on the development of the child, parent, and family. (Chandler & Yun, 2006, p. 2)

For example, parents state that they really want their 20-month-old son, Ezra, to walk. The goal or outcome written collaboratively on the IFSP states, "By age 23 months, Ezra will walk independently from his bedroom to the kitchen." The therapist could take Ezra out of his mother's arms and work with him on a therapy ball for strengthening and balance work for an intermediate goal of independent sitting. The therapist focuses on the foundations for walking by first working on trunk strength in sitting. Ezra cries when removed from his mother, but the therapist believes that she's addressing separation and independence. Did that therapist assess Ezra's level of emotional development as closely as she assessed his motor development so that she could address the emotional foundations of sitting and walking along with the motor foundations? If Ezra is delayed in the emotional realm, he may not yet be ready to maintain only a visual contact with his mother for reassurance. He may be ready to leave direct bodily contact but still require proximity for periodic touch reassurance. An alternative treatment scenario may be that Ezra's mother holds the therapy ball from the front, maintaining visual and touch contact with him, "feeling" how the ball is adjusted to challenge Ezra's skills. She can then later play with him in this same manner.

Typically developing young children are emotionally ready to leave their parent's lap around the same time that they are physically ready to leave. The therapist must be sensitive to emotional differences for a child who is not physically ready to leave or separate. "Parents orchestrate, or direct and structure, their children's engagement within occupations (Primeau, 1998) and, thus, play a significant role in the child's development" (Chandler & Yun, 2006, p. 2.)

> Through the endless repetition of having their parents respond to their needs (e.g., being fed when hungry or swaddled when cold), babies come to trust and love their parents. . . . The reciprocal interaction between parent and infant is essential to the infant's physical, cognitive, social and emotional development, as well as to his self regulation abilities. (Green, 1994, p. 5)

The most important relationships motivate young children. Sharing information, whether through social referencing or pointing and joint attention, is not solely communication skills; it is a primary example of relationship-driven emotional communications.

Temperament

Within our practices or within our own families, we see different types of temperament. One child is "easy," but another is not. Often, these descriptions are applied shortly after birth and the child lives up to the description. Although probably even cave men (and women) could tell differences in the temperaments of their offspring, in-depth study of temperament by means of a scientific process has occurred only recently. Stella Chess and Alexander Thomas, New York psychiatrists, are credited with the first comprehensive study of temperament, in which they followed more than 100 children for the first 3 years of their life (the New York Longitudinal Study [NYLS]; Thomas, Chess, & Birch, 1970). They defined *temperament* as the behavioral style of a person, or the "how" of behavior, and identified nine characteristics, or dimensions, of temperament, which could be scored as medium, high, or low (Table 3.2). Three clusters were then identified through factor analysis: the easy child (40%), the difficult child (10%), and the slow-to-warm-up child (15%). Of note, 35% of the children (according to the characteristics of how they behaved) did not fit well in to any of the three clusters (Thomas, Chess, Birch, Hertzig, & Korn, 1963). Thomas et al. (1970) found that temperament traits are evident very early in life (the first months) and are relatively stable to adulthood. Temperaments allow children to modify their responses as they grow and learn.

Carey and McDevitt (1995), following the work of Thomas et al. (1963, 1970), stated that each of the nine temperament dimensions has a positive and a negative aspect. For example, a child who is observant may have been distractible as a baby. A stubborn toddler may be persistent in his studies later in school.

It is generally accepted that temperament may be influenced by biological or environmental factors. The environment includes both human (e.g., relationships with primary caregivers) and nonhuman aspects (e.g., noise, light) and influences how a child's temperament is expressed (Gowen & Nebrig, 2002). "Goodness of fit" between a child's temperament and his parents' caregiving practices is crucial for positive outcomes in emotional development (Thomas & Chess, 1977; Williamson & Anzalone, 2001). The temperament of both parent and child can significantly influence the relationship and attachment that the child has to the parent. If there is not a goodness of fit between the parent and the child, attachment may be negatively affected. Learning Activity 3.3 provides an opportunity for readers to reflect on their own temperament and its influences on their behavior and choices.

Attachment

The work of psychoanalysts John Bowlby, Mary Ainsworth, and others provides a foundation for our current understanding of attachment behaviors. Bowlby (1969) broke with both traditional psychoanalysis and the genetic view of infant and child psychological development by developing a new theoretical approach, now known as *attachment theory,* to describe the young child's drive to seek comfort and

Table 3.2. Temperament Traits

Trait	Description
Activity level	Level and extent of motor activity
Rhythmicity	Degree of regularity of functions such as eating, elimination, and the cycle of sleeping and wakefulness
Approach or withdrawal	Response to a new object or person in terms of whether the child accepts the new experience or withdraws from it
Adaptability	Adaptability of behavior to changes in the environment
Sensory threshold	Sensitivity to stimuli
Quality of mood	General disposition, whether cheerful or given to crying, pleasant or cranky, friendly or unfriendly
Intensity of reaction	Energy level of responses
Distractibility	Distractibility from what he is doing
Persistence and attention span	Persistence in an activity and span of time on activity

Source. Thomas, Chess, and Birch (1970).

security when in a challenging situation. Mary Ainsworth (1973; Ainsworth, Blehar, Waters, & Wall, 1978), a theoretician in her own right, carried out seminal clinical research that supported Bowlby's early theories. Essentially, Bowlby theorized that the infant's ability to discriminate strangers from familiar people, along with the infant's emotional connection to his or her mother or parent, established the foundation for understanding that person's current and later emotional life. Attachment theory helps us understand some children's aggression toward others or other children's excessive clinginess or withdrawn behavior. It also provides an explanation of how we learn to establish and maintain intimate relationships and how we pass on our parenting style to our children.

Bowlby (1969) suggested that the child's tie to his or her mother is the result of a preadapted, genetically based motivational system. In this viewpoint, both infants and parents are predisposed to respond to each other's signaling as a way of ensuring physical proximity and care needs. As a newborn, these signals go out to all adults initially but soon become directed to specific people. Within this context, the attachment bond develops as the infant's physical and interactive needs are met and

Learning Activity 3.3. Role of Temperament in One's Life

Consider your own temperament.

- How has it influenced how you behaved as a child? Was your temperament different from that of your sibling(s) or parent(s)?
- How do you see your basic temperament reflected in your actions as an adult?
- If you are a parent, think about your temperament and the temperament of your child or children.
- In what ways does a person's basic temperament influence therapeutic interactions?
- In what ways does it influence therapeutic use of self?

he or she feels physically and emotionally safe and secure. Bowlby suggested that this attachment system is activated by the presence of an unknown person or some other threat. This theory explains why an infant cries, crawls rapidly back to his or her mother, or is clingy when in a new situation that holds threat signals. When the infant perceives that the threat is gone, he or she feels safe to explore but will check back in with the mother either physically or visually to ensure his or her safety and security. This is termed *safe base* or *secure base* behavior (Landy, 2009). Through these repeated experiences, by approximately age 1 year, the infant develops an internal model of his or her mother as a "safe base." This internal model is imbued with emotional meaning that is based on the quality of responsive caregiving he or she has experienced.

As the child matures, he or she maintains the internalization of his or her parent as a safe base. This safe base model allows the child to eventually separate from his or her mother and promotes the development of independence. Infants who have had consistent, sensitive caregiving are thought to have an internal model of the parent as warm and responsive and of themselves as worthy of love. Infants who have had parents who are inconsistent or nonresponsive to their needs are thought to develop internal models of themselves as unworthy of love and support (Holloway, 1998).

In the early 1960s, Mary Ainsworth (1973; Ainsworth et al., 1978) carried out research at Johns Hopkins University that supported Bowlby's theories. She followed children at home, measuring their mother's style of feeding, smiling, eye contact, and response to distress. She then watched them in what she termed a "strange situation." At approximately age 1, mothers and their infants came to her clinical setting, where Ainsworth observed the infants' responses when a stranger entered the room, when the mother left the stranger and baby alone in the room, and when the mother returned. From her observations, Ainsworth was able to demonstrate different types of attachment—what she termed *secure attachment* or *insecure attachment*. These types of attachment were postulated as setting the scene for an infant's healthy emotional development (vs. development of low self-esteem and impaired future relationships).

The "strange situation" experiments yielded information about the behavior of infants with different types of attachment. Generally, infants who are securely attached to their parent or other important adult express some distress when separated from that person and then seek comfort when reunited with him or her. The securely attached infant is able to respond appropriately to comforting. An infant who has an insecure attachment of an anxious or resistant nature shows intense upset when separated and cannot be immediately comforted by the reappearance of his parent. In anxious–avoidant (or ambivalent) attachment, the child does not show any upset when separated from the parent and so shows little need for closeness or comfort when the parent returns. The child with a disorganized–disoriented attachment style demonstrates a mixture of these insecure attachment behaviors (Landy, 2009). These types of attachments describe behavioral styles, much like the temperament descriptors.

Although Bowlby's and Ainsworth's early work was controversial, it began a new direction in the understanding of early emotional development and its impact on later life. Since that time, a variety of attachment researchers have continued this work with increased application to both child and adult psychological intervention. The growing body of research that explains different aspects of child development has helped to further define and promote understanding of the role of attachment in children's behaviors and skill development. The complexity of attachment processes is being revealed as research yields more specific information about disorders of attachment.

We include this attachment discussion to remind readers that when providing early childhood services, occupational therapists must look at all possible contributors to a young child's behavior. For example, a therapist observes that a child is clingy during therapy and does not want to let go of his father's arm when placed on a climbing apparatus. It appears that he really needs his dad to help him cope. A therapist with a background in sensory processing might wonder whether that child has some gravitational hyperresponsivity that contributes to this behavior. A therapist who comes from a neurodevelopmental treatment background might question the child's postural and motor control. Using a social–emotional development background, another therapist might wonder about attachment, knowing that clinginess is typical for a young child of a certain age and that for an older child, it may suggest immature or delayed emotional development. It is incumbent on each therapist to draw from all possible perspectives when developing an intervention plan with any young child and parent.

This chapter presents just a brief introduction to the topic of attachment. For a more in-depth discussion and information related to early intervention, see Landy (2009) and Foley and Hochman (2006).

The Primary Relationship: Feeding as a Metaphor for Parent as Nurturer

A discussion of feeding, a common reason that occupational therapists are called upon to work with children, serves as an illustration of these concepts in an important area of parent–child co-occupation.

The importance of eating goes well beyond nutrition. To be hospitable, we offer our guests something to drink or eat when they visit our home. To build group solidarity, we may go out after work for drinks with our coworkers. Types of foods, food preparation rituals, and food sharing have culturally based meaning and status. Our vocabulary has food-based words: That child is *spoiled rotten;* that's a *half-baked* idea; he's all *steamed up*. One of the first and most primary ways in which a parent nurtures and provides for his or her child is through his or her ability to feed that child. What might it mean to a parent when his or her child is unable or unwilling to be fed?

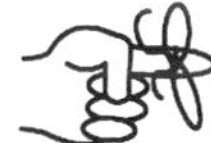

Remember this. . . .
One of the first and most primary ways in which a parent nurtures and provides for his or her child is through his or her ability to feed that child.

Eating or feeding is a significant daily occupation. Feeding times cannot be ignored; they routinely take place several times each day. We are all aware that a child's growth and development require appropriate nutrition. For many parents, feeding is the ultimate expression of their ability to nurture their child. Feeding one's child is filled with personal meaning and, potentially, stress. For the young child with special needs, this stress may be heightened. If parents perceive that they are unsuccessful feeding their child, what does that feeling imply to them about their ability to nurture and their self-perception of what it means to be a good parent? We can see how difficult feedings—whether based in neuromotor dysfunction, medical limitations, or other issues—may influence the child–parent relationship and thus affect all aspects of development. From multiple perspectives, addressing feeding is a microcosm of all areas of occupational therapy concern.

Occupational therapists encounter children with feeding challenges in a variety of contexts—from the NICU to preschool snack time to family celebrations. It is important for the occupational therapist to begin by understanding the range of concerns that influence the child's ability to eat successfully. It is equally important to appreciate the parent's vision of how the child's ability to participate in family and community life is influenced by eating or being fed.

Feeding in the Neonatal Intensive Care Unit

Feeding for most infants in the NICU relates to supporting maturational processes while taking physical stability and medical recovery into account. Typically, by the end of the hospitalization, the occupational therapist and nursing staff are able to feed the infant, mostly by mouth and occasionally by tube. The NICU staff, however, will not be accompanying the child home to become a family member. The parent needs to be equally, if not more, competent at feeding the baby. In addition, as the infant's needs change, the parent will have to be able to identify how the changes influence feeding and be able to problem solve without the immediate feedback of a professional.

Price and Miner (2008) described one approach that the occupational therapist can use to facilitate this process. They emphasized the occupational therapist's use of mentoring and scaffolding strategies to train parents in feeding techniques while exploring with the parents their own vision of parenting the infant and enabling them to move forward. Why is this important? It is the parent who structures the environment outside of the NICU to promote the family life into which the infant enters. The mutuality and reciprocity inherent in the parents' successful feeding of their infant is a reflection of the experience each child requires throughout the first years of life.

Transition to Oral Feeding

Some children are fed by means of gastrostomy tube or nasogastric tube over prolonged periods of their early lives. This situation may be caused by the child's medical condition, such as poor cardiorespiratory reserve to support the work of feeding; poor neuromuscular coordination and control; or a conditioned aversion caused by, for example, repeated negative experiences related to feeding or the functioning of the gastrointestinal tract. Almost from the beginning, there is an additional component to poor feeding: the emotional component. Eating can be a highly emotionally charged activity for a family and child. The emotional component of eating may influence the child's ability to transition from tube to oral feedings even if there is no medical reason to continue nonoral feedings. The child may be ready to feed from medical and oral–motor perspectives, but prior negative experiences for either the child or the parent may produce anxiety that spills over into mealtime.

One may may hear a health or early childhood professional mention a behavioral component to the feeding difficulty. The term *behavioral* often has a negative connotation, as though the young child is just spoiled. If we understand cognitive and emotional development, however, we understand that some children who are labeled negatively in this way are not cognitively or emotionally mature enough to be able to be spoiled. The "behaviors" that are observed by the occupational therapist should be interpreted as the child's communication of distress, an emotional response.

Strong Food Preferences or Aversions

Occupational therapists hear this refrain all too often: "Why won't he just eat?" Strong food preferences that influence the rhythm of family life or that limit a child's food repertoire, thereby putting that child at nutritional risk, are another feeding-related area in which occupational therapists are involved. Often, this type of feeding challenge is frustrating to family and professionals alike. This frustration may arise from what appears to be the inconsistent nature of the child's eating. Parents may ask, "Why does he refuse soft foods but love smooth and crunchy foods?" or "Why will he only take his bottle in the middle of the night, when he's asleep?" Often this situation is related to inefficient sensory processing; that is, difficulties with sensory modulation or discrimination. It is also necessary to determine with the parents in what ways their reactions to their child's preferences or aversions are influencing the child's choices. No toddler can drive himself to the fast-food joint for chicken nuggets.

Young children often appear to feed better for one parent than the other. Parents are often fatigued by this process—at times, they are literally sleep deprived. Their concern that their child is not growing may be compounded by the threat of tube feedings with possible surgery. Such a step would further influence the parents' perception of themselves as failing to be able to feed their child.

These multifactorial feeding challenges require the occupational therapist to use a broad lens in examining all factors that contribute to the situation. This lens necessarily includes the child's level of emotional development as well as the emotional stressors involved in the feeding situation and how they flow into the rest of the child's and family's life. What is the threat to the ongoing relationships between parents; between parent and child; and even among siblings, whose every meal focuses on the "problem eater"?

Infant Mental Health

Infant mental health has developed into accepted practice and influenced programs and services for all children. The field emerged from research in the 1970s with infants who were blind (Fraiberg, 1980) and is supported by continuing research on brain growth and development, emotional and affective states, attachment, environmental influences, and the importance of the quality of the parent–infant relationships for optimal development. "Babies on the couch" is the phrase that the *Ann Arbor News* once used to describe infant mental health (Waters, 2004). The focus of the interventions, however, is not on "baby pathology" but on helping parents develop positive, nurturing relationships with their infants.

> Extensive research has shown that the quality of experiences in the first 3 years of life has a profound impact on later development, including how children perform in school and their ability to form satisfying relationships with teachers, friends and others. Having caring relationships with sensitive parents or other primary caregivers is the most important factor in determining later outcomes. (Center on Infant Mental Health and Development, 2009)

Infant mental health has multiple definitions. The World Association of Infant Mental Health defined infant mental health as follows:

> The ability to develop physically, cognitively, and socially in a manner which allows [infants] to master the primary emotional tasks of early childhood without serious disruption caused by harmful life events. Because infants grow in a context of nurturing environments, infant mental health involves the psychological balance of the infant–family system. (Osofsky & Fitzgerald, 1999, p. 25)

Zero to Three (2008) defined infant mental health as follows:

> The healthy social and emotional development of a child from birth to 3 years and a growing field of research and practice devoted to the
>
> - Promotion of healthy social and emotional development;
> - Prevention of mental health problems; and
> - Treatment of the mental health problems of very young children in the context of their families.

Infant mental health services are provided by professionals who have the knowledge and skills, by virtue of their professional education and their specific focus on the parent–infant relationship, to support parents in their relationship with their baby. Weatherston (2000), a leader in infant mental health, described the infant mental health professional as "someone with a distinct set of core beliefs, skills, training experiences, and clinical strategies who incorporates a comprehensive, intensive and relationship-based approach to working with young children and families" (p. 5).

A parent and child could benefit from infant mental health services for many reasons. Many of the children occupational therapists treat have biologically based issues that make it difficult to soothe them or to interpret their behavior. These challenges can be very distressing or confusing to parents, particularly first-time parents, and can disrupt the parent–infant relationship. In other circumstances, parents may have a substance abuse problem, be under stress because of poverty or housing issues, or simply not know how to respond positively and appropriately to the infant, often repeating the negative ways in which they themselves were treated as a child. Fraiberg (1980) referred to the influence of negative memories of childhood on one's parenting style as "ghosts in the nursery."

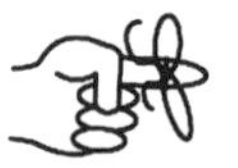

Remember this. . . .
"The home environment is the family's place and space where the surroundings are familiar and extended family may be present. Available resources are known or seen. Normal routines can be used as the process of intervention" (Chandler & Yun, 2006, p. 1).

Infant mental health services are best provided in the setting in which most infant–parent interaction occurs: the home. Chandler and Yun (2006) stated, "The home environment is the family's place and space where the surroundings are familiar and extended family may be present. Available resources are known or seen. Normal routines can be used as the process of intervention" (p. 1). Fraiberg (1980) referred to this approach as "kitchen table therapy." Is it easy to see the link to the ways in which early intervention services are to be provided.

The infant mental health definitions presented earlier speak to the importance of the early years, to the multiple influences on a developing child, and to the primacy of the parent–child relationship. According to Weatherston (2000), the dimensions of infant mental health services are concrete assistance, emotional support, developmental guidance, early relationship assessment and support, advocacy, and infant–parent psychotherapy. Occupational therapists working from an infant mental health perspective rely heavily on their therapeutic interaction skills (Chandler & Yun, 2006). Maslow's (1954) seminal work on the needs of humans and the hierarchy of needs addressed infant mental health needs. Basic needs must be met before other needs can be addressed. Often, the concrete assistance that families need involves shelter, food, clothing, and transportation. Weatherston (2000) suggested that advocacy involves giving the family a voice to get what it needs. Advocacy also involves giving a voice to what the therapist perceives to be the baby's perspective to help the parent interpret the child's behavior.

Consider this scenario: A 2-year-old is having a meltdown at the park after unsuccessfully trying to climb a new piece of equipment. His mother witnessed his attempt but said, "That's too hard, sweetie, try something else." The child, being 2, replies "NO!" and continues to tantrum. His mother is trying to contain the tantrum and, appearing increasingly frustrated and embarrassed, tells him, "Calm down, you want to play here more, don't you?" Again, the 2-year-old says, "No!" She attempts to pick him up to leave, but he has a death grip on the equipment.

Advocacy for the child might take the form of a kindly occupational therapist at the park with her own kids, who vocalizes for him, "I'm frustrated, I want to climb up." Mom catches on, allows him to use her hand as a leverage point, and enables him to climb. The tantrum stops—infant mental health in action.

Emotional support is essential to the infant mental health approach and involves being cognizant of and responsive to the emotional state of clients; it involves paying attention to explicit and tacit expressions of emotion. The *Occupational Therapy Practice Framework: Domain and Process, 2nd Edition* (American Occupational Therapy Association [AOTA], 2008) allows occupational therapists the latitude to consider young children and other people within their environment as clients. It explicitly states, "The term *person* includes others who also may help or be served indirectly, such as caregiver, teacher, parent, employer, or spouse" (p. 652).

Pilkington (2006) stated that "as occupational therapy practitioners interact with and care for parents and other caregivers, so will parents and caregivers treat their children," suggesting that role-modeling interaction styles that promote positive communication skills and behavioral management strategies will assist families in seeing the value in those skills and learning how to use them. Infant mental health professionals often use dyadic assessment and intervention strategies when working with families. Pilkington (2006) encouraged occupational therapists to consider each stage of the child's emotional development to create effective intervention activities and to engage the parent and child in nurturing, contingent, and empathetic interactions.

Infant mental health approaches view infant–caregiver relationships as crucial contexts for child development. Evidence for this approach is compelling. Some studies have examined the patterns of infant–caregiver relationships as predictors of infant development, whereas others consider the effects of the infant–caregiver relationship as strategies to moderate biological risk factors, such as prematurity (Landry, Smith, & Swank, 2006; Minde, 1993).

Weatherston (2000) referred to nondidactic developmental guidance as an important aspect of infant mental health services. In this guidance, the therapist helps the parents learn to

- Sensitively respond to the child's needs for care,
- Accurately understand the child's specific abilities,
- Recognize what the baby is doing, and
- Anticipate the next step of development or skill that will emerge.

Weatherston (2000) referred to early relationship assessment and support and recommended using the therapeutic relationship with the parents to help them develop and nurture their relationship with their infant. Observing real-time interactions of parents with their infants and using "in the moment" comments to reinforce positive interactions or identify infant responses that parents might misinterpret are examples of early relationship assessment and support (Chandler & Yun, 2006).

Babies and young children thrive when they are cared for by adults who are crazy about them—in other words, when they have adults who are responsive to them (Bronfenbrenner, 1976). The work and writings of Stanley Greenspan (Greenspan et al., 1997; Greenspan & Wieder, 1998) provide guidance and examples of how occupational therapists and other early childhood specialists can incorporate the body of knowledge about infant mental health, emotional development, and early relationships into their work with young children and their families.

Weatherston's (2000) dimensions of infant mental health service suggest a variety of ways to meet the mental health needs of very young children and their families. Learning Activity 3.4 provides an opportunity to specifically identify ways in your practice that you do or could use these languages of infant mental health.

Conclusion

Young children cannot survive on their own. They need the attention and nurturance of people who care for and about them. This chapter has briefly examined relationships, emotional development, and the field of infant mental health. It has emphasized the importance of primary relationships between caregivers (usually parents) and young children. Occupational therapists must always bear these relationships in mind when working with families with young children.

To promote optimal participation means that occupational therapists must engage with parents in their daily parenting experience and their relationship with their child as a focus of therapy and not focus only on the child. Occupational therapists should consider the following points when working with young children and their parents (Holloway, 1998):

- Parents and caregivers are the mediators of the child's sensory and affective experiences.
- Always observe the child and the child and parent spontaneously interacting when assessing emotional development.
- Always consider how emotional development influences all aspects of development, interaction, and intent.

Learning Activity 3.4. Infant Mental Health in Practice

- Identify two examples of each of the dimensions of infant mental health.
- Discuss how you see these practices as related to and reflected in the *Occupational Therapy Practice Framework* (AOTA, 2008).
- Identify four different circumstances when you used infant mental health practices with your clients.
- With a learning group, identify five different articles on infant mental health from five different journals. Discuss the content of the articles and its application to occupational therapy practice with infants and their parents.

- The family's daily routines set the stage for providing a variety and richness of experiences that the infant needs.
- Therapeutic intervention should acknowledge and support the parents' observations of the child's behavior and include parent education.
- The child's emotional state should guide therapeutic activities as well as the intervention goals.
- Always seek to engage the parent and child in mutually positive interactions.
- The timing and rhythm of therapeutic activities must incorporate the dynamic cycling of parent–infant interaction.
- Occupational therapists must focus on their internal affective state and the type and timing of expression as well as the physical distance from the infant.

Providing family-centered care requires relationship-based approaches at all levels of early childhood service, from the public policy level to the individual level of working with families and colleagues, especially service coordinators. The importance of working with and collaborating with families cannot be stressed enough. We end this chapter by listening to the voice of a parent who writes of her experiences and perspectives of and contemplations on being a mother—a mother who has a child without disabilites, has lost a child, and had a child with special needs for almost 8 years. Vicki Forman graciously gave permission for her essays to be included here (Boxes 3.1–3.3). They are included to remind readers to listen to the parents' experience first, then attend to the parent–child relationship while addressing the child's development. All of this information leads the occupational therapist to establish a therapeutic relationship with the child and parent as well as to support the parent–child relationship. These relationships enable occupational therapy to promote developmental progression as well as the child's participation in family life, one of the most important occupations of early childhood. Learning Activity 3.5 refers to Box 3.1, and Learning Activity 3.6 refers to Box 3.2.

The family, not the individual, is the real molecule of society, the key link in the social chain of being.

—Robert Nisbet (1975, p. 260)

Box 3.1. Bravery and Fear

My son hates to have his teeth brushed or his nails trimmed. Each is a struggle that results in violent cries and tears; both require that he be pinned down, either between my legs or with someone else holding him while I do the job. I have learned that the best place to do either is in his car seat while he's strapped in. And so I trim my son's nails and brush his teeth in the parking lot of his school, the theory here being that since he loves school, no matter how hard he screams he will recover, knowing that he is on his way into the classroom. "It's okay, Evan," I'll tell him, as I snip at his nails or shove the toothbrush in his mouth, "as soon as you're done we're going to see Mr. Chase" (or Miss Myrna or Miss Lesley or Miss Kami or Miss Judy, depending on which day it is and which service provider's turn it is with him.). I have yet to be questioned about this Draconian abuse; most assume that if I am the mother, I can't be hurting him too awfully. Most assume that there must be a purpose to my cruelty, snipping off those nails while he's strapped in, brushing his baby teeth around those awful cries.

I'm not sure when and how I developed the talent to pin my son down and endure these terrible moments; in the hospital, certainly, during the six months after he was born and I witnessed IV pokes and arterial cut downs and extubations and reintubations. From the pediatrician, too, who has to immobilize Evan with his thick forearms during examinations. I remember one dentist teaching me the more sophisticated technique of holding his head between my legs and pinning his legs between my own. "That's how to get his teeth brushed," the man told me. "And you can do it all by yourself!" What I do know is this: When it's time to put Evan into a human straight jacket, mama knows best.

~

One day, a few weeks ago, I snipped a bit of Evan's pinky finger along with his nail, precision being a tricky thing with a child who is professionally squirming out of one's grasp. In a flash, the blood trailed down his hand, all the way to his forearm. I got him into the classroom and enlisted the help of his teacher in applying a band aid. The cries that began with the nail clipping only grew worse once the band aid was on. I consoled him as best I could, then left for work.

Half an hour later, the phone rang. "Evan's in the nurse's office. He took his band aid off and his finger's bleeding and we need you to come put it back on."

"You need me to do what?"

"We're afraid to do it ourselves. He's so upset. We don't want to get him angrier."

Back at school, I explained to the nurse, who knows Evan but who typically hands over duties like this to me, how to immobilize my son. "You put his legs between yours like this, then clamp down his hands like this, then strap your legs across his chest like this. . . ." When I was done, and the band aid reapplied, I looked into the nurse's eyes and said, "Now you know how I do it. Now you'll be able to do it yourself."

"Sure," she said, but on her face I could see what she really thought. No way am I ever pinning a child down like that. I could lose my job.

~

I have become a master of motherly acts that go beyond brave: I can shove medicine into my son's clamped mouth; pin him down for any task, from doctor's appointments to teeth-brushing; ignore his cries in the middle of the night when I know there is no consoling him, when I have already tried and failed. The memories of my older, typical daughter taking a fall or crying in the middle of the night are like phantom ghosts, pale shadows of the bravery I now know. I have seen my son into nearly a dozen surgical rooms, heard from specialists that he will never see, that he very well might not talk, that his seizure disorder has the potential for devastating outcomes. I have learned to hear it all, and to do it all. And now, rarely, does my heart even stop. I pin him down, I change the band aid, and not once do I stop to think about what I have learned to do.

But I also learned that bravery is impossible without fear, and that in so many ways these two qualities are inextricably bound. From the day Evan was born I have been faced with primordial fear: of his future, of all those surgeries, the hard facts of his disability. Of how my life has changed. I bless the truths these fears have taught me, the friends I have gained along the way and the courage I have learned. But the fears are still there, frequent, just a hair's breath [*sic*] beyond the bravery. For every moment I muster the strength to pin my son down, there is another moment when my breath catches in my throat and I recognize that fear.

Fear that the doctors might be right, or that I will always be the only one strong enough to trim his nails, brush his teeth and change the band aid. That someday even my own strength and bravery won't be enough. Fear of my son's future, of the day our beautiful, typical daughter leaves the house for college and my husband and I are alone, in the quiet, with our son.

If I am the bearer of pain to my son in the form of toothbrush and nail clippers, my husband provides the joy. He loves to play bongos with Evan, who giggles with him in these nightly drum sessions as loudly as he cries with me in the morning over the toothbrush.

One night, while Evan laughed and my husband drummed, I shared with him this fear of being alone with Evan with Josie gone, of how it might exaggerate for me the reality of Evan's disabilities.

"I will be so sad when Josie leaves, and it's just you, me, and Evan."

"You mean, you, me, Evan, and the bongos."

"I guess. . . ."

Cliff drummed louder, and Evan laughed hard. "Listen to that," my husband said. "You won't be sad. You'll be happy."

I hope my husband is right, and that I will be happy when it's just him, me, Evan, and the bongos. Right now I don't feel very brave about that inevitable day. But in my time as Evan's mother I have come to learn that like fear, which can sometimes feel endless, bravery has a way of showing its own boundless nature, too.

Source. From "Bravery and Fear," by Vicki Forman, April 22, 2007. Copyright © by Vicki Forman. Retrieved January 21, 2010, from www.literarymama.com/columns/specialneedsmama/archives/2007/bravery_and_fear.html. Used with permission.

Learning Activity 3.5. Serving Clients With Multiple Needs

Reflection: Think of one of your clients who has multiple needs. Consider all the daily caregiving activities that the parents must do with him or her.

- How many and which of these activities are typical and atypical for a child his or her age?
- How many and which of these involve skills that most parents never have to learn or do?
- What does that parent feel while carrying out those actions?
- What might others think?
- What is our responsibility in this realm, because self-care is a daily occupation?
- How should we be helping parents to find "ways that work" that, perhaps, are not so stressful for parent and child?

Box 3.2. Special-Needs Siblings

When my daughter was 4 years old, she received an end-of-the-year scrapbook from her preschool teachers. There, amidst the anecdotes of prereading Max & Ruby stories, the child-created observations of flower growth in the classroom garden, and reports of endless water play with friends, I read the following: "During the year, Josie has shown enormous anger at the illness of her baby brother, as well as guilt and remorse over that anger. . . ." The sentence went on but I could not read any more. Instead, I closed the book, my hands trembling, and I thought, not about the teacher, but about myself, *"How could you not see this? You fool."*

The next time my daughter asked to see the scrapbook, I had blacked out those words. Because even if they were true, I did not want them there for her to see. This brother of hers, with his illness and complications, had to be more than a source of anger and guilt. Her sibling experience needed to count for more than that.

I grew up in a large family, two brothers and a sister. For me, the sibling experience was practically totemic in its necessity, and I knew as soon as my daughter was born, it would be important for her to have the same. A brother or a sister, someone to keep her company after we were gone, a legacy of shared genes and memories. That quest for another child brought us our son and gave our daughter a very atypical sibling experience, eliciting the editorial comments from her preschool teacher, and marring an otherwise perfect scrapbook with my daughter's difficult reality.

I have several friends who have one typically developing child, and another with special needs. One of my friends will say, apropos of her typical son, "Look, none of us signed up for this. He's dealing with it the way we all are, he's coping."

I appreciate my friend's candor and her honesty. But my own journey as the mother of both a typical child and a special-needs child is more conflicted (as I'm sure my friend's is, too). I feel guilty about my daughter's embarrassment at her brother's many behavioral outbursts, his blindness, lack of speech, delayed development; guilty that a typical sibling experience is not in the cards for her; and, finally, guilty that I can't always acknowledge those challenges. Like the words in that preschool scrapbook, sometimes I have to black them out and turn away.

At night, in bed, my daughter will ask me a lot of questions about my own siblings, their pet names for me, the things we did together growing up. I sometimes wonder if she's trying to imagine not only the life I had growing up but also the life she might have had, if her brother had not been born 17 weeks early, weighing only a pound.

The life of a special-needs sibling is unlike any other. My oldest Special Needs Mama friend has two daughters, one a typically developing 3-year-old, the other a 7-year-old with cerebral palsy. Recently, when the 3-year-old started preschool and was having a hard time being without her mother, she used an outrageous set of excuses as to why they should call her mother to take her home. "I'm having seizures," she said. "I need to go to the hospital. My G-tube is leaking!"

One Christmas, when my son was still in the NICU and my daughter was 3 years old, the doctors offered to let her inside the unit to visit—a very rare occurrence for siblings her age. Josie gave me a long look and asked me, "Why?" Why would she want to go in there and see Evan? What difference did it make? "But Santa's in there," I said, indicating through the glass door an older man in a beard and Santa Suit, leaning over Evan's isolette.

"Santa doesn't belong in the NICU," she said.

It takes enormous reason—and outsized coping skills—for a child to navigate these waters, those of seizures and G-tubes and visits from Santa in the NICU. Logic, and solid sense of self, have carried my daughter through some tough years with her brother spent in doctors' offices and hospitals, therapy sessions, and clinics. I still don't know that I agree with her preschool teachers about all that anger and guilt, but I do know that she has adapted to this strange world as only a child can, going so far as to use rubber gloves as toys or G-tube adapters for water play. Every once in a while, she'll come to me with some device she's found in Evan's room—an empty syringe, perhaps, or a nebulizing cage—and ask, "Mommy, can I use this?"

Just like my friend's 3-year-old with her outgrown excuses, the seizures and the need to go to the hospital, my daughter copes by expanding her own horizons as a child to incorporate this special-needs world. Last week, she went through a therapy session blindfolded, "To see what it was like," she said, "to be Evan."

It would be easy to stay in the place of guilt, where being a special-needs sibling is simply a raw deal. Sure there is the surreality of seizures, G-tubes, and therapy sessions. But then I remember Piaget's concepts of assimilation and accommodation and marvel at how beautifully my daughter has mastered these concepts. Often, after spending the day at a friend's house, one where a typical younger brother resides, my daughter will come home to report, "I'm so glad I don't have a sibling *like that.*" In other words, one who follows the girls around, throws a punch or two, demands the TV remote. A typical brother.

And then there are the basics: My daughter is growing up with an extra measure of compassion and the knowledge that the world is not perfect. She knows that some people don't walk or talk but that this doesn't always interfere with other abilities. She is the first to take pride in her brother's achievements, and because she is human, she is also the first to say, at the end of a long evening of "Evan's annoying Pooh CD," as she calls it, "Isn't it time for Evan to go to bed?"

Beyond the coping and the jealousy and the simple challenge of navigating these waters, there is, finally, my pride in my daughter and her own journey. She is a marvel of a person, neither false in her affection for her brother, nor unstinting in her praise of him.

"He said hello!" she announced the other night, after reading a communication log from Evan's school. "Mommy, did you read this? Evan said 'hello' at school today!"

Finally, she is simply her own person, which is the best accomplishment of all. After reading about Evan in this column one morning, Josie came to me and asked softly, "Are you going to write about me some day?"

I can't imagine, in my own growing up, having to compete with a child like Evan for my mother's attention. I know of adults with special-needs siblings who themselves remember times in their teen years that they resented their siblings, the stress it caused their families, the responsibility they feel for their brother or sister in adulthood. I try not to think about this future as I tell my daughter, "Yes, yes, I'm going to write about you. What would you like me to say?"

Source. From "Special-Needs Siblings," by Vicki Forman, October 7, 2007. Copyright © by Vicki Forman. Retrieved January 21, 2010, from www.literarymama.com/columns/specialneedsmama/archives/2007/special_needs_siblings.html. Used with permission.

Learning Activity 3.6. Silent Partners

Reflections: Siblings are often the "silent partners" of a child with special needs.

- What does the essay "Special-Needs Siblings" say to you about the experiences of a child with a brother or sister with special needs?
- What kind of "special" time, help, attention, or guidance might a parent consider giving to a sibling? What does a sibling need?

Box 3.3. Letter to a Therapist

The following is a letter to a therapist that Vicki Forman posted on her blog. Although it is not directed to any one of us, it gives one pause to think about situations where it may have been directed to a therapist we know or with whom we work. We hope not, but . . . how do we always be sure that we have respected the parents' perspective?

Dear Nameless and Shameful Therapist,

I am writing to express my deep disappointment and frustration with your refusal to write a letter of medical necessity for my son, Evan, for a collapsing, adaptive stroller. You have suggested that said stroller is not medically necessary for Evan due to his high level of "functional" walking. When I asked you how Evan was supposed to walk through the supermarket, or Descanso Gardens, or Target or Borders or any of the other places we go as a family on a regular basis, how he was meant to cane his way up and down the aisles so that I might buy groceries, for example, you said, "He is capable of doing that, he just refuses." You said, "He can do all those things on a functional level, it's his behavioral issues that hold him back."

And I said, "Nameless and Shameful Therapist, Evan is new to walking. If you had a 2-year-old typical child, would you expect that child to do all those things you are asking of Evan? Would you describe that child's inability to walk all the way around Target as a 'behavioral' issue? Or would you (naturally) assume that that child was, in fact, simply tired and worn out after a period of walking? Would you call that child's fatigue 'behavorial' or would you praise the child for all the walking he had already done and promptly reward him by putting him a stroller?"

And you said, "Well, I know exactly what you're saying but I still can't write the letter. And my supervisor said no as well."

NST, nowhere in the copious goals and expectations that we have written together for Evan does it say he must walk through the supermarket or, as you suggested yesterday, Disneyland. Nowhere has anyone suggested that having given up his walker a mere three months ago, Evan should now be able to walk everywhere, all the time. Yes, he walks from the car to physical therapy, or from the car to his classroom, or from the car to the pool. And guess what? All those trips take twice as long as they would with a typical child. And yes, when he gets to his destination, he is tired. And here's another thing—have you looked at his gait lately? It's wobbly and precarious, and even when walking he's something of a hazard. This is the child you expect to walk through the store or Disneyland? Not quite.

Evan has taught us all quite a bit about hard work and determination. He has proven himself capable of doing all the things we have asked of him and more. So how does it help him not to support those gains? And what right do you, or anyone else, have to decide that those gains do not warrant the support of something so fundamental as the ability to get around?

It saddens me to think that your view of my son and his needs are so narrow and absolute. It even makes me wonder if you are, in fact, the right therapist for my child.

Yours,

Vicki Forman

Source. From "Dear Nameless and Shameful Therapist," by Vicki Forman, September 6, 2006. Copyright © by Vicki Forman. Retrieved June 16, 2010, from www.vickiforman.com/?p=475. Used with permission.

How Very Far We Have Come: Little School (1958–1959)

Lydia was tireless in her efforts to get the county school system to admit Danny. They were equally adamant that they could not do so because state law prohibited it.

Lydia realized quickly that she could not "win" acceptance to the public school immediately for Danny and that she had to find a way for him to be educated. She was convinced that although he had some physical disabilities, he was not mentally retarded. Working with other parents whom she had met at the National Association of Parents and Friends of Mentally Retarded Children and building on what they had done in a larger town, she and three other mothers in her county "established" a school for their children with disabilities.

Initially, it met every Wednesday, rotating from one house to the next. With no formal training as teachers but drawing on what their other children were doing in school, a curriculum was developed, lesson plans were created, and classes were held. It was only a half-day at first, but within a year four other children had joined, and the need for something more formalized was evident. The ages of the children ranged from 6 to 12, and their needs were varied.

The pastor of the largest local church was approached about using the church basement during the week for classes in exchange for cleaning and lawn maintenance of the church. There was opposition at first among parishioners because the school was not part of the mission of the church, but the pastor was supportive. Few knew that he had an older brother with profound mental retardation living in a state institution.

It was a little school, but it was school! They named it Main Street School because that was the address of the church. It also sent a not-so-subtle message: that the children attending the school belonged on "Main Street" as much as anyone else.

Questions

1. How could states exclude children with disabilities from public school? What was the rationale?
2. What kind of challenges would the running of such a school face? What opposition?
3. Did the Supreme Court's ruling in *Brown v. Board of Education of Topeka* (1954) have any bearing on the operation of these parent-supported schools?

References

Ainsworth, M. (1973). The development of infant–mother attachment. *Chld Development Research, 3,* 1–93

Ainsworth, M. D. S, Blehar, M. C., Waters, E., & Wall, S. (1978). *Patterns of attachment: A psychological study of the Strange Situation.* Hillsdale, NJ: Erlbaum.

American Occupational Therapy Association. (2008). Occupational therapy practice framework: Domain and process (2nd ed.). *American Journal of Occupational Therapy, 62,* 625–683.

Barrera, M. (1986). Distinctions between social support concepts, measures, and models. *American Journal of Community Psychology, 14,* 413–441.

Bowlby, J. (1969). *Attachment and loss. Volume I: Attachment.* New York: Basic Books.

Brazelton, T. B., & Greenspan, S. (2000). *The irreducible needs of children.* Cambridge, MA: Da Capo Press.

Bronfenbrenner, U. (1976). *The ecology of human development.* Cambridge, MA: Harvard University Press.

Brown v. Board of Education of Topeka, 347 U.S. 483 (1954).

Bruder, M. B., & Dunst, C. J. (December 1999/January 2000). Expanding learning opportunities for infants and toddlers in natural environments: A chance to reconceptualize early intervention. *Zero to Three, 20,* 34–36.

Carey, W. B., & McDevitt, S. C. (1995). *Coping with children's temperament.* New York: Basic Books.

Center on Infant Mental Health and Development. (2009). *What is infant mental health?* Retrieved December 12, 2009, from http://depts.washington.edu/chdd/uceddcimhd_3/3_cimdhmain.html

Chandler, B. E., & Yun, A. R. (2006). Defining occupational therapy's role in infant mental health. *School System Special Interest Section Quarterly, 13*(4), 1–4.

Foley, G. M., & Hochman, J.D. (Eds). (2006). *Mental health in early intervention.* Baltimore: Brookes.

Fraiberg, S. (1980). *Clinical studies in infant mental health: The first year of life.* New York: Basic Books.

Gowen, J., & Nebrig, J. (2002). *Enhancing early emotional development.* Baltimore: Brookes.

Green, M. (Ed.). (1994). *Bright futures: Guidelines for health supervision of infants, children, and adolescents.* Arlington, VA: National Center for Education in Maternal and Child Health.

Greenspan, S. I., Kalmanson, B., Shanook, R., Wieder, S., Williamson, G. G., & Anzalone, M. (1997). Assessing and treating infants and young children with severe difficulties in relating and communicating. *Zero to Three, 17,* 55–64.

Greenspan, S. I., & Weider, S. (1998). *The child with special needs: Encouraging intellectual and emotional growth.* Boston: Addison Wesley.

Hanft, B., Rush, D., & Shelden, M. (2004). *Coaching families and colleagues in early childhood.* Baltimore: Brookes.

Holloway, E. (1998). Early emotional development and sensory processing. In J. Case-Smith (Ed.), *Pediatric occupational therapy and early intervention* (pp. 163–197). Woburn, MA: Butterworth-Heinemann.

Howard, J. (1978). *Families.* New York: Simon & Schuster.

Humphry, R. (1989). Early intervention and the influence of the occupational therapist on the parent–child relationship. *American Journal of Occupational Therapy, 4,* 738–742.

Hurth, J. (1998, December). Service coordination caseloads in state early intervention systems. *NECTAS Notes, 8.* Chapel Hill, NC: National Early Childhood Technical Assistance System. Retrieved September 8, 2009, from www.nectac.org/~pdfs/pubs/nnotes8.pdf

Individuals With Disabilities Education Improvement Act of 2004, Pub. L. 108–446, 20 U.S.C. § 1400 *et seq.*

Landy, S. (2009). *Pathways to competence: Encouraging healthy social and emotional development in young children.* Baltimore: Brookes.

Landry, S., Smith, K., & Swank, P. (2006). Establishing early foundations for social, communication, and independent problem solving skills. *Developmental Psychology, 42*(4), 627–642.

Lillas, C., & Turnbull, J. (2009). *Infant/child mental health, early intervention, and relationship-based therapies.* New York: Norton.

Markowitz, J. (2001). *Synthesis brief: Part C service coordination: State policies and models. Project forum.* Alexandria, VA: National Association of State Directors of Special Education.

Maslow, A. (1954). *Motivation and personality.* New York: Harper.

Mattingly, C., & Fleming, M. (1994). *Clinical reasoning: Forms of inquiry in a therapeutic practice.* Philadelphia: F. A. Davis.

McWilliams, R. A, & Scott, S. (2001, November). Therapy ain't tennis lessons. *Integrating Therapy Into the Classroom, 1,* 5. Individualizing Inclusion in Child Care Project. Retrieved March 27, 2007, from www.fpg.unc.edu/~inclusion/IT.pdf

Minde, K. (1993). The social and emotional development of low-birthweight infants and their families up to age 4. In S. Friedman & M. Sigman (Eds.), *The psychological development of low birthweight children: Advances in applied developmental psychology* (pp. 157–185). Norwood, NJ: Ablex.

National Early Childhood Technical Assistance Center. (2008). *Document 1: Mission and key principles for providing early intervention services in natural environments*. Retrieved January 10, 2010, from www.nectac.org/topics/families/families.asp

National Early Childhood Technical Assistance Center. (2009a). *Family-centered principles and practices*. Retrieved March 12, 2009, from www.nectac.org/topics/families/famctrprin.asp

National Early Childhood Technical Assistance Center. (2009b). *Family-centered services: Family-centered principles*. Retrieved January 5, 2010, from www.nectac.org/topics/families/families.asp

Nisbet, R. (1975). *The twilight of authority*. New York: Oxford University Press.

Osofsky, J. D., & Fitzgerald, H. E. (Eds.). (1999). *World Association of Infant Mental Health handbook of infant mental health: Perspectives on infant mental health* (Vol. 1, p. 25). Southgate: Michigan Association for Infant Mental Health.

Philbin, A. (1996). *Capacity building in social justice organizations*. Detroit: Ford Foundation.

Pilkington, K. (2006). Side by side: Transdisciplinary early intervention in natural environments. *OT Practice, 11*(6), 12–17. Retrieved January 5, 2010, from www.aota.org/Pubs/OTP/1997-2007/Features/2006/f-040306.aspx

Pletcher, L., & McBride, S. (2000). *Family-centered services: Guiding principles and practices for delivery of family-centered services*. Des Moines: Iowa Departments of Education, Human Services and Public Health. Retrieved September 8, 2009, from www.extension.iastate.edu/culture/files/FamlCntrdSrvc.pdf

Price, M., & Miner, S. (2008). Mother becoming: Learning to read Mikala's signs. *Scandinavian Journal of Occupational Therapy, 16,* 1–10.

Rush, D., & Shelden, M. (2005). Evidence-based definition of coaching practices. *CASEinPoint, 1*(6), 1–6. Retrieved April 28, 2010, from www.fippcase.org/caseinpoint.php

Shonkoff, J. P., & Phillips, D. A. (2000). *From neurons to neighborhoods: The science of early childhood development*. Washington, DC: National Academies Press.

Thomas, A., & Chess, S. (1977). *Temperament and development*. New York: Brunner & Mazel.

Thomas, A., Chess, S., & Birch, H. (1970). The origin of personality. *Scientific American, 223*(2), 102–109.

Thomas, A., Chess, S., Birch, H., Hertzig, M., & Korn, S. (1963). *Behavioral individuality in early childhood*. New York: New York University Press.

Waters, R. (2004). The baby brain connection. (2004, November 14). *San Francisco Chronicle,* p. CM–16.

Weatherston, D. (2000). The infant mental health specialist. *Zero to Three, 21,* 3–10.

Webb, N., & Jaffe, L. (2006, September). Coaching model in early intervention: An introduction. *Developmental Disabilities Special Interest Section Quarterly, 29*(3), 1–4.

Williamson, G. G., & Anzalone, M. E. (2001). *Sensory integration and self-regulation in infants and toddlers: Helping very young children interact with their environment*. Washington, DC: Zero to Three.

Winnicott, W. D. (1964). *The child, the family, and the outside world*. London: Penguin Press.

Zemke, R. & Clark, F. (1996). *Occupational science: The evolving discipline*. Philadelphia: F. A. Davis.

Zero to Three. (2008). *Early childhood mental health*. Retrieved March 12, 2009, from www.zerotothree.org/site/PageServer?pagename=key_mental#2

CHAPTER 4

Models and Process of Service Provision in Early Childhood

Joanne J. Foss, PhD, OTR/L

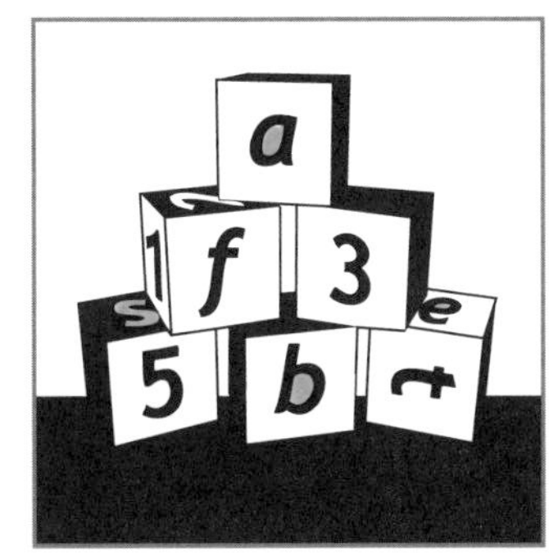

Learning Objectives

After reading this material and completing the examination, readers will be able to

- Delineate the roles and functions of health and human service care provider teams in service provision to young children;
- Delineate the roles and functions of development-, health-, and education-oriented teams in service provision to young children;
- Delineate the role of federal and state legislative and regulatory requirements and their influence on the delivery of early childhood services;
- Delineate the philosophy and application of family-centered approaches in early childhood as part of team orientation, process, and function; and
- Delineate the goals and process of transition planning and apply them to early childhood transitions.

Occupational therapists who work in early childhood do so in a variety of settings and with a variety of other people. Settings may include the child's or relative's home, child care facilities, public and private preschools, charter schools, and inpatient and outpatient clinics. The primary focus of this chapter is team structure and function in the provision of effective and evidence-based early childhood (birth through age 5) health, developmental, and educational services.

The organization of services that evaluate and intervene to promote occupational engagement and performance in early childhood is supported by federal and state legislation and regulation, best practice guidelines, community characteristics, and professional preparation. Well-planned and well-coordinated multidisciplinary systems of care and education for children with disabilities and their families are the result of years of advocacy and incremental changes in health, developmental, and educational services. These systems of services, which usually follow initiatives for children without disabilities and reflect the increasingly acknowledged equal rights of all citizens, and the people who work in them have transformed the experiences and expectations of children with disabilities and their families. From the establishment of the first state program for handicapped children in Minnesota in 1893 to the widespread adoption of the Uniform Newborn Screening Panel in 2006–2007 (Maternal and Child Health Bureau, 2009), efforts to promote uncompromised health and development for all children and to prevent disabilities are ongoing.

The roles of professionals, parents, and others in the provision of health, developmental, and early educational services are varied—sometimes discrete and sometimes blended, depending on the program and the child's need. The purpose, structure, and funding of a program with which a child and family may be involved determines the composition of teams who will provide the services. The individualized plan or program designed for each child determines the service model, team members, and intervention services required.

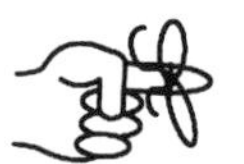

Remember this. . . . **Pediatric "best care" practice is defined by a collaborative approach that delivers intervention within the context of the child's family, environment, and community.**

Pediatric "best care" practice is defined by a collaborative approach that delivers intervention within the context of the child's family, environment, and community. The context of the services for each young child determines the model of care, the dynamics of the team of professionals involved, and the intervention approaches. According to the domains of occupational therapy practice,

> Occupational therapists and occupational therapy assistants provide services to children, families, caregivers, and educational staff within a variety of programs and settings. Regardless of where the evaluation and intervention services are provided, the ultimate outcome is to enable the child to participate in the activities of daily living, education, work, play, leisure, and social interactions. (American Occupational Therapy Association [AOTA], 2004, p. 685)

Occupational therapy is a primary service in early intervention, a related service in preschools operating under the Individuals With Disabilities Education Improvement Act of 2004 (IDEA 2004), and a possible service in Head Start and Early Head Start programs. The category of service determines the parameters of service models and team membership. State guidelines and local government interpretations of guidelines can also influence practice. It is vitally important that practitioners be knowledgeable about federal legislation and regulations and state and local guidelines to provide effective and ethical practice and to advocate successfully for children and their families.

Service Models in Early Childhood

Service models reflect the condition or needs of the child and determine the focus of the family and intervention goals. The three models discussed here are commonly referred to as medical/health, developmental, and educational models of care and services.

The *medical/health model* of service delivery occurs in hospital and inpatient settings or primary care outpatient clinics or offices that provide intervention for children with acute care needs or well-child checkups for services such as immunizations and developmental monitoring. Because inpatient services focus on care of the sick, premature, or developmentally delayed child in need of inpatient services, the role of the team is diagnostic and symptom focused. Teams working under the medical model seek to manage the secondary medical problems associated with prematurity and other congenital conditions that place children at risk for developmental delay. Primary care services focus on well-child checkups at predetermined ages, symptoms of illness, or symptoms that place a child at risk for future developmental problems (e.g., slow growth, especially head circumference).

The primary treatment goal in the medical/health model is to stabilize the child's health and to meet the immediate developmental needs of the child. Clinicians must work hard to function together as a multidisciplinary team and to provide effective short-term intervention. The emphasis is on discharge preparation and referral to other appropriate community services. Team members usually work directly with the child or caregiver. Because the team approach is more often multidisciplinary in hospital- or clinic-based services, families communicate with each team member directly during intervention sessions.

Developmental practice models include the Infants and Toddlers With Disabilities Program (hereinafter referred to as *early intervention*) under Part C of IDEA 2004, Early Head Start (Administration for Children and Families, 2008) and, to a lesser extent, child care facilities and centers. The notion of services provided in the natural environment, which can be seen philosophically as a further descriptor of the least restrictive environment, and family-centered service are key concepts of Part C of IDEA 2004. Both Early Head Start and early intervention include as primary goals the promotion of the development of the family's capacity to meet the child's needs and foster growth and learning. Central to these structures is the belief that the neurodevelopmental process is facilitated by early environmental experiences. The child's home and family are a micro context in which the child resides during early development. This environment provides the experiences that facilitate the foundation for later development. Early childhood intervention programs, such Early Head Start and early intervention, deliver home- and center-based services. The primary role of the family characterizes these early intervention models. Parents are encouraged to participate to the extent to which and in the manner in which they feel most capable. The team, which is most often transdisciplinary, follows the family's lead.

Educational practice models for young children include preschools, both public and private, and some child care centers. Preschool programs vary in location from local school campuses to churches and day care centers; they vary in nature from state to state depending on fiscal support and the demands for educational outcomes. Programs such as Head Start and Smart Start focus on children 3 to 4 years old. Services support the child's developmental growth and ability to participate in the preschool learning experiences. The team approaches most often seen in school or preschool settings are multidisciplinary or interdisciplinary.

Team Approaches to Service Provision

Whether receiving services in a clinical, home-based, educational, or community-based setting, children benefit the most from the perspectives of parents and professionals who function as a team. The team members should be determined according to the setting, the child's needs, the child's age, and the complexity of problems presented by the child's disabilities. For example, an infant newly discharged from a neonatal intensive care unit (NICU) may need a team that includes a physician, a nurse, and an audiologist as well as occupational and physical therapists, whereas a toddler with an acquired head injury may require additional team members, such as an early childhood educator, social worker, and speech–language pathologist (SLP). The team composition will change with the developing needs of the child and can require the participation of additional professionals during times of transition or family or medical crises. Primary decision making or team facilitation and leadership can also change on the basis of the child's immediate needs or as the child moves from one model to another. Under the medical/health model, the physician may be the primary team leader, especially in acute care settings, whereas the occupational therapist may be the primary team leader in the developmental model; the preschool teacher or other educational specialist may be the primary team leader in an educational model.

Team assessment and planning ensure a more comprehensive approach and prevent a perspective limited by the point of view of one professional discipline (Snell & Janney, 2000). Team planning and service delivery depend on the collaboration and communication skills of the team members. Effective team skills are essential to service delivery in any pediatric setting and can be as important as any of the therapeutic techniques or skills unique to occupational therapy (Case-Smith, 2005). Interactions among professionals and with the family can determine the success or failure of an intervention program and the ability of the team to facilitate comprehensive outcomes (Shortell, 2004).

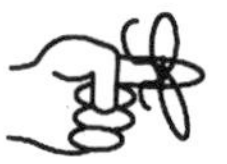

Remember this. . . .
A goal of the team process, no matter what the service model is, is to ensure collaboration in planning, developing, and monitoring a comprehensive and individualized plan for intervention.

A goal of the team process, no matter what the service model is, is to ensure collaboration in planning, developing, and monitoring a comprehensive and individualized plan for intervention. Team collaboration begins with the planning of the evaluation process and continues through the child's service transitions (Muhlenhaupt, 2000). An effective team coordinates the establishment of realistic goals and objectives, appropriate strategies for intervention, and accountability for achievement of a child's expected outcomes. Achieving this level of cooperation and coordination requires communication and a team of professionals that interacts well (Shortell, 2004). Poor team collaboration may present one of the largest barriers to effective intervention planning for children (Muhlenhaupt, 2000).

Traditionally, three team approaches have defined the roles and perspectives of team members in pediatric service delivery: multidisciplinary, transdisciplinary, and interdisciplinary. Except for the transdisciplinary approach, team roles are generally agreed on and distributed among the members to avoid duplication, address specific needs and priorities, facilitate timeliness, and reduce the stress on the family and the child (Snell & Janney, 2000).

Learning Activity 4.1 assists readers in identifying and reflecting on past and present team membership.

Team Composition Models

Multidisciplinary Team Approach

In the *multidisciplinary model,* the child is evaluated by each team member individually, and the child's intervention plan is composed of the goals and treatment

Learning Activity 4.1. Teams in Your Practice

- Identify the types of teams that you have been part of in your practice.
- Identify what you liked and did not like about the teamwork.
- Hypothesize how you could have changed something about the teamwork or your own actions that may have enhanced the team's functioning.
- In what ways did the team composition best serve the needs of the clients (parents and children)? In what ways did it not?

---

approaches selected by each team member. Evaluation and intervention procedures are delivered by each discipline in a parallel manner, and communication is often limited to formal conferences in which team members share results and plans (Carrasco et al., 2007) or through medical or bedside rounds in hospital-based settings. Informal communications are often conducted by telephone or, more recently, secure e-mail. Although each discipline contributes a unique perspective, setting priorities for intervention goals is often left to overwhelmed and conflicted parents (Vergara & Bigsby, 2004).

The priorities and concerns of the parents are paramount to all multidisciplinary team members; under the team approach, however, parents often must serve as the care coordinators. The professionals involved in the child's care may individually communicate their concerns and plans, leaving the parents to synthesize the comments and suggestions of each practitioner. Parents often must set aside large blocks of time to communicate with team members from each of the disciplines involved in their child's care (Vergara & Bigsby, 2004). Navigating and negotiating the health care system under this model can be overwhelming to parents already under the significant stress of caring for a child with special needs.

The multidisciplinary team approach is common in acute care or hospital-based settings, where the medical model of service delivery is primary. Third-party payer requirements and medical model hierarchies dictate the composition of multidisciplinary teams in these settings. The team leaders and primary decision makers are most often primary care nurses or social workers. Physicians dictate, through referral, the other disciplines involved and the primary care provided. Communication and shared decision making among all disciplines in a medical model setting and on multidisciplinary teams is generally considered ideal. These practices are gradually becoming more standard as team members become educated about the expertise of other professionals and are expected to communicate with each other and with parents during the decision-making process.

Interdisciplinary Team Approach

The *interdisciplinary model* involves greater collaboration and integration among team members (Case-Smith, 2005). Each member must possess expertise in his or her own discipline as well as a general knowledge of the roles and functions of the disciplines represented by the other team members. Although evaluations may be conducted by individual team members or by members working together, identifying goals and planning are a group process that represents a more collaborative approach to intervention than does the multidisciplinary model (Jackson, 2007).

Team members may intentionally, as agreed on in the planning process, reinforce the intervention goals and approaches of other team specialties. Interdisciplinary team members must communicate more often to coordinate a child's intervention effectively. In addition to formal team meetings, informal communication among individual team members or small groups of the team is often necessary.

Teams of professionals located in educational or school-based settings are most often interdisciplinary. In an interdisciplinary team in the educational environment, coordination of team meetings and other forms of formal communication among members are often accomplished through the special education teacher or another professional who functions as the educational services coordinator. The team is responsible for preparing a comprehensive program (and individualized education program [IEP]) that reflects a high level of integration and coordination in the evaluation and planning process. This plan also must reflect the input of the family as team members, although the focus is education. As team members, parents attend all team meetings and provide guidance concerning the family's priorities for their child.

Transdisciplinary Team Approach

In the *transdisciplinary team* approach, the initial evaluation is usually performed by one or more representatives of the team, and those assigned assess the child's abilities in all areas of development. This model bypasses the traditional disciplinary boundaries. After establishing the appropriate goals, the intervention is delivered by the team member whose expertise most closely fits the child's needs. The other team members provide ongoing consultation, sharing skills and knowledge that can be incorporated into the intervention (Case-Smith, 2005). Because the family interacts primarily with one team member, communication with the family is more consistent and assistance is provided to that team member in establishing intervention priorities. Transdisciplinary teams are most often found delivering early intervention services to young children in the home environment. This model requires a great deal of communication and coordination and can be logistically complicated to implement.

Learning Activity 4.2 asks readers to identify the approaches in which those teams appeared and to compare the strengths and weakness of both the model and the team approach.

Table 4.1 provides basic information about team members common in early childhood settings. The composition of teams will vary state to state, especially in early intervention programs. Table 4.2 compares service models and settings with the typical team approach; it summarizes the information presented on these subjects in this chapter.

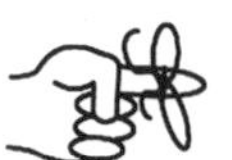

Remember this. . . .
Research has confirmed that collaborative teaming facilitates children's attainment of outcome measures (Barnes & Turner, 2001).

Team Collaboration and Interaction Skills

Research has confirmed that collaborative teaming facilitates children's attainment of outcome measures (Barnes & Turner, 2001), and successful team interaction has been found to be essential for effective intervention services (Bose & Hinojosa, 2008; LaGrossa, 2002; Muhlenhaupt, 2000). Collaboration can take several forms, depending on the child's needs and the model of intervention. In early intervention, problem solving and monitoring of a child's progress is an ongoing process that does not

Learning Activity 4.2. Strengths and Weaknesses of Service Models and Teams

Think about the various teams of which you have been a member (refer to the teams you identified in Learning Activity 4.1).

- Specifically, how did the team function according to the commonly accepted roles?
- What are the strengths of each model resulting from its use in a specific service setting?
- What are the drawbacks in terms of coordination, time commitment, communication, and perhaps licensure or regulatory issues?

Table 4.1. Medical/Health, Developmental, and Educational Team Members

Professional	Team Member and Role
Audiologist	Specializes in the identification, evaluation, and treatment of children with hearing disabilities
Dietitian	Specializes in the identification of nutritional needs and provides services to schools, children, and families
Early childhood specialist	Professional with a certification or associate's degree in early childhood education; credentials and titles vary from state to state
Educational diagnostician	Educator with advanced training in assessments and measurement
Head Start educator	Teacher with an advanced degree in early childhood education; specializes in young children with or at risk for developmental delay
Hearing specialist	Certified to provide assessment and intervention services to children with hearing impairments
Nurse	Provides preventative, symptomatic, and restorative interventions on the basis of the child's medical and health needs; may be in a medical facility or health department
Occupational therapist	Promotes engagement in occupations that are age appropriate and of value and meaning to the child
Parent/caregiver	Considered the unique source of knowledge and the primary source of care for children
Physical therapist	Evaluates and treats children with physical and motor issues
Physician	Medical clinician; can be in a general practice (general practitioner or pediatrician) or specialist practice (e.g., neonatologist, orthopedist, neurologist)
Psychologist	Provides psychological and behavioral assessment and intervention for children and families
Respiratory therapist	Administers inhalation intervention for respiratory issues
Service coordinator	Serves as the main contact for families and team professionals in the coordination of assessment and intervention services for children and families; credentials and required competencies vary significantly from state to state
Social worker	Assists families in maximizing social support, competency, and resources; usually organizes discharge planning from medical facilities; may also be involved in judicial custody and advocacy as part of Department of Social Services and court procedures
Speech–language pathologist	Specializes in the development of language, communication, and speech production; provides assessment and intervention in speech delay and disorders
Teacher	Provides formal instruction, usually in a group setting
Vision specialist	Certified to provide assessment and intervention services to children with visual disabilities

Table 4.2. Models, Settings, Approaches, and Teams

Service Model	Typical Settings	Typical Team Approach	Possible Team Members
Medical	Neonatal intensive care unit, pediatric intensive care unit, acute hospital settings, outpatient clinic settings	Multidisciplinary	Primary or specialty care physician, nurse, social worker, occupational therapist, physical therapist, audiologist, dietician, lactation consultant, respiratory therapist, social worker
Developmental	Natural environments, such as home-based care, day care, Smart Start, home or community programs	Transdisciplinary	Parents or caregiver, early childhood educator, occupational therapist, physical therapist, speech–language pathologist, developmental care coordinator, dietician, developmental pediatrician
Educational	Head Start programs, private or state preschool programs	Interdisciplinary	Parents or caregiver, Head Start educator or teacher, psychologist, speech–language pathologist, occupational therapist, physical therapist

rely on formal meetings for collaboration or logistical planning. Team members, however, often communicate informally as well as formally. As a result, communication may be fragmented except at the specially designated review times. Episodic required formal reviews or changes in individualized family service plans (IFSPs) require meetings and documentation. Therefore, effective teaming depends on the quality of the team interactions and communication and is extremely important to address as the transdisciplinary model gains greater acceptance in early intervention. The reality is that professionals may be members of 20 or more different teams, and the communication and coordination can be challenging.

In services provided under Part C of IDEA 2004, the collaboration of service providers, which is facilitated by service coordinators, should provide reasonable accommodations, prohibit discrimination, and ensure coordination and smooth transitions across agencies, facilities, and programs (AOTA, 2004). Part C assigns early intervention teams the sole responsibility for eligibility decisions and identification of family priorities and desired outcomes. The family is an equal partner in team decisions. The regulations also hold all team members mutually responsible for the outcomes of those decisions and implementation of the commitments made by each team member (U.S. Department of Education, 2007; 34 C.F.R. § 300.344)

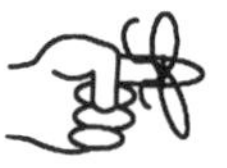

Remember this. . . .
For a team to collaborate successfully to meet the needs of the child, it must operate as a cohesive unit.

The interpersonal communication skills needed by team members differ from those needed to communicate with children and, often, from those we use in our everyday life. Team membership requires skills in negotiation and compromise with a family and child focus rather than a discipline-specific concentration (Friend, 2000). According to Friend (2000), team interactions are characterized by voluntary participation, the equal status of all team members, and the common goal of facilitating the child's progress.

For a team to collaborate successfully to meet the needs of the child, it must operate as a cohesive unit. *Team* can be defined as a small number of people with complementary skills who are committed to a common purpose, performance goals, and common approach. Collaborative teams hold themselves mutually accountable

(Shortell, 2004). Highly effective teams have been found to have the following characteristics:

- Team members have mutual goals that are focused on the needs of the child and the support of the family.
- Team members believe that each member has equally valuable resources to contribute and value each other as equals (Shortell, 2004).
- Team members are willing to share resources, strategies, authority, and accountability (Friend & Cook, 2003).
- The team social environment is mutually supportive (Willis & Case-Smith, 1996) and collegial and fosters open expression of ideas and perspectives (Friend & Cook, 2003).
- Mutual respect among members fosters conflict resolution and productive, creative problem solving (Shortell, 2004).
- The team places high value on joint problem solving and mutual respect of each member's expertise and supports the continued learning and growth of each team member (Giangreco, 2001).

Because successful service delivery depends on the occupational therapist' ability to develop and maintain productive team relationships (Jackson, 2007), initial preservice education and continuing professional education in collaboration and communication skills should be part of the professional development plans for all early intervention providers (Bose & Hinojosa, 2008).

Family-Centered Approaches

Early childhood services are built on the premise that the child is a member of a family system. The needs of the family and the relationship of those needs to the child's need for intervention services expand the typical client-centered approach to a family-centered approach. Under Part C, IDEA 2004 defines the *early intervention client* as the infant or toddler with a disability and his or her family (34 C.F.R. §300.24(a)).

Evidence supports the success of family-centered approaches. Early Head Start successfully involves parents in their child's outcomes; through its community partnerships, the program has succeeded at assisting families to become more self-sufficient (Isaacs & Roessel, 2008). A growing body of research has provided support for the positive effects of early childhood education on improvement of children's cognitive skills and, ultimately, school-related outcomes, such as prereading and math skills (Isaacs, 2008; Zero to Three, 2005). Isaacs and Roessell (2008) found that children in Head Start programs were less likely to exhibit behavioral problems and that parents of children in Head Start programs increased the average number of times they read to their child and were less likely to spank their children.

An important function of the occupational therapist is to assist the family in fostering the optimal development of age-appropriate occupations built on age-appropriate sensorimotor processes and neurobehavioral and cognitive skills. The training and education of occupational therapists make them ideal for addressing the occupational issues of the developing child and the child's family (AOTA, 2008a). Promoting the match or "goodness of fit" between the child's capacities and his or her physical environment, social community, family dynamics, and parental expectations greatly enhances the child's competent occupational performance and the emotional well-being of the child and the family. Building the capacity of the family to focus on the quality of the child's environment and promotion of developmentally appropriate experiences during critical stages of the child's development can be vital to the child's future well-being. (See Chapters 2 and 6 for further information on the interaction of development and learning.)

Families as Collaborators—Team Members

Early intervention services may be the family's first experience with intervention services (Carrasco et al., 2007), or they may represent the movement from the complexity of hospital care to the demands of care of a child in the home. As discussed previously, all team members are responsible for including the parents in the team process and affording the parents the same regard as others for their contributions to the team.

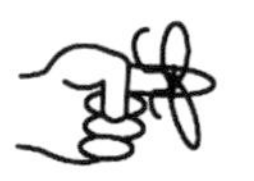

Remember this. . . .
As with all members of the team, parents share equally in the responsibility for the planning and implementation of effective interventions.

As with all members of the team, parents share equally in the responsibility for the planning and implementation of effective interventions. Under IDEA 2004, the focus of family-centered services is not simply a matter of meeting the needs of the family but of seeking to strengthen the family's capacity to meet the child's needs. As part of a team, family members identify what is important to them and what resources are needed to strengthen and enhance the function of the family in support of their child. Parents have the right to agree or to disagree with the recommendations of professionals—only those services that they agree to can be implemented (34 C.F.R. §§ 300.519–300.529).

As members of the team, family members typically contribute in the following ways (Jackson, 2007):

- Designate family priorities and concerns for the formation of intervention goals and outcomes
- Provide information about family routines and community participation to enable the child's integration into those activities (AOTA, 2006a)
- Identify and provide information about the services and resources needed by the family
- Identify specific priorities for family support and goals related to the child's intervention plan
- Participate in the development of and consent to the implementation of the IFSP and IEP.

Early Childhood Programs

Early childhood programs are designed to enhance the child's development and assist the child and the family in laying an effective foundation for the child's future. Family-centered care is accepted as the best model for effective care for infants and young children (Carrasco et al., 2007). Family-centered intervention is based on the principle that young children depend on their family and caregivers for daily physical care and emotional needs (Stephens & Tauber, 2005). The family's environment nurtures and supports the young child through the initial, critical periods of development.

Brain Development and Early Intervention

Service delivery models for infants and young children are based on research regarding brain development in young children. (Refer to Chapters 2 and 6 for more specific information on early brain development.) The literature suggests that the foundation for efficient and effective brain functioning is established early in a child's life. Dynamic interactions of environmental conditions and early experiences have a significant effect on the brain's architecture (National Scientific Council, Center on the Developing Child at Harvard University, 2007b). The quality of the child's environment and appropriate experiences at the critical stages of development appear to be crucial to determining how well the child will be able to think and regulate emotions. An early environment that promotes growth and positive social interactions with caregivers not only enhances the normal development process but also plays a role in shaping the brain's capacity. A healthy pre- and postnatal environment allows the brain to develop to its full genetic potential (Weaver et al., 2004). Early intervention services for infants and toddlers who are experiencing developmental delays or who are at risk for delays can increase the chance of positive outcomes (National Scientific Council, Center on the Developing Child at Harvard University, 2007a, 2007b).

Although a child's brain is genetically wired to form its circuitry, his or her experiences mold how that formation occurs. From early infancy, children are motivated to reach for warm, clear, and dependable responses from caregivers. Those responses allow them to feel pleasure and reward in their accomplishments. Children develop well in a stimulating environment in which the caregivers respond in a warm and caring manner. An environment that is not responsive or, worse, neglectful or abusive, can result in lifelong impairments in learning and behavior. Social participation in a warm and caring environment and stimulation of learning through interactive play promotes healthy development and later achievement. If early learning lays the architectural foundation for later learning, the window of opportunity for influencing the child's developing brain focuses on the first 3 or so years of a child's life. The most constant influence in the child's life at this time is his or her family. Therefore, it is imperative to expand the capacity of the family to support positive environmental circumstances and reciprocal interactions.

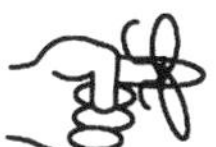

Remember this. . . .
If early learning lays the architectural foundation for later learning, the window of opportunity for influencing the child's developing brain focuses on the first 3 or so years of a child's life.

The unique role the family plays in facilitating the growth and development of children is essential to the legal foundation of early intervention legislation. Part C of IDEA 2004 requires identification of the supports and services that the family needs to build its capacity to meet the developmental needs of the child. In a review of the original federal statutes and the history of reauthorizations, it is clear that Congress intended for families to play a collaborative role in the planning and implementation of services for their child. Over time, the multiple reauthorizations of the IDEA legislation have directed services to strengthen the authority of and encourage the participation of families in meeting the needs of their children (34 C.F.R. 303.12(c)).

Family-Centered Service Provision

Family-centered care requires that parent–professional interactions be those of collaborative partners (Pilkington, 2006). This concept is not new to occupational therapy practitioners, who have always viewed the person seeking assistance or guidance as a collaborative partner in the process. Pilkington (2006) stated, "Occupational therapy practitioners can bring their 'therapeutic use of self' to *all* team and family interactions" (p. 13). Families and practitioners can identify the family's typical daily activities that will reinforce previous occupations and behaviors or facilitate new learning. Adapting routines or environments can enhance the child's experience and facilitate family function. Opportunities to model interactions with the child or strategies that create successful experiences in the parent–child relationship can occur when the practitioner and parent are engaged in "side-by-side" collaboration (Pilkington, 2006).

Family-centered interventions using what is called *coaching* or *modeling* motivate parents and caregivers to carry through many aspects of the intervention during daily routines, providing reinforcement and enhancing the possibility of positive interaction and healthy development for the child. *Coaching* fosters the development of skills through mutual reflection, observation, practice, and feedback (Rush, Shelden, & Hanft, 2003). Early intervention professionals can facilitate a dynamic conversation that results in the implementation of strategies that allow families to adapt to new situations, people, and settings (Rush et al., 2003) and solve challenges that occur because of the barriers children with special needs face. In a coaching situation, the parent becomes an adult learner and the child directly benefits from the skills and strategies developed (Kaiser & Hancock, 2003).

Offering needed support to parents and young children includes recognizing the strengths and needs of the child and the family. By developing the parents' confidence to access information, design strategies, and reach solutions, coaching assists the family in enhancing the child's development and participation in family and community activities. After establishing trust and communication, early intervention professionals often assist parents in working through many issues, such as family routines or schedules, discipline, everyday care activities, and transportation (Rush et al., 2003). Coaching in early intervention practice is a means of providing support to the family in its natural setting.

The modeling of strategies within the learner's environment provides examples of strategies that are easier to generalize and implement (Kaiser & Hancock, 2003). During interactions with the child and the family, team members can display or model strategies and behaviors that can be copied by caregivers during their own interactions with the child. Caregivers can add to their behavioral repertoire actions they have actually watched therapists successfully use.

Coaching and modeling strategies are familiar to occupational therapists. Increasing recognition of the value of these types of interventions is leading to their increased implementation in early childhood programs.

Working in a natural environment, side by side with the parent or other caregivers, is a familiar aspect of practice for many occupational therapists. Evidence is emerging that this perspective in practice models enhances developmental outcomes and empowers families to function more effectively (Bruder & Dunst, 1999–2000; Pilkington, 2006). Occupational therapists receive education and training in clinical reasoning, observation techniques, task analysis, and therapeutic use of self; these basic skills of occupational therapy practice are being recognized and used in early childhood programs across the nation. (Refer to Chapter 3 for more information on the implementation of family-centered practices, building family capacity, and coaching.)

Occupational Therapy and Early Intervention

In early intervention, an occupational therapist may be functioning as a service coordinator, an evaluator as part of the initial eligibility process or subsequent evaluations, a provider of occupational therapy services, or a primary provider of all early intervention services. Occupational therapy helps children participate in activities of daily living (ADLs) through intervention services that promote social–emotional, physical, cognitive, communication, and adaptive behaviors. Occupational therapists identify the effects of delays on the child's participation and design interventions that promote healthy development, promote skill development, and reduce environmental barriers through modification or assistive technology (AOTA, 2006b). Intervention services in early intervention might include fostering the development of feeding skills, play skills, language and communication skills, motor and postural development, self-regulation and other aspects of social–emotional development, sensory awareness, neurobehavioral development, and parent and child interactions (AOTA, 2006a; Bruder & Dunst, 2000), helping the family and child engage in occupations that are meaningful and of value to them (Opp, 2008).

Occupational therapy at the early intervention level focuses on the family. Evaluation and intervention identify concerns on the basis of the needs and priorities recognized by the family. Pilkington (2006) described how occupational therapists can encourage families of a child with or at risk for a disability known to contribute to developmental delay to identify activities that can be done throughout the day as part of the normal routine that will enhance and reinforce skills, improve sensory processing, and enable new learning. Moreover, Opp (2008) emphasized the support and encouragement occupational therapists supply to parents and the importance of that support to the parent–child relationship. The reinforcement of skills and their application to the child's natural context is vital to the child's ultimate intervention outcomes.

Occupational therapists can provide families and caregivers with information about their child's development and, by their presence, provide modeling or coaching that assists parents in enhancing their child's skills and forming mutually satisfying and nurturing relationships with their children. In all of those areas, communication with the family and other team members is essential.

Transitions

Transitions in service may occur as a result of a change in program or facility, the child's age, disability status, or family needs or location. Some transitions can be anticipated, such as eligibility changes from Part C to Part B services or from home to center- or school-based locations. Anticipated transitions are planned for and documented in the initial IFSP. Transition planning identifies changes in the continuum of services received by the child (34 C.F.R. §300.29). IDEA encourages a planning continuum that coordinates changes or movement between programs and ensures that movement between programs, grades, or schools goes smoothly.

One of the 16 core requirements of a state's Infants and Toddlers With Disabilities Program is the requirement related to transition. Chapter 1 contains specific information about the legal requirements of the transition process. Each state must establish policies and procedures regulating how services for children from ages 3 to 5 are to be implemented. Individualized planning, the hallmark of IDEA-based service delivery requirements, requires that the early interventionists and early childhood professionals meet with the family to plan for a transition between environments and the change in services. To effectively plan for the child's smooth transition, parents and professionals need to agree on timelines, goals, and a process to identify barriers to success. Families and professionals need to be aware of the changes in policy and service delivery that will result from the service changeover. To provide accurate information and to understand the responses of children and families, professionals must be knowledgeable of the services provided on both sides of the transition. Lillie and Vakil (2002) stressed that "parents and professionals need to be cognizant of the nature of transition as a process rather than a product to adapt each transition to the specific needs of the child" (p. 54).

The perspective of an occupational therapist can be especially valuable for transition planning. Occupational therapists can assist the child in preparing for the challenge of changes in expectations, routines, and social environments. An emphasis on the promotion of independence, functional abilities, and participation in daily routines can be important for successful transition (AOTA, 2008b).

Transitions between service provision levels can be stressful. Parents and caregivers often must leave behind professionals with whom they have formed a bond and begin to deal with others who may not be as familiar with their child's care. In addition, an unfamiliar environment with unfamiliar people may cause a regression of skills. In the preschool setting, parents will be separated from their child, and the environment may not facilitate the same level of everyday involvement. Preschool may be the first time their child is among his or her typically developing peers, providing a contrast that is emotionally unsettling to parents as well as to the child.

Collaboration and early planning are needed to make sure services and supports are in place before the child's arriving in the environment. A lag in services causes delays and frustration and may lead to a temporary (one hopes) loss of skills, along with the pain caused by an unsuccessful integration in the new setting. Occupational therapists, along with other team members, can assist with the transition from early intervention services to a preschool environment by

- Preparing the family and the child for changes in routine and role,
- Preparing the school staff for the unique developmental needs of the child,
- Facilitating the modification and adaptation of environments and activities for full participation,
- Collaborating with school staff concerning any needed assistive technology, and
- Supporting and enhancing the child's social skills and self-confidence in the school environment (AOTA, 2008b).

The transition from family-centered to child-centered approaches can be challenging for parents. Although family involvement is essential to the early intervention model (Part C), in the educational model of Part B, the school assumes a primary role (Johnson, 2001). As advocates for their child, parents may find that their priorities may not match those of the educational focus mandated under this model. The interdisciplinary team, however, through effective planning, preparation, and communication, can smooth the path to this level. Again, communication is essential.

IDEA requires that a conference with the parents be convened 3 to 6 months before the child turns 3 years old (34 C.F.R. §300.29). This time period can easily be filled with the official process of the preparation of paperwork and documentation and mandatory meetings. The team members need to be aware that this process may not provide all the steps necessary to ensure an effective transition for the child and the parent (Lillie & Vakil, 2002). Some steps that can be implemented to support the child and the family and smooth this transition are as follows:

- The parents and the child should visit the school and meet with the teachers and other staff before the formal transition meeting. Such meetings can help the family feel more comfortable and familiar with the environment and personnel. Parents may also want to bring the early intervention team member they are the closest to (such as the developmental care coordinator or developmental specialist) so that they have someone with whom to discuss the visit (Bruns & Fowler, 2001; Johnson, 2001).
- Arrange frequent opportunities for consistent and effective communication. The early intervention team might designate a member to provide follow-up communications after school visits and after meetings with the team. Parents often have questions or concerns after they have time to think through their experiences. Parents form trust in the people caring for their child over time, and making sure they feel that their input is valued and consistently regarded is key to developing open and effective communication. Follow-up phone calls or weekly written reports encourage parents to clarify information and ask questions (Johnson, 2001; Lillie & Vakil, 2002).
- Reestablish team roles and expectations for the new model. Parents need to know what is expected of them and what to expect of the school (Johnson, 2001; Lillie & Vakil, 2002). Clear boundaries and responsibilities help parents feel competent and valued.
- Establish programs at the school for parents. Support groups (Johnson, 2001) and parent workshops can facilitate an atmosphere in which the parents feel comfortable on the school campus and can provide opportunities to share valuable information with parents (Bruns & Fowler, 2001). Support and assistance provided in the groups can help parents reinforce program goals and skills and foster the child's development and growth at home.
- Provide flexible programs with flexible schedules. Young children with developmental delays may not be initially ready for a full preschool

experience, and parents might feel a schedule that phases in attendance would be more successful. Under some programs, a combination of school and home-based services might be an option (Johnson, 2001).

Taking the time to formulate a plan that includes the formal mandated transition process along with a series of more informal options to increase the comfort level of the child and the parents can be well worth the initial effort. Ineffective transitions can waste the efforts of parents and school personnel (Lillie & Vakil, 2002). Reestablishing trust with the child and the family, restoring self-confidence, and making up for lost time in outcome achievement can cost valuable time and divert efforts from more positive efforts.

Professionals involved in the child's early care also benefit from viewing transitions as a multistep process. Professionals often feel a bond with the child and the family. Many times, as a team, the professionals and the family have shared an experience that has many ups and downs and challenges and successes. The process of smoothing the way for child's next challenge can assist them in passing their roles and responsibilities to the education personnel at the preschool setting. Pride in ensuring that the child's transition is as successful and as uneventful as possible can be satisfying to everyone involved (Johnson, 2001).

Table 4.3 summarizes the benefits of regarding transitions as a process rather than an outcome. The extra work for the team can pay dividends in the end for the child, the parents, and the professionals involved.

The following case study applies the information concerning models of early childhood service delivery and team interaction as discussed in this chapter.

Case Study

Melvin Jesse (called MJ by his family) was born 7 weeks premature and spent 7 weeks in the NICU with oxygen support and oral tube feeding. MJ received occupational therapy in the NICU primarily for feeding support. MJ's mother, Sonja, is single. MJ is now 3 years old and his mother's only child. Sonja has always been at home, in a rural area, full time with MJ. Some support is offered by his maternal grandparents who live nearby. Initially, MJ received early intervention services at home through the local Infants and Toddlers With Disabilities Program and Early Head Start. The occupational therapist and the early childhood specialist worked with Sonja to assist MJ with feeding and developmental activities and to promote her occupational role as a caregiver and nurturer. An SLP provided several visits to coach Sonja on strategies to help MJ increase vocalizations during everyday routines.

At 19 months (adjusted age of 17 months, 1 week), MJ was reevaluated at Sonja's request because of concerns about his play skills, language development, and feeding. At the time, he was able to crawl, but he showed little mobility or active play. He was referred for continued home-based services by the transdisciplinary early intervention team (social worker, psychologist, early childhood specialist, physical therapist, occupational therapist, SLP, and the parent). Early childhood specialists visited the home twice a week to work with Sonja to provide developmental play activities to stimulate social–emotional, mobility, cognitive, communication development, and adaptive behaviors. The occupational therapist continued

Table 4.3. Benefits of Successful Transitions

For Children	For Parents	For Professionals
Continuity of services (Johnson, 2001); continued progress on occupational performance and educational goals	Trust and confidence in service continuity and the commitment of the service providers	A sense of pride in their efforts to affect the lives of children and their families (Johnson, 2001).
Trust, openness, and self-confidence with new experiences (Johnson, 2001) and a new environment	Self-confidence in their ability to communicate with other team members and advocate for their child in this new environment (Johnson, 2001)	Increased family and community support (Johnson, 2001)
Enhanced community participation	Increased knowledge and skills to facilitate child's growth and education	Increased knowledge of the roles and responsibilities of preschool professionals and the programs they provide
New social relationships with peers and adults	Networking relationships with other parents and families	Increased knowledge of children and families; enhanced ability to meet their needs

to work with MJ and his mother in relation to self-feeding and acceptance of solid foods. To increase MJ's preparation for preschool, coaching strategies were implemented to encourage MJ to express his needs through words and signs.

In preparation for transition to preschool and to determine his eligibility for Part B services, MJ was referred for evaluation for Head Start preschool at age 2 years, 6 months. The transdisciplinary team (Head Start educator, service coordinator, SLP, occupational therapist, dietitian, and physical therapist) designated the occupational therapist to perform a comprehensive developmental assessment based on MJ's history of receiving occupational therapy services and his familiarity with the occupational therapist, feeding, and mobility concerns.

MJ has few toys available at home. Sonja has been reluctant to accept toys from the lending library because of concerns about germs. For the same reason, she is hesitant for him to be out in the community. For safety reasons, MJ plays in his crib or playpen. Sonja was very directive in play with MJ and expressed concern that he does not know how to play with his toys correctly. MJ has no regular contact with other children or adults other than his grandmother. Sonja is also concerned about his everyday activities and his transition to preschool. MJ is still unable to eat table food; he eats only semisolid foods and demonstrates aversive facial responses to textured foods such as crackers and applesauce; he is not drinking from a cup or using a spoon. His expressive language is limited, and he is unable to clearly express his needs.

MJ wears bilateral ankle–foot orthoses. He cruises and walks independently for short distances, but he prefers to crawl. He consistently initiated and engaged the therapist and his mother in play. MJ's abilities reflected the following age ranges on the developmental assessment used: receptive language, gross motor, and cognitive skills in the 12- to 15-month range; expressive language in the 9- to 11-month range; and fine motor skills in the 10- to 11-month range.

MJ began attending a Head Start program at 3 years old. Because of concerns about his health and endurance, Sonja prefers 3 half-day sessions per week at this time. Sonja attends several parent group activities each month and volunteers once a week during outside play and group activity sessions in a classroom for 4-year-olds. Intervention activities include stimulation of social, language, motor, and play developmental skills. MJ's IEP goals include developmentally appropriate instructional activities geared toward increasing his participation in all ADLs in school learning environments. The team has identified MJ's need to increase participation in peer and community-based activities to encourage literacy, communication, social skills, and endurance.

Planning for MJ's transition to kindergarten has begun. The team has already collaborated with the teachers to modify the classroom environment to increase MJ's participation in all activities. The team has identified the need to plan services to assist MJ with integrating successfully to kindergarten. Areas of concern include assistance with school mobility, preparing Sonja for changes in daily routines and roles, and enhancing social communication skills.

Although the composition and orientation of the teams that supported MJ in his early years varied from the medical model in the NICU to the developmental and health model in early intervention to the educational model in preschool and used different models of teaming, MJ's needs and his mother's priorities were always part of the consideration and decision-making processes.

Conclusion

This chapter focuses on the structure and provision of effective early childhood services through teams. Although the needs of each young child determine the model of care, the dynamics of the team of professionals involved, and the intervention approaches (Katzenbach & Smith, 1986), services are dictated by federal and state legislation and regulation, best practice guidelines, community characteristics, and professional preparation.

Occupational therapy is a primary service in early intervention. It is a related service in preschools operating under IDEA and a possible service in Head Start and Early Head Start. Working in a variety of settings, occupational therapists provide a unique perspective to the care of young children. Occupational therapists evaluate and intervene to promote occupational performance in early childhood, helping children grow, learn, play, and interact—fulfilling their occupational roles and providing a firm foundation for the future.

How Very Far We Have Come: Danny Goes to School (1959–1965)

Danny loved going to the Main Street School. His mother taught there 2 days a week, and she picked up two other children who lived in their part of the county. The same system was used for covering the teaching and transportation the other days, with the "lead teacher" transporting those who lived close to her and other mothers and teachers bringing the rest of the children. At least four women were in the classroom each day, teaching a total of 12 children initially.

When he was 7 and 8 years old, Danny missed a lot of school because he had several surgeries to lengthen muscles that had contracted and to receive therapy to help him learn to walk. He was now going to a university-affiliated hospital in his state. He also attended the hospital school while he was there. His teachers felt that he had a slight learning disability but that he was not at all mentally retarded and, in fact, was a rather sharp little fellow. It was hard for Danny to be away from home for long periods of time, but it was deemed best by the doctors who could closely monitor his care.

Danny eventually learned to walk with crutches, but his gait was awkward and slow, and he had difficulty with balance. He used a wheelchair at times when he was fatigued or recovering from surgery or from an injury sustained when he was walking with his crutches. He called them his "trip mes," because he often tripped on them. The crutches were supplied by the hospital. A wheelchair was not supplied because walking was the goal for Danny. Wheelchairs cost a lot of money, which the family did not have. At first, Danny's grandfather had made a wheelchair from bicycle tires and the seat from a kitchen chair. It was rather awkward, but it was needed when Danny needed to go long distances.

Eventually, Danny's family obtained a wheelchair from what became known as the "underground wheelchair network." Essentially, equipment was passed on from one family to another, sometimes directly, often indirectly through a home health nurse or therapist who knew of needs across the county.

Questions

1. Why did Danny need to stay in the hospital rather than be followed at home postsurgery?
2. Danny attended the hospital school while recovering from surgery at the university-affiliated hospital. What does *university affiliated* mean? Why were his teachers able to better determine his learning abilities?
3. With all of the assistive technology now available, why is there still a need for "underground wheelchair networks," lending closets, and the like?

References

Administration for Children and Families. (2008). *About the office of Head Start.* Retrieved December 12, 2008, from www.acf.hhs.gov/programs/ohs/about/index.html

American Occupational Therapy Association. (2004). Occupational therapy services in early intervention and school-based programs. *American Journal of Occupational Therapy, 58,* 681–685.

American Occupational Therapy Association. (2006a). *Occupational therapy for children: Birth to 3 years of age.* Retrieved November 27, 2008, from www.aota.org/Practitioners/Resources/Docs/FactSheets/Children/38516

American Occupational Therapy Association. (2006b). *Occupational therapy in preschool settings.* Retrieved November 27, 2008, from www.aota.org/Practitioners/Resources/Docs/FactSheets/School/38510

American Occupational Therapy Association. (2008a). Occupational therapy practice framework: Domain and process (2nd ed.) *American Journal of Occupational Therapy, 62,* 625–683.

American Occupational Therapy Association. (2008b). *Transitions for children and youth: How occupational therapy can help* [Fact sheet]. Bethesda, MD: Author.

Barnes, K., & Turner, K. (2001). Team collaborative practices between teachers and occupational therapists. *American Journal of Occupational Therapy, 55,* 83–89.

Bose, P., & Hinojosa, J. (2008). Reported experiences from occupational therapists interacting with teachers in inclusive early childhood classrooms. *American Journal of Occupational Therapy, 62,* 289–297.

Bruder, M., & Dunst, C. (December 1999/January 2000). Expanding learning opportunities for infants and toddlers in natural environments: A chance to reconceptualize early intervention. *Zero to Three, 20,* 34–36.

Bruns, D., & Fowler, S. (2001). *Transition is more than a change in services: The need for a multicultural perspective.* Retrieved January 30, 2009, from www.clas.uiuc.edu/techreport/tech4.html

Carrasco, R., Skees-Hermes, S., Clark, G., Polichino, J., Ralabate, P., Thomas, L., et al. (2007). Occupational therapy service delivery to support child and family participation in context. In L. Jackson (Ed.), *Occupational therapy services for children and youth under the IDEA* (3rd ed., pp. 89–128). Bethesda, MD: AOTA Press.

Case-Smith, J. (2005). Teaming. In J. Case-Smith (Ed.), *Occupational therapy for children* (5th ed., pp. 32–52). St. Louis, MO: Elsevier/Mosby.

Friend, M. (2000). Myths and misunderstandings about professional collaboration. *Remedial and Special Education, 21,* 130–132.

Friend, M., & Cook, L. (2003). *Interactions: Collaboration skills for school professionals.* New York: Allyn & Bacon.

Giangreco, L. (2001). Interactions among program placement and services in educational planning for students with disabilities. *Mental Retardation, 39,* 341–350.

Individuals With Disabilities Education Improvement Act of 2004, Pub. L. 108–446, 20 U.S.C. §1400 *et seq.*

Isaacs, J. (2008, September). *Impacts of early childhood programs* (Research Brief 1: State prekindergarten). Washington, DC: Brookings Institution. Retrieved September 9, 2009, from www.brookings.edu/papers/2008/~/media/Files/rc/papers/2008/09_early_programs_isaacs/09_early_programs_brief1.pdf

Isaacs, J., & Roessel, E. (2008). *Impacts of early childhood programs* (Research Brief 3: Head Start). Washington, DC: Brookings Institution. Retrieved September 9, 2009, from www.brookings.edu/~/media/Files/rc/papers/2008/09_early_programs_isaacs/09_early_programs_isaacs.pdf

Jackson, L. (2007). Legislative context of occupational therapy practice in schools and early childhood settings. In L. Jackson (Ed.), *Occupational therapy services for children and youth under the IDEA* (3rd ed., pp. 1–22). Bethesda, MD: AOTA Press.

Johnson, C. (2001). Transition: Making it a process rather than an event. *Educational Audiology Review, 18*(3), 5–11.

Kaiser, A., & Hancock, T. (2003). Teaching parents new skills to support their young children's development. *Infants and Young Children, 16*(1), 9–21.

Katzenbach, J., & Smith, D. (1986). *The wisdom of teams.* Boston: Harvard Business Review Press.

LaGrossa, J. (2002). School-based OT: Could yours qualify as a best practice? *Advance for Occupational Therapy Practitioners, 18*(2), 16–19.

Lillie, T., & Vakil, S. (2002). Transitions in early childhood for students with disabilities: Law and best practice. *Early Childhood Education Journal, 30*(1), 53–58.

Maternal and Child Health Bureau. (2009). *MCH timeline: History, legacy, and resources for education and practice.* Retrieved September 9, 2009, from http://mchb.hrsa.gov/timeline/

Muhlenhaupt, M. (2000). OT services under IDEA 97: Decision-making challenges. *OT Practice, 5*(24), 10–13.

National Scientific Council, Center on the Developing Child at Harvard University. (2007a). *A science-based framework for early childhood policy: Using evidence to improve outcomes in learning, behavior, and health for vulnerable children.* Retrieved September 9, 2009, from www.developingchild.harvard.edu/content/downloads/Policy_Framework.pdf

National Scientific Council, Center on the Developing Child at Harvard University. (2007b). *The timing and quality of early experiences combine to shape brain architecture* (Working Paper 5). Retrieved August 27, 2008, from www.developingchild.net/pubs/wp/Timing_Quality_Early_Experiences.pdf

Opp, A. (2008). *Occupational therapy in early intervention: Helping children succeed.* Retrieved September 26, 2008, from www.aota.org/Consumers/WhatisOT/CY/Articles/40021.aspx

Pilkington, K. (2006). Side by side: Transdisciplinary early intervention in natural settings. *OT Practice, 11*(6), 12–17. Retrieved January 8, 2010, from www.aota.org/Pubs/OTP/1997-2007/Features/2006/f-040306.aspx

Rush, D., Shelden, M., & Hanft, B. (2003). Coaching families and colleagues: A process for collaboration in natural settings. *Infants and Young Children, 16*(1), 33–45.

Shortell, S. (2004). The role of perceived team effectiveness in improving chronic illness care. *Medical Care, 42,* 1040.

Snell, M., & Janney, R. (2000). *Collaborative teaming.* Baltimore: Brookes.

Stephens, L., & Tauber, S. (2005). Early intervention. In J. Case-Smith (Ed.), *Occupational therapy for children* (5th ed., pp. 771–793). St. Louis, MO: Elsevier/Mosby.

Vergara, E., & Bigsby, R. (2004). *Development and therapeutic interventions in the NICU.* Baltimore: Brookes.

Weaver, I., Cervoni, N., Champagne, F., D'Alessio, A., Sharma, S., Seckl, J., et al. (2004). Epigenetic programming by maternal behavior. *Nature Neuroscience, 7,* 847–854.

Willis, K., & Case-Smith, J. (1996). Perception and experiences of occupational therapists in rural schools. *American Journal of Occupational Therapy, 50,* 370–378.

U.S. Department of Education. (2007). Title 34: Education. Part 300—Improving the academic achievement of the disadvantaged; Individuals With Disabilities Education Act (IDEA); Final rule (72 FR 17748). 34 C.F.R. § 300 *et seq.*

Zero to Three. (2005). *The national evaluation of Early Head Start: Early Head Start works.* Herndon, VA: Author. Retrieved November 28, 2008, from www.zerotothree.org/site/DocServer/ehs.pdf?docID=565

CHAPTER 5

Evaluation, Assessment, and Outcomes in Early Childhood

Gloria Frolek Clark, PhD, OTR/L, BCP, FAOTA

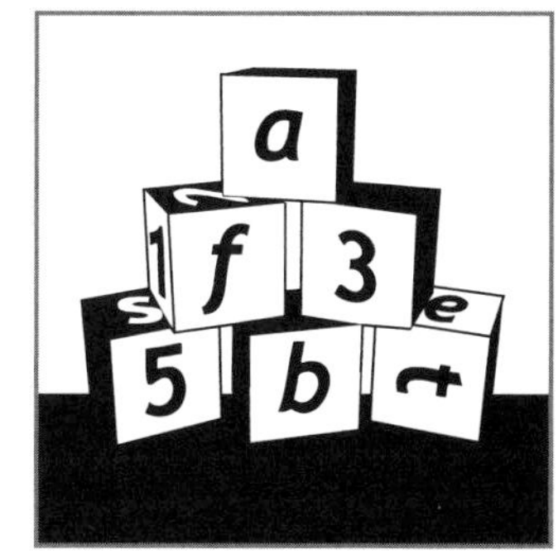

Learning Objectives

After reading this material and completing the examination, readers will be able to

- Identify the primary purposes of evaluation and appropriate tools for each purpose;
- Recognize alternative methods of evaluating children birth to age 5;
- Identify the parent, child, and occupational therapist roles in evaluation and use of assessments;
- Identify the child and parent outcomes (early childhood outcomes) for the Infants and Toddlers With Disabilities (ITD) program; and
- Delineate how the multidisciplinary evaluation for eligibility in the ITD program is structured and the types of assessment most useful for this purpose.

Occupational therapy addresses the physical, cognitive, psychosocial, sensory, and other aspects of occupational performance of people to support engagement in everyday life activities (American Occupational Therapy Association [AOTA], 2004; Moyers & Dale, 2007). The occupational therapist works in early childhood to support the child's health, development, and participation through engagement in *occupations,* defined as "daily activities that reflect cultural values, provide structure to living, and meaning to individuals; these activities meet human needs for self-care, enjoyment, and participation in society" (Crepeau, Cohn, & Schell, 2003, p. 1031, as cited in AOTA, 2008b, pp. 628–629).

Through the process of evaluation, the occupational therapist views and facilitates the interactions among the person, activities and occupations, and environment and context to determine the supports and barriers to the person's engagement and participation (AOTA, 2008b). Services may be provided to many different entities, including the child, family or caregivers, educational and child care staff, and district committees.

This chapter discusses evaluation and assessment guidelines from national, state, and local perspectives. Several key points are highlighted, including the importance of engaging parents as active team members in the process to identify their child's strengths and needs, determine the purpose of the evaluation, select the methods or tools of assessment to provide reliable and valid results, and determine the location and time of the evaluation to capture the child within the natural environment and appropriate routines. The chapter closes with a focus on various roles of the occupational therapist in early childhood practice. Occupational therapy evaluation of adaptive, physical, communication, social–emotional, and cognitive and learning development, including typical assessment tools used in early intervention and preschool practices, is covered as well. Finally, the early childhood outcomes of the U.S. Department of Education's Office of Special Education Programs (OSEP) are reviewed with respect to occupational therapy practice.

Evaluation and Assessment Considerations

American Occupational Therapy Association

AOTA publishes professional guidelines and resources that contain information for occupational therapists about evaluation and assessment. Some of the common guidelines and pediatric resources from the association are highlighted in the following sections for occupational therapists to use as companions to this chapter.

Standards of Practice

The *Standards of Practice for Occupational Therapy* (AOTA, 2005) defines *evaluation* as "the process of obtaining and interpreting data necessary for intervention. This [definition] includes planning for and documenting the evaluation process and results" (p. 89). *Assessment* is defined as "specific tools or instruments that are used during the evaluation process" (p. 89). Occupational therapists are required to adhere to the standards in the *Standards of Practice* document. Box 5.1 contains the standards related to screening, evaluation, and reevaluation.

The Individuals With Disabilities Education Improvement Act of 2004 (IDEA 2004) and the occupational therapy professional literature now use the terms *evaluation* and *assessment* consistently as they relate to initial eligibility evaluations (Polichino, Clark, Swinth, & Muhlenhaupt, 2007). *Evaluation* is the process of obtaining and interpreting information (e.g., full and individual initial and subsequent evaluations), whereas *assessments* are the specific tools or instruments used to gather data about the student's strengths and needs (AOTA, 1995). The terms *assessment* or *assessments,* however, are used elsewhere in the law to refer to the process of evaluation. These terms are often used interchangeably in early childhood literature.

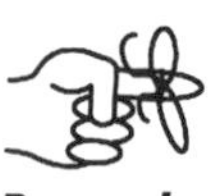

Remember this. . . .
Older literature and other professionals tend to define the terms *assessment* and *evaluation* differently, which may cause confusion for occupational therapists.

Older literature and other professionals tend to define the terms *assessment* and *evaluation* differently, which may cause confusion for occupational therapists. The

Box 5.1. *Standards of Practice for Occupational Therapy:* Standard II—Screening, Evaluation, and Reevaluation

1. An occupational therapist accepts and responds to referrals in compliance with state laws or other regulatory requirements.
2. An occupational therapist, in collaboration with the client, evaluates the client's ability to participate in daily life activities by considering the client's capacities, the activities, and the environments in which these activities occur.
3. An occupational therapist initiates and directs the screening, evaluation, and re-evaluation process and analyzes and interprets the data in accordance with law, regulatory requirements, and AOTA documents.
4. An occupational therapy assistant contributes to the screening, evaluation, and re-evaluation process by implementing delegated assessments and by providing verbal and written reports of observations and client capacities to the occupational therapist in accordance with law, regulatory requirements, and AOTA documents.
5. An occupational therapy practitioner follows defined protocols when standardized assessments are used.
6. An occupational therapist completes and documents occupational therapy evaluation results. An occupational therapy assistant contributes to the documentation of evaluation results. An occupational therapy practitioner abides by the time frames, formats, and standards established by practice settings, government agencies, external accreditation programs, payers, and AOTA documents.
7. An occupational therapy practitioner communicates screening, evaluation, and re-evaluation results within the boundaries of client confidentiality to the appropriate person, group, or organization.
8. An occupational therapist recommends additional consultations or refers clients to appropriate resources when the needs of the client can best be served by the expertise of other professionals or services.
9. An occupational therapy practitioner educates current and potential referral sources about the scope of occupational therapy services and the process of initiating occupational therapy services.

From "Standards of Practice for Occupational Therapy," by the American Occupational Therapy Association, 2005, *American Journal of Occupational Therapy, 59,* p. 664. Copyright © 2005 by the American Occupational Therapy Association. Used with permission.

reader is cautioned to consider the date of an article and the perspective of the authors when reading. For example, Salvia and Ysseldyke (1995; remedial and special education) defined *assessment* as "the process of collecting data for the purposes of making decisions about students" (p. 5). Bagnato, Neisworth, and Munson (1997; early intervention) noted that assessment is a comprehensive procession of data collection and "integrates both quantitative and qualitative data that are translated into treatment-based terms" (p. 4). Peterson (1987) defined *evaluation* as a "process of making judgments about a child's behavior or development, an instructional procedure, a program, or anything else about which conclusions are to be drawn" (p. 282); this definition was more in line with how evaluation and assessment are defined in occupational therapy literature. Peterson defined *assessment* as the "ongoing activity of collecting data for purposes of evaluation" (p. 282).

The terms *formative evaluation* and *summative evaluation* are also being used in current literature. Formative evaluation occurs at the initiation of a research, intervention, or work process and can be thought of as "present level of performance." Data are collected throughout the program or instruction. Summative evaluation

formative - like weekly tests
Summative - Final exam

Learning Activity 5.1. Terminology

1. Think about the way AOTA uses the terms *evaluation* and *assessment.* Does this usage cause confusion when talking with professionals outside of occupational therapy?
2. Think about the way your agency has defined the terms *evaluation* and *assessment.* Which term tends to refer to the overall process and which one refers to the tools being used?
3. Review the language in IDEA 2004 to clarify the use of these terms in early intervention and preschool services.

---

occurs at the end of or at designated points in the process of intervention (i.e., the level of performance after intervention) and compares pre–post functioning to determine outcomes, need for ongoing services, and the like (Bagnato et al., 1997). Learning Activity 5.1 emphasizes the use of terminology and invites the reader to think about how these terms are being used.

The Guide to Occupational Therapy Practice

The second edition of *The Guide to Occupational Therapy Practice* (Moyers & Dale, 2007) continues to provide the occupational therapy profession with information about the scope and process of occupational therapy. During the evaluation process, "the occupational therapist uses theories and evidence to frame the client's occupational performance problems and concerns" (p. 22). As data are collected, client–child priorities and desired outcomes should be determined, goals to achieve these outcomes should be written, and interventions should be implemented to achieve those goals and desired outcomes. In a client-centered approach, occupational therapists and clients collaboratively establish client goals and priorities (e.g., desired outcomes).

The *Occupational Therapy Practice Framework: Domain and Process* (AOTA, 2008b) defines the term *outcome* as "the end-result of the occupational therapy process and describe what occupational therapy intervention can achieve with clients" (p. 660). *Outcomes* are what actually occurred. Laws, agencies, and payment sources may use this term differently and may have specific goals, objectives, or outcomes that must also be met through interventions. In Part B of IDEA 2004, the term *measurable goal* is used to describe what the child will be able to do after or as a result of intervention or special education; Part C uses the term *outcomes* (rather than goals) to describe what is desired and expected for the infant or toddler and the family as a result of early intervention services. Occupational therapists should be aware of the terms and requirements in their agency for developing and documenting client priorities and desired end results.

Because occupational engagement and social participation are the results of many factors interacting dynamically, an occupational therapy evaluation must consider many factors to address family and child concerns. The evaluation process should yield outcomes for the child that enhance health and participation in valued occupations. For example, evaluating only physical function (e.g., developmental milestones, fine motor skills) is not a complete measure of performance in occupation. Rather than just list the physical functions, the occupational therapist analyzes the impact on the child's participation and sets intervention goals and desired outcomes to enhance that engagement. "Outcome measures reflect performance as influenced by client factors, context and environment, performance patterns and skills, and activity demands" (Moyers & Dale, 2007, p. 47). For example, an outcome for a young child with cerebral palsy may be to enable independent participation in classroom art projects rather than to stabilize his arm and hand. Stabilizing his arm and hand is a means to the desired outcome of participation in classroom art projects.

Occupational Therapy Services for Children and Youth Under IDEA

The AOTA publication *Occupational Therapy Services for Children and Youth Under IDEA* (3rd ed.; Jackson, 2007) assists occupational therapists in preparing and positioning themselves to effectively meet the needs of children and youth under IDEA. Occupational therapists working specifically in early childhood settings and schools may find the evaluation data beneficial because the book emphasizes specific aspects of IDEA in relation to evaluation requirements and expectations. The text highlights specific areas of occupation and their relationship to IDEA Parts B and C and compares occupation-based and component-based approaches in evaluations under IDEA (Polichino et al., 2007). It also presents detailed information about the occupational therapy decision-making process (Handley-More & Chandler, 2007).

State Regulatory Laws for Occupational Therapy

Occupational therapists should review state practice acts to identify screening, evaluation, and assessment activities permitted within that state. Some states allow screening activities and ongoing screening, whereas others require an evaluation before the occupational therapist can make any recommendations. The role of the occupational therapy assistant in screening, evaluation, and assessment also varies considerably from state to state and should be carefully identified. If occupational therapy services are being considered, the decision on provision of occupational therapy services and determination of frequency and duration are typically the responsibility of the occupational therapist or the referring physician. If the occupational therapist, as part of the team, evaluates the child and documents the results and recommendations, this structure should not be an issue. Conflict and potential licensure violations occur when the occupational therapist is not part of the team that makes decisions about occupational therapy services. The state practice act or state occupational therapy regulatory board should be consulted for guidance on this issue.

Federal and State Education Laws and Regulations

Multiple federal laws affect occupational therapy practice in early childhood (see Chapter 1 for a review of the laws and the programs they authorize). IDEA 2004 has specific requirements for screening, evaluation, and assessments to identify children with a disability for specific services under this law. Other laws and programs (e.g., Early Head Start) may specifically identify requirements for children who are able to attend the program (e.g., family income) but may not have such specific requirements to receive occupational therapy services.

Infants and Toddlers With Disabilities Program

The Infants and Toddlers With Disabilities (ITD) program (Part C of IDEA 2004) is a discretionary (voluntary) federal program for infants and toddlers who meet specific eligibility criteria established by each state. States can choose to participate in this program. If they do so, they must apply for the funding and meet certain requirements in doing so. Under § 1435(a)(1), IDEA allows each state to determine a rigorous definition of developmental delay. Occupational therapists working in early intervention programs should know their state's definition of developmental delay because the definition establishes eligibility for services.

> Most states have established quantitative criteria for a delay, such as a percentage of delay (typically 20% or 25% delay, with some states as high as 50%) or as a standard deviation below the mean on a norm-referenced instrument (typically 2.0 or 1.5 standard deviations). (Clark, 2008, p. CE–2)

In addition to appropriate diagnostic instruments or procedures, children may be determined to be eligible if they have established conditions, such as Down syndrome, extreme prematurity, or intrauterine growth retardation, or on the basis of informed clinical opinion (Bagnato, 2006; Shackelford, 2002). Establishing eligibility on the basis of informed clinical opinion means that both quantitative and qualitative data are used to form a determination. A child may not meet the state's established quantitative criteria (test score) for eligibility; however, the occupational therapist may use information from the parent interview and observation of the child during play to determine that the child's performance is atypical and has a high probability of causing a delay in development without intervention.

For example, an infant may have been born full term and may be developing appropriately but could be gagging and choking when drinking from a bottle. This inability to coordinate suck, swallow, and breathe may result in the child's avoidance of the bottle and, consequently, weight loss. Early intervention services may be necessary for the child to develop an efficient drinking pattern.

Another example may be that of a child with low muscle tone who is able to complete tasks but uses atypical patterns of movement and grasp. If the team believes the child's movement and grasp patterns could interfere with the child's ongoing development, informed clinical opinion could be used to entitle the child to services under Part C.

Informed clinical opinion should be based on multiple sources of data and data that are collected across multiple settings and methods (Bagnato, 2006) and should be documented to provide a baseline for measuring progress (Shackelford, 2002). Documentation of informed clinical opinion is necessary to identify that procedural safeguards were applied during the process of determining eligibility. Documentation could include an identification of the child's functioning level, structured method of collecting the data, and a consensus decision making by people who know the child (Bagnato, 2006). Learning Activity 5.2 invites readers to review their state's eligibility criteria. Readers who have never considered using informed clinical opinion to determine eligibility may find the documents informative.

Learning Activity 5.2. Determining Eligibility Using Your State's Definition or Informed Clinical Opinion

- How is developmental delay defined in your state for eligibility purposes for the Infants and Toddlers With Disabilities (ITD) program?
- How is the level of developmental delay determined in your state?
- Are children who are at risk eligible for the ITD in your state? If so, how is *at risk* defined and determined?

Read more about informed clinical opinion. Two documents on this topic can be obtained on the Internet:

Shackelford, J. (2002). *Informed clinical opinion* (NECTAC Notes No. 10). Chapel Hill: University of North Carolina, FPG Child Development Institute, National Early Childhood Technical Assistance Center. Retrieved March 8, 2009, from www.nectac.org/~pdfs/pubs/nnotes10.pdf

Bagnato, S. (2006). Formalizing informed clinical opinion assessment procedures is more likely to yield accurate results. *Endpoints, 2*(3), 1–2. Retrieved September 16, 2009, from www.dec-sped.org/uploads/docs/conference/2008_handouts/ASM199%20W22_Research%20Foundations_CJ%20for%20EI%20Eligibility.pdf

- How can you use this information within your practice to determine eligibility for children in a systematic way?
- How is this different from or similar to how you use this type of information in other clinical settings?

IDEA Part C § 635 requires, at a minimum, timely, comprehensive, multidisciplinary evaluation of the unique strengths and needs of the child to assist the team in developing the individualized family service plan (IFSP). The IFSP must contain a statement of the child's current levels of development, based on objective criteria, in the following five areas:

1. Physical development (which includes hearing and vision), which is often described in terms of fine motor and gross motor skills
2. Cognitive development
3. Communication development
4. Social or emotional development
5. Adaptive development.

The occupational therapist also evaluates the child's ability to functionally participate in his or her family's routines and desired settings (e.g., home, park, library, day care, church). Combining quantitative information (from the test) with the qualitative information collected during observation, interview, and record review provides a comprehensive view of the child's functioning within the family role. In addition to the evaluation of the child, Part C, 20 U.S.C. §1436(a)(2), requires "a family-directed assessment of the resources, priorities, and concerns of the family and the identification of the supports and services necessary to enhance the family's capacity to meet the developmental need of the infant or toddler." The occupational therapist can and, as appropriate, should participate in this assessment. If other members of the team conduct the family-directed assessment, the occupational therapist should use the information to guide occupational therapy service needs for the child and family.

The evaluation and a written IFSP must be completed within 45 calendar days from the date the child was referred to the local ITD program. OSEP requires 100%

compliance with this requirement. The only exceptions allowed are family-based reasons (e.g., the child was medically ill and could not be tested, parents declined further evaluation). Agency-based delays (e.g., understaffing, staff on maternity leave) are not excused and are counted as incomplete evaluations. States must track these data and report them on an annual basis to OSEP through their state performance plan and annual performance report (20 U.S.C. § 1416(b)(1)).

Evaluations conducted by the occupational therapist should include information about the child's current level of performance in his or her natural environment. Information about the family's routines and activities is highly beneficial because it is a measure of the child's ability to participate in daily routines and provides the therapist with a method for embedding interventions during natural routines and environments.

Occupational therapists serving children on an IFSP should use evaluation and assessment data when participating in the development of transition plans. IDEA requires that these transition plans be developed no less than 90 days (and, in many places, no more than 9 months) before the child's third birthday. Evaluation data should support the recommendations being made. Recommendations may include Part B preschool services, other federal programs, discharge (if the child does not meet Part B eligibility requirements), or discharge from Part C to community-based programs for parent services. See Chapters 1 and 4 for further information about transition services.

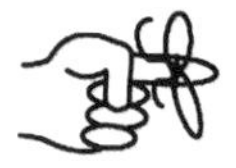

Remember this. . . . **Evaluations conducted by the occupational therapist should include information that indicates the child's ability to participate in appropriate activities.**

Part B Preschool

Part B of IDEA 2004 is a federally mandated program for preschool- and school-age children. Part B details procedures that must be completed before special education and related services (e.g., occupational therapy) can be provided to a child with a disability. Note that occupational therapy under Part C is defined as a primary developmental service. Under Part B, however, occupational therapy is a "related" service; that is, it is related to the child's specially designed instruction as defined in the individualized education program (IEP). A full and individual initial evaluation must be completed "within 60 calendar days of receiving the parental consent for evaluation" (20 U.S.C. § 1414 (a)(1)(C)(I)). Specific requirements of the law under 20 U.S.C. § 1414(b)(2)(A–D) are listed in Box 5.2.

Evaluations conducted by the occupational therapist should include information that indicates the child's ability to participate in appropriate activities. This information may be gathered through informal and formal methods. Interviewing the parent or teacher will provide the therapist with information about the child's strengths and needs. Observation of the child in the natural environment provides information about supports and barriers to participation and the interaction of the child with the environment. Observation in the preschool routine provides the therapist with knowledge about the curriculum (or lack of one) and the instruction being provided. Standardized and nonstandardized tests may be used to support or refute hypotheses that the therapist develops during the interview or observation.

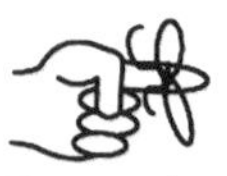

Remember this. . . . **Observation of the child in the natural environment provides information about supports and barriers to participation and the interaction of the child with the environment.**

In conducting evaluations, occupational therapists must be aware of their state education laws. Learning Activity 5.3 will help readers explore their state's legislation and regulations.

Box 5.2. IDEA 2004 Requirements Related to the Evaluation and Use of Assessment Tools Under IDEA Part B

20 U.S.C. § 1414(b) states the following:

(2) Conduct of evaluation

In conducting the evaluation, the local educational agency shall—

(A) use a variety of assessment tools and strategies to gather relevant functional, developmental, and academic information, including information provided by the parent, that may assist in determining—

(i) whether the child is a child with a disability; and

(ii) the content of the child's individualized education program including information related to enabling the child to be involved in and progress with general education curriculum, or, for preschool children, to participate in appropriate activities;

(B) not use any single measure or assessment as the sole criterion for determining whether a child is a child with a disability or determining an appropriate educational program for the child; and

(C) use technically sound instruments that may assess the relative contribution of cognitive and behavioral factors, in additional to physical or developmental factors.

(3) Additional requirements.

Each local educational agency shall ensure that—

(A) assessments and other evaluation materials used to assess a child under this section—

(i) are selected and administered so as not to be discriminatory on a racial or cultural basis;

(ii) are provided and administered in the language and form most likely to yield accurate information on what the child knows and can do academically, developmentally, and functionally, unless it is not feasible to so provide or administer;

(iii) are used for purposes for which the assessments or measures are valid and reliable;

(iv) are administered by trained and knowledgeable personnel; and

(v) are administered in accordance with any instructions provided by the producer of such assessments.

Head Start Programs

Many occupational therapists work in Early Head Start or Head Start programs or Head Start branches (e.g., Migrant and Seasonal Program, American Indian–Alaska Native Program). These programs have income qualifications and a requirement that children with disabilities may attend. Occupational therapists identify the child's need for occupational therapy services, using input from parents, teachers, and evaluation data. For example, a child may attend an Early Head Start program as one of the identified services on the IFSP to assist in meeting the desired outcomes. The child may participate in occupational therapy at the Early Head Start program toward those same ends or outcomes. Learning Activity 5.4 provides more information about Head Start and provides links to Head Start partnerships.

Learning Activity 5.3. Your State's Special Education Laws

Access the education and special education laws through your state's Web site or agency resources.

- How are occupational therapy services defined in these laws?
- How do these definitions compare with the definition in your state regulatory/licensure law?

Learning Activity 5.4. Head Start Partnerships

Go to www.nhsa.org, the National Head Start Web site. This site provides information about initiatives for children. Click on the Programs tab to read about the partnerships with various resources such as the Center on the Social and Emotional Foundations of Early Learning and programs such as Healthy Kids.

Recommended Practices From National Early Childhood Associations

Whereas professional organizations have developed their standards and best practice documents on early childhood evaluation and intervention, two major early childhood organizations have published extensive professional standards in early childhood. Summaries of those standards are included here.

Council for Exceptional Children: Division for Early Childhood

The Council for Exceptional Children has worked to develop and field validate the assessment standards published by its Division for Early Childhood. Neisworth and Bagnato (2004) categorized these standards into 10 overarching standards (Box 5.3).

Bagnato (2007) summarized the standards according to two fundamental elements. First, developmentally appropriate procedures must be followed. The location and content must match the interests and capabilities of early childhood. The second fundamental element is the active cooperation with parents. Including the parents as active, collaborative team partners allows the examiner to gather data that would otherwise not have been accessible. Parents have information about the child that teams must be willing to gather, even when the data are discrepant from the information that the professionals have gathered. These fundamental elements serve as a guide for occupational therapists working with early childhood teams.

National Association for the Education of Young Children

The National Association for the Education of Young Children (NAEYC) and the National Association of Early Childhood Specialists (NAECS) in State Departments of Education coauthored a joint position statement in 2003 titled *Early Childhood Curriculum, Assessment, and Program Evaluation: Building an Effective, Accountable System in Programs for Children Birth Through Age 8*. This document provides an overview of relevant trends, guiding principles, and the rationale for each recommendation made in the joint position statement.

The document states that ethical principles would be used by professionals to drive assessment practices (e.g., decisions would not be based on one assessment). The term *assessment* is used in this context because these standards are from the early childhood literature and discuss the use of various assessment tools in practice. Assessment tools should be used for the purpose for which they were designed (e.g., screening tools are not used for diagnostic purposes). Assessment tools must be appropriate for the age, socioeconomic status, abilities, disabilities, and language of the children being tested and should be valid and reliable. Assessments should be aligned with the state's early learning standards and program's curriculum. Multiple sources of evidence should be gathered in a variety of settings over several days.

Box 5.3. Council for Exceptional Children's 10 Developmentally Appropriate ?ractice Assessment Standards

. *Utility:* Usefulness for intervention
Acceptability: Social worth and agreement
Authenticity: Natural methods and contexts
Equity: Adaptable for special needs
Sensitivity: Fine measurement of gradations
Convergence: Synthesis of ecological data
'ollaboration: Parent–professional teamwork
ongruence: Special design, field validation, evidence base
chnology: Portable, computer-based observations, recordings, and reporting
'utcomes: Assessed content aligned to state or federal outcome benchmarks.

Source. From *Authentic Assessment for Early Childhood Intervention* (p. 24), by S. Bagnato, 2007, New York: Guilford Press. Copyright © 2007 by the Guilford Press. Adapted with permission.

Standardized tools and norm-referenced assessments have limited data and are more useful for diagnostic purposes than for program planning, curriculum design, and accountability. Families are seen as part of "a community that sees assessment as a tool to improve outcomes for children" (NAEYC & NAECS, 2003, p. 11).

Because this statement was coauthored by specialists in state departments of education, occupational therapists should be aware of its content and reflect on their practices within the context of the document. Occupational therapists' ongoing awareness of and participation in early childhood organizations is important to development of strong services to children and families. Learning Activity 5.5 provides more in-depth information about two major early childhood organizations.

Collaborating With Parents

Guided by the previously mentioned documents and their knowledge and skills, occupational therapists providing services in early intervention and early childhood practices identify the recipient of service as the family and young child, not just the child (Dunn, 2000; Hinojosa, Sproat, Mankhetwit, & Anderson, 2002; Schultz-Krohn

Learning Activity 5.5. Comparing Standards for Early Childhood Evaluation

Visit the Web sites of two early childhood organizations to learn about them and the resources that they offer:

- Division of Early Childhood: www.dec-sped.org/
- National Association for the Education of Young Children: www.naeyc.org/.

Activities

- Compare and contrast the purpose of the organizations.
- Describe how you could use their work in early childhood as part of the guidance for your practice in early childhood.
- Identify specific practices in relation to a child and family with whom you work.

& Cara, 2000). Occupational therapists collaborate with the family to determine the child's strengths and needs. The family-centered model in early intervention requires the occupational therapist to enter into a relationship with the family to understand their resources, priorities, and concerns (Hinojosa et al., 2002; Schultz-Krohn, 1997). When children are in child care or preschool programs, therapists must work with the families and the child's caregivers to identify the child's needs and current developmental performance to participate in everyday routines and activities.

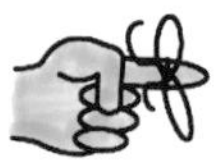

Remember this. . . .
The only members of the team with a long and in-depth knowledge of the child are the parents or caregivers.

The only members of the team with a long and in-depth knowledge of the child are the parents or caregivers. The term *caregivers* includes the variety of people who may care for a child. Caregivers may include family members, foster care parents, or child care providers. Limiting involvement to asking parents and caregivers questions and having them complete a checklist may be missing their unique contribution to the evaluation and assessment of the child. Best practices in developmental services now encourage parents to become active and collaborative partners with the team. Parents can and should facilitate their child's performance during testing, describe the routines of the day that are working or not working, and have a role in decision making. Bailey and colleagues (1998) identified characteristics of collaborative relationships, including trust, mutual respect, open and clear communication, a collaborative attitude, follow through, and interpersonal skills. In collaborative relationships, the parent may be included in all aspects of the evaluation process. Although parents have the opportunity to participate, some parents may choose to have limited involvement. Partners in a collaborative relationship would not judge this decision but would accept the parents' choice.

McLean and Crais (2004) listed several reasons for facilitating collaborative efforts among all members of the team, especially the parents:

- Families have an essential position in the child's life and development. Supporting and encouraging parents to have an active role in their child's assessment strengthens their position in their child's life.
- Families have knowledge about the child that others do not have. Involving the family means that assessment activities will be directly linked to the families' concerns, priorities, and resources.
- Families can assist with assessment activities, including completing tools about the child; identifying routines, settings, or strategies for assessment; contributing to intervention planning; and improving the validity of assessment by acknowledging the child's typical performance.
- Families should be provided with opportunities to participate in the assessments to convey the message that they are important members of the team. If early childhood professionals take a lead role, parents may take a passive role and not feel supported in their knowledge of their own child.

"Misrepresenting children through mismeasuring them denies children their rights to beneficial expectations and opportunities" (Neisworth & Bagnato, 2004, p. 198). Models that encourage family and child care and preschool staff involvement provide more accurate measurement of children. The following questions, among others, can guide teams:

- How can professionals understand family and staff concerns about the child?
- How are the family and staff concerns, priorities, and resources used to shape the assessment process?
- How are the family and staff being asked to communicate the child's strengths and needs?
- How does the location and time of day contribute to or hinder the child's performance?
- How is the family being made aware that they could invite other people significant in the child's life to be present and contribute to this evaluation process?
- During the evaluation, how is the family's role as active participants supported?
- How do the professionals ask family and staff to identify routines that are problematic and those that support performance?
- How were family and staff asked their impressions of the child's performance?
- How valid and authentic (natural routines and contexts) are the data that were collected using this approach?
- How are the data used as basis for determining decisions such as eligibility and program planning?

According to McLean and Crais (2004), "the more active families and caregivers are *during* the assessment planning and implementation, the more likely they are to take an active part during the sharing of the results and the intervention planning" (p. 55). They identified several roles for parents during the assessment, including interpreter of their child's behavior, participant in their child's assessment, validator of the assessment and results, and identifier of the family concerns.

Facilitating families to be active members of the evaluation process encourages a collaborative partnership in goal setting and implementation. Working together to plan the evaluation, implement the activities, review the results, and make decisions empowers families and enhances "the capacity of families to meet the special needs of their infants and toddlers with disability" (20 U.S.C. § 1431(a)(4)) and to meet the needs of their older child as well. Learning Activity 5.6 encourages readers to reflect on their perceptions about the parent's role in the child's evaluation and assessment process.

Learning Activity 5.6. Empowering Parents to Participate in Evaluation and Assessment

- How are you encouraging parent participation in evaluations and assessments?
- Are you comfortable with parents as active members of the team? If so, what helped you to develop your comfort level? If not, what might be causing your discomfort?
- How can you start to address those issues?
- Discuss with parents who take an active role their reasons and strategies for doing so.

Initial and Ongoing Evaluation and Assessment Practices

Professionals "must use assessment tools that are individually, culturally and linguistically appropriate, and that measure children's strengths, developmental status, progress and needs" (Rous & Townley, 2006, p. 3). The results of an assessment often lead to high-stakes decisions, such as eligibility or program planning. Bagnato and colleagues (1997) wrote that the focus should be not on test scores (the result of a specific assessment tool) but on the quality of decisions.

IDEA provides guidance for evaluation, which aligns with much of the early childhood information covered in this chapter. For instance, 20 U.S.C. § 1414(b) deals with evaluation procedures and provides several overarching ideas:

- Use a variety of assessment tools and strategies to gather relevant functional, developmental, and academic information, including information provided by the parent.
- Do not use any single measure or assessment as the sole criterion for determination of eligibility or of the appropriate educational program.
- Use technically sound instruments.
- Use instruments for the purposes for which they are valid and reliable.

Occupational therapists should collect data from more than one person to gain a comprehensive view of the child's performance. Using records review, interviews, observations, and various tools can reveal patterns or inconsistencies in performance. Assessing across various settings, locations, and times of the day also provides a comprehensive view of the child's and family's routines and areas of strength and need. Readers are encouraged to use Learning Activity 5.7 to more closely review their own practices.

Purpose of the Evaluation and Assessment

Purposes underlying evaluation and assessment may include screening, diagnosis, program (intervention) planning, and program evaluation (see Table 5.1). Professionals misuse assessments when they fail to match the purpose or need with the tool chosen. For instance, screening tools are used primarily to identify areas of concern that may need to be further evaluated. Using a screening tool to determine eligibility for federal programs is not appropriate and conflicts with the law (20 U.S.C. § 1432(5)(A)(i)), which defines an *infant or toddler with a disability* as one "who needs early intervention services because the individual is experiencing developmental

Learning Activity 5.7. Evaluating Your Evaluations

Review your most recent three evaluations to see how your practices align with the recommendations given in the text.

- If you are using these practices in your evaluation process, how did you develop the skills, and what assists you in using the skills in your practice?
- If you aren't using these assessment practices, identify reasons (barriers) for not using them, and identify which one could you start to use in your practice.

Table 5.1. Purposes of Evaluation and Assessment Under IDEA 2004

Descriptors	Answers What Question	Part C	Part B
Screening	Is there a problem?	Determine the need for further evaluation	Determine the need for further evaluation
Diagnostic	What is the problem?	Determine eligibility	Determine eligibility and educational need
Program planning	What can I (we) do about the problem?	Determine the unique strengths and needs of the infant and toddler, and identify services appropriate to meet such needs Perform family-directed assessment of the resources, priorities, and supports Determine the appropriate transition services for the infant or toddler (at least 90 days before child's 3rd birthday)	Determine educational needs of child Determine the appropriate transition needs related to training, education, employment, and, where appropriate, independent living skills
Program evaluation	Did we make a difference? What is the outcome of intervention? Has the child met the desired goal or outcome?	Ongoing assessment to determine progress toward outcomes Determine ongoing eligibility for program (as appropriate)	Ongoing assessment to determine progress toward outcomes Determine ongoing eligibility for program (as appropriate)

delays, as measured by appropriate diagnostic instruments and procedures. . . ." Diagnostic instruments tend to be standardized and are used to determine the significance of the delay. Table 5.1 guides readers through various purposes of evaluation and assessment under IDEA's Part C and Part B. Box 5.4 provides information for occupational therapists to consider when gathering information.

Different types of assessments have been used in early intervention and early childhood (Table 5.2). Some assessments are actual tools or instruments, whereas others may be a method (e.g., portfolio or observation). Most commonly used assessments include norm-referenced assessments (used primarily for diagnostic purposes) and criterion-referenced assessments (used to measure a child's mastery of skills). Problems have occurred over the years in relying on norm-referenced (e.g., standardized test) assessments. McLean and Crais (2004) identified one dilemma: "[T]he use of norm-referenced instruments to evaluate change in a child as a result of motor intervention . . . is not appropriate in that these measures are typically designed to be discriminative in nature" (p. 330). Standardized tests are designed to be discriminative in nature and thus are not appropriate for measuring the rate of progress over time. In early childhood and early intervention, there has been a move toward the use of criterion-referenced assessment—specifically, toward criteria linked to curriculum, referred to as *curriculum-based assessment* (CBA). These curriculum-based measures are used in general and special education programs for decisions ranging

Box 5.4. Reasons for Evaluation

Occupational therapists need to be clear about *why* they are evaluating a child and what information they need to gather. Answering these questions will lead them to choose the appropriate assessment tools.

Using the same series of assessments on every child is not efficient or productive. For example, the evaluation purpose may be to determine whether a preschool child needs occupational therapy services to participate in activities in the classroom (i.e., why the child was referred) that require fine motor skill (coloring, cutting with scissors, buttoning). Because the concern is to determine how fine motor skills may be hindering the child from participating in the classroom, the occupational therapist must first work with the teacher to identify which activities in the classroom are problematic (i.e., what information needs to be gathered).

The occupational therapist must analyze the curriculum, instruction, and environment to determine the supports or barriers to participation (e.g., the child has no experience with using crayons, is unable to follow two-step commands, and did not understand areas to color and not to color; crayons are too thin and child is unable to grasp them). Observation of the child in the natural setting may lead the occupational therapist to other questions regarding the child's skills and performance. The therapist may use various assessment methods to answer these questions. For example, a screening of in-hand manipulation skills of this child and several preschool classmates would indicate how this child is performing, on the basis of peer standards and whether the in-hand manipulation skills are interfering with fine motor performance and, thus, class participation.

Reflection

Think about the assessment tools you are using. Why are they being used? Do you have tools to use for each different purpose?

from eligibility to progress monitoring (Macy, Bricker, & Squires, 2005; McLean, 2005; Neisworth & Bagnato, 2004; Slentz & Hyatt, 2008).

Instead of using specific assessment tools or instruments, the evaluation process may include data from alternative assessment models. Losardo and Notari-Syverson (2001) provided examples of alternative approaches for gathering information about young children. They classified the approaches into three major categories of assessment: embedded models, authentic models, and mediated models.

The first category, *embedded models,* may be either naturalistic or focused assessments. *Naturalistic assessment* may be embedded in child-initiated and routine activities or may provide the child with several opportunities to perform skills. An example is that of the ecological approach, in which the context of the assessment depends on the child's routine, schedule, and environment. Teaching and testing are closely linked. *Focused assessment,* in contrast, uses adult-structured interventions to elicit child behaviors. These activities may or may not be part of the daily classroom routines. Play-based assessments are a type of focused assessment.

The second category of assessment models is that of *authentic models,* which include performance assessment and portfolio assessment. *Performance assessment* focuses on the child's strengths, strategies, and processes. A wide range of methods and products, including observation, videotaping, photographs, and work samples, is used to document the child's performance. Tasks could be part of the daily routine or specific activities for the assessment. Although the portfolio may contain performance-based work, it is used to document the child's performance over time. "It is an assessment tool to be used for a purpose; it requires a clear process and evaluation criteria and the child's active involvement" (Losardo & Notari-Syverson, 2001, p. 101). Occupational therapists tend to collect samples of the child's performance as a method of documenting the child's progress.

Table 5.2. Types of Early Childhood Assessment Methods

Method		Descriptions	Examples
Norm-referenced assessment		Compares child's performance to a normative group of children; standardized	Battelle Developmental Inventory (Newborg, 2004)
Criterion-referenced assessment		Indicates child's performance on specific skills	Carolina curriculum for preschoolers with special needs (Johnson-Martin, Jens, Attermeier, & Hacker, 1990)
Alternative Approaches			
Embedded	Naturalistic	Embedded in child's routine, schedule, and environment	Ecological-based assessment
	Focused	Adult-structured interactions to elicit child behaviors; activities may not necessarily be authentic	Play-based assessment
Authentic	Performance	Actual products gathered from the child during tasks of the daily routine or specific activities for assessment	Videotapes, photographs, work samples
	Portfolio	Has a clear process and evaluation criteria; child is actively involved in gathering tasks for the portfolio	May contain performance-based work but also would include a rating scale or other method of evaluation
Mediated	Dynamic assessment	Test–teach–retest method of learning that supports predictions about child's response to interventions and future performance	Anecdotes
	CBA	Specific type of criterion-referenced assessments that directly align with curricular content and provide programming suggestions	Hawaii Early Learning Profile (Parks et al., 1994)
IGDIs		A general outcome measure, indicators that are conceptually parallel	Dynamic Indicators of Basic Early Literacy Skills (Kaminski & Good, 1996)

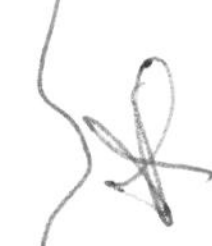

Note. CBA = curriculum-based assessment; IGDI = individual growth and development indicator.

Occupational therapists working in early childhood have probably encountered the term *authentic assessment.* This term is used to describe data collected through the evaluation process that are actually produced as part of the child's natural routine and activities rather than from a contrived activity for an assessment tool (e.g., the child's actual art project would be used rather than scoring the child's performance on a test form where a circle is drawn). Authentic assessment may be used as part of the evaluation process and has long been a part of the occupational therapy evaluation process, although perhaps not identified by this term.

Many early childhood organizations and leaders have advocated authentic assessment. Grisham-Brown, Hemmeter, and Pretti-Frontczak (2005) wrote that authentic assessment is sometimes called *play-based assessment, functional assessment, standards-based assessment,* or *performance assessment.* Authentic assessment may be used for typically developing children as well as for children with delays.

Grisham-Brown et al. (2005) listed several recommended practices of an authentic assessment model. Assessment should

1. Be ongoing and used for decision making;
2. Include all relevant areas of development and learning;
3. Be conducted in natural and authentic settings and routines;
4. Result in information for identification, intervention, and monitoring; and
5. Involve multiple observations, multiple approaches, and multiple interviews.

The third assessment model, *mediated models,* includes dynamic assessment and CBA. This model uses the term *assessment* to describe a specific type of evaluation process or model (note that the model uses "assessment" differently from either the *Framework* [AOTA, 2008b] or IDEA). Dynamic assessment is used to determine both what the child has learned and what the child is capable of learning with scaffolding and mediation. This method is a test–teach–retest model that allows the examiner to facilitate the child's performance during the assessment. This dynamic method of assessment supports predictions about the child's response to interventions and future performance. When writing goals, the supports and modifications used to facilitate skills should be included. CBA links the assessment to the curriculum and provides programming suggestions. A child is not "taught the task"; rather, the curriculum becomes the skills that the child is taught. Activities in the curriculum that are strengths or needs are outlined for the child and serve as a guide for interventions. Ongoing data are collected to monitor changes in a child's performance.

Another type of assessment is emerging. Individual growth and development indicators (IGDIs) identify children who are not responding to instruction and monitor children's progress over time. IGDIs were recently developed and supported by research evidence (Greenwood, Carta, Walker, Hughes, & Weathers, 2006). Strong links exist among assessment, intervention, and measurement of progress. IGDI scores are graphed and allow the team to visually compare skills to peers, observe the child's rate of growth over time, and monitor the child's response to intervention. "IGDIs are a form of progress monitoring assessment for children younger than kindergarten" (Greenwood et al., 2008, p. 536). The development and use of IGDIs is supported by the trend toward response to intervention, CBA, and progress monitoring. IGDIs are designed for use in home, child care, and preschool settings.

Teachers should align what they are teaching with their evaluation practices. This alignment ensures that they are using the assessments to guide instruction for the child. Basing decisions about instruction on student performance rather than standardized instruments allows the teacher to focus instruction on functional skill development in the natural context of the program. Occupational therapists need to be aware of the different methods of assessments being used by teachers and review them as part of the child's records. Learning Activity 5.8 offers readers an opportunity to reflect on these different types of assessment.

Role of the Occupational Therapist in Evaluation

Occupational therapy has a long history of evaluating a person's occupational performance within the natural environment and context. Slentz and Hyatt (2008) stated that the most valuable information about child performance is not produced

Learning Activity 5.8. Types of Assessments

Review the different types of assessments that were summarized.

- How familiar are you with these different types of assessments?
- Differentiate how the term *assessment* is used for both a specific tool and for a specific way of evaluating.
- How are or can you use a variety of assessments in your practice?

---

during a contrived testing situation but rather by observation of spontaneous performance during natural routines. This observation fits with the idea of alternate assessments and authentic assessment described in the previous section. Early childhood literature may use the term *assessment* similar to the way that occupational therapy literature uses the term *evaluation.* Neisworth and Bagnato (2004) wrote that assessment in early childhood should be authentic—occurring in the child's natural, everyday routines—to document the child's real capabilities. This is the heart of occupational therapy evaluation in early childhood education and early intervention. "Engagement in occupation as the focus and objective of occupational therapy intervention involves addressing both subjective and objective aspects of performance. Occupational therapists understand engagement from this dual and holistic perspective" (AOTA, 2008b, p. 628). Occupational therapists schedule their assessments within the child's natural routines (e.g., feeding during snack or lunch; self-care as the child is dressing for recess or leaving for home; play within the area of the home where the family encourages the child to play). Learning Activity 5.9 includes additional information about the use of evaluation practices.

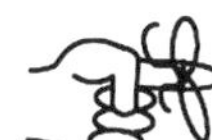

Remember this. . . .
"Engagement in occupation as the focus and objective of occupational therapy intervention involves addressing both subjective and objective aspects of performance. Occupational therapists understand engagement from this dual and holistic perspective" (AOTA, 2008b, p. 628).

Using the *Framework* to Guide the Evaluation Process

The *Occupational Therapy Practice Framework* (AOTA, 2008b) describes two parts to evaluation: (1) the occupational profile and (2) the analysis of occupational performance. The occupational therapist uses the occupational profile to begin the evaluation process. The analysis of the occupational performance focuses on data collection and interpretation to determine areas needed for intervention (AOTA, 2008b).

Collaborating With the Client to Develop the Occupational Profile

The occupational profile focuses on gathering information about the person seeking assistance (client). In the case of early childhood, adults (e.g., family, teacher,

Learning Activity 5.9. Using Evaluation Results

- Evaluation within the natural environment or context includes spontaneous performance during natural routines. What are the barriers and the supporting factors that allow you to evaluate within the child's natural environment or routines?
- How have or will you prepare yourself to practice in an authentic way?
- Identify the benefits of evaluation within the natural environment, routines, and contexts.
- How will you use the data derived from the evaluation process for decision making?
- How will you participate in reconciling any differences in recommendations among team members?

---

caregiver, agency, other professionals) are generally the clients seeking assistance for the child. The child is also the client, because services are provided to the child and the family.

The various perspectives on the child's occupational performance, the child's strengths and needs, the resources available, and the environmental supports or barriers to health and participation are important information for the occupational therapist to consider. The priorities, concerns, and desired outcomes communicated by the person seeking assistance guide the therapist in identifying areas to be evaluated, assessment methods or tools to use, activities and occupations to assess, and the environment and context for the evaluation. Generally, this data collection is ongoing throughout the service delivery process (AOTA, 2008b).

Analyzing the Occupational Performance

The occupational therapist uses the data from the occupational profile to determine the focus of the second part of the evaluation, the analysis of occupational performance. Influenced by the concerns, priorities, and needs of the practice setting, information is collected that leads the occupational therapist to identify factors that support or hinder the child's occupational performance. Therapists working in natural settings do not need to run every child though a battery of tests to make inferences about performance. The occupational therapist should be able to observe the child's performance during the natural routine and observe, if available, his or her peers' performance during this activity. Is there a discrepancy? Is it significant?

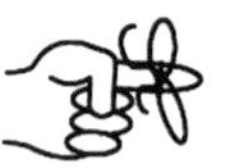

Remember this. . . .
Occupational therapists are trained to analyze various factors of the environment, activity, and person to determine a hypothesis.

Occupational therapists are trained to analyze various factors of the environment, activity, and person to determine a hypothesis. This hypothesis is then supported or refuted on the basis of the data collected. For example, if a child were unable to drink efficiently from a bottle, the occupational therapist would observe the caregiver feeding the child using the typical materials (e.g., bottle, formula). The therapist would then analyze various factors of the environment (e.g., noise that distracts the child), the activity and materials (e.g., drinking from the bottle, the bottle, the type of nipple), and the child (e.g., ability of child to suck, interaction with the caregiver).

If necessary, additional data would be gathered through other assessments to interpret the information correctly and identify strengths and barriers. Validating the information with the family, caregiver, teacher, or other significant adults in the child's daily life is important. Gathering data from multiple people and multiple methods allows the occupational therapist to determine whether the data are valid and reliable. If the parent stated that the infant was only drinking 2 to 3 oz but the day care provider stated that the child was consuming 6 to 7 oz, the therapist would have to gather additional data to determine, for instance, whether different nipples were being used, different techniques were being used, or someone was force feeding the infant.

Evaluating performance in any of the areas of occupation includes focusing on the activities and occupations that have been identified by the family, school, and child. Tables 5.3 and 5.4 list the various aspects of the occupational therapy evaluation, as outlined in the *Framework* (AOTA, 2008b). Because of the developmental expectations of early childhood, occupational therapists working in early

Table 5.3. Using the *Framework* as a Guide for Evaluating Occupations

Areas of Occupation (AOTA, 2008b)	Early Childhood Examples
Activities of daily living	Washing hands, dressing, eating, feeding, getting into sitting position, cleaning glasses, blowing nose, using toilet
Instrumental activities of daily living	Care of pet, using computers, putting toys away, riding in the car seat, or riding in the seat in the grocery cart
Rest and sleep	Ability to relax during rest time, sleeping through the night, return to sleep by self if awaken, ability to self-soothe
Education	Developmental skills, preliteracy (looking at books)
Work	Functional work tasks (e.g., sorting, matching, stacking)
Play	Using a variety of toys and equipment
Leisure	Free time use, ability to play by self
Social participation	Interactions with family, peers, educational staff, and others

Note. AOTA = American Occupational Therapy Association.

Table 5.4. Using the *Framework* as a Guide for Evaluating Performance Areas

Performance Areas (AOTA, 2008b)	Early Childhood Examples
Activity demands	Rules of game, steps to form letters of name, noise in the room, need to zip up coat
Performance skills	Manipulating objects, timing the movement, controlling anger, sequencing tasks to complete puzzle, using gestures and signs to communicate
Performance patterns	Morning routine to get dressed, avoiding task by self-stimulating
Context and environment	Community day care, significant others, instruction and curriculum
Client factors	Memory, awareness of body position and space, strength and endurance, eye–hand coordination

Note. AOTA = American Occupational Therapy Association.

childhood settings will find their focus more on activities of daily living, play, social participation, and education.

Performance Skills

During evaluation, occupational therapists should consider the child's performance skills, performance patterns, context and environment, activity demands, and client factors and how these tend to support or inhibit occupational performance.

Performance skills are learned, goal directed, and observable. To evaluate performance skills, therapists must consider the context, activity demands, and the individual body structures and functions (AOTA, 2008b). Performance skills include sensory–perceptual, motor and praxis, emotional regulatory, cognitive, and communication and social skills. These skills underlie occupational engagement and should be addressed when necessary. Table 5.5 provides examples of performance skills.

Table 5.5. Examples of Performance Skills

Performance Skills (AOTA, 2008b)	Early Intervention Examples of Activities and Occupations	Preschool Examples of Activities and Occupations
Emotional regulation	• Calming self • Displays appropriate emotions such as laughing or smiling	• Expressing regret if someone else is hurt • Responding to other people's feeling
Motor and praxis	• Manipulating spoon to bring food to mouth • Squatting down to retrieve a toy	• Coordinating body to climb on playground equipment • Drawing shapes
Sensory–perceptual	• Locating parent's voice in a crowd • Discerning hot and cold food temperatures	• Identifying rough and smooth objects • Selecting correct piece to fit into puzzle
Cognitive	• Anticipating events that occur frequently • Identifying familiar toys	• Sequencing tasks to complete three-step commands
Communication and social	• Imitating other people's actions • Gesturing to make needs known	• Taking turns during play with others • Fulfilling the role as "line leader"

Note. AOTA = American Occupational Therapy Association.

Performance Patterns

Performance patterns include the habits, routines, and rituals that people use when engaging in activities or occupations. Specific, automatic behaviors, such as removing a coat and hanging it on the classroom hook, are considered a *habit*. Habits may support performance, may need to be established, may dominate behaviors (e.g., compulsive needs), or may be inappropriate (e.g., tossing coat on floor after removal).

Routines are established sequences that provide structure. Families may have a routine for getting children ready for bed or for eating meals. To effectively work on skills, occupational therapists must be aware of the routines and the sequence of performances that occurs within them. Research has shown improved performance in children when parents implemented interventions during natural routines in the home (Dunst et al., 2001; Wetherby & Woods, 2006; Woods, Kashinath, & Goldstein, 2004). A lack of routines can lead to chaos and ineffective performance. Chapter 6 provides an in-depth discussion of routines.

Rituals are routines with special meaning to a person. Rituals may be culturally based and personal.

Contexts and Environments

Performance occurs within a social and physical environment. This environment influences the adult's and child's performance and must be considered during the evaluation process. Assessments that are completed in a clinic may yield different results from assessments completed within the family's home and the child's natural routine.

Contexts have been described as cultural, personal, temporal, and virtual. For example, certain activities or occupations may be performed in the morning (temporal) rather than in the afternoon. When gathering data, therapists should determine the influence of the environment (e.g., the ergonomic factors of the seating or work areas) and the context (e.g., language spoken in the room, location of the activity) as a support or barrier to occupational performance. For example, I found that a child who was unsuccessful in completing a task in a room with 15 other children was able to perform the task at a small table with one or two peers. The child had the skills to complete the task, but the physical and temporal environments were too distracting to do so without a simple location change. Setting up work areas in quieter locations allowed the child to be successful in the preschool setting.

Activity Demands

Activity demands refers to the specific aspects of an activity, such as the objects, physical space, social demands, actions or skills needed, and required body functions and structures. The type and amount of effort required to perform the activity are analyzed to determine how they fit with the person's capacity. Because activity demands are specific to each activity and are influenced by the environment and context, the occupational therapist must carefully analyze and document strengths and deficits for the child on the basis of the activity.

Client Factors

Client factors relate to body structures and body functions that reside within the client and influence occupational performance. "Despite their importance, the presence or absence of specific body functions and body structures does not necessarily predict a client's success or difficulty with daily life occupations" (AOTA, 2008b, pp. 631–633). Body structure and function need to be considered with the activity demands, the environment and context, and the client's performance skills and performance patterns. For example, a 4-year-old child may be independent and age appropriate in her daily life occupations despite having a medical diagnosis of cerebral palsy. This child would not require educationally based occupational therapy services in preschool. Parents may seek medical-based occupational therapy services to work on the speed and quality of movements.

Develop and Refine Hypothesis

The *Framework* (AOTA, 2008b) encourages the occupational therapist to review evaluation data that have been gathered; observe the child's performance in activities and occupations within the natural routines and environments; administer assessment tools, as needed, to gather specific information about performance skills and performance patterns; and analyze data to determine supports and barriers to performance. From this information, the therapist develops or refines a hypothesis to guide professional thinking. This hypothesis is based on the knowledge, skills, and experience of the therapist as well as frames of reference within the profession (see Table 5.6). "Frames of reference provide the 'what' and 'how' of treatment, and the theoretical perspectives provide the 'why'" (Handley-More & Chandler, 2007, p. 68). Kramer and Hinojosa (1999) is a valuable resource for pediatric occupational therapists who would like to know more about a variety of frames of reference

Developing a hypothesis on the basis of a frame of reference is a critical step because the hypothesis serves as a guide for goal development and intervention planning. For instance, the concern expressed by the teacher is that Joey (a 4.5-year-old preschooler) is unable to cut across paper with scissors. This problem could be the result of any of the following reasons:

Table 5.6. Common Tools and Methods for Early Childhood Assessment

Assessment	Ages
Screening	
Ages and Stages Questionnaire, 2nd ed. (Squires, Potter, & Bricker, 1999)	4–60 months
Ages and Stages Questionnaire Social–Emotional (Squires, Potter, & Bricker, 1997)	3–60 months
Denver II (Frankenburg et al., 1990).	Birth–6 years
Diagnostic (Norm Referenced/Standardized)	
Battelle Developmental Inventory, 2nd ed. (Newborg, 2004)	Birth–8 years
Bayley Scales of Infant Development, 3rd ed. (Bayley, 2005)	1–42 months
Beery VMI (5th ed.; Beery, Buktenica, & Beery, 2006)	2–18 years
Developmental Assessment of Young Children (Voress & Maddox, 1998)	Birth–5.11 years
Developmental Test of Visual Perception (Hammill, Pearson, & Voress, 1993)	4–10 years
Miller Function and Participation Scales (Miller, 2006)	2.6–7.11 years
Peabody Developmental Motor Scales, 2nd ed. (Folio & Fewell, 2000)	Birth–5 years
Pediatric Evaluation of Disability Inventory (Haley, Coster, Ludlow, Haltiwanger, & Andrellos, 1992)	6 months–7 years
Sensory Integration and Praxis Test (Ayres, 1989)	4.0–8.11 years
Sensory Profile (Dunn, 1999)	3–10 years
Infant/Toddler Sensory Profile (Dunn, 2002)	Birth–26 months
Sensory Profile School Companion (Dunn, 2006)	3–11 years
Test of Gross Motor Development, 2nd ed. (Ulrich, 2000)	3.0–10.11 years
Test of Visual–Perceptual Skills (Martin, 2006)	4–19 years
Vineland Adaptive Behavior Scales–II (Sparrow, Balla, & Cicchetti, 2007)	Birth–adult
Programming (Criterion Referenced)	
Assessment, Evaluation, and Programming System (Bricker, 2002)	Birth–6 years
Assessment of Motor and Process Skills and School Assessment of Motor and Process Skills (Fisher, 2005)	3 years–adult 3–12 years
Carolina Curriculum for Infants and Toddlers With Special Needs, 3rd ed. (Johnson-Martin, Attermeier, & Hacker, 2004)	Birth–36 months
Carolina Curriculum for Preschoolers With Special Needs, 2nd ed. (Johnson-Martin et al., 2004)	24–60 months
Creative Curriculum for Early Childhood (Dodge, Colker, & Heroman, 2002)	Preschoolers
Creative Curriculum for Infants, Toddlers, and Twos (Dodge, Rudick, & Berke, 2006)	Birth–3 years
Hawaii Early Learning Profile: Birth to 3 (Furuno et al., 2004)	Birth–3 years
Hawaii Early Learning Profile for Preschoolers (VORT Corporation, 1995)	3–6 years
Learning Accomplishment Profile, 3rd ed. (Hardin & Peisner-Feinberg, 2004)	36–72 months
Early Learning Accomplishment Profile (Hardin & Peisner-Feinberg, 2001)	Birth–3 years
Oregon Project Curriculum for Preschool Children Who Are Blind or Visually Impaired, 6th ed. (Anderson, Boigon, Davis, & deWaard, 2007)	Birth–6 years
Alternative Measures	
Embedded: Naturalistic and Focused	
Choosing Outcomes and Accommodations for Children, 2nd ed. (Giangreco, Cloninger, & Iverson, 1998)	3–21 years
Knox Preschool Play Scale (Knox, 1997)	Birth–6 years
Observation of child during natural routines	All ages
Transdisciplinary Play-Based Assessment (Linder, 1993)	Birth–6 years
Authentic: Performance and Portfolio	
Documentation of amount of food ate, liquid drank	All ages
Portfolio of key work	All ages
Videotapes	All ages
Mediated: Dynamic and Curriculum Assessment	
Assessment, Evaluation, and Programming System (Bricker, 2002)	Birth–6 years
Carolina Curriculum for Infants and Toddlers With Special Needs, 3rd ed. (Johnson-Martin et al., 2004)	Birth–36 months
Carolina Curriculum for Preschoolers With Special Needs, 2nd ed. (Johnson-Martin et al., 2004)	24–60 months
Hawaii Early Learning Profile: Birth to 3 (Furuno et al., 2004)	Birth–3 years
Hawaii Early Learning Profile for Preschoolers (VORT Corporation, 1995)	3–6 years
Oregon Project Curriculum for Preschool Children Who Are Blind or Visually Impaired, 6th ed. (Anderson et al., 2007)	Birth–6 years

- Joey has not had experience doing the task and needs to be taught how to hold the scissors (occupational, developmental).
- He has not been positively reinforced to complete this activity, and he hates to do it (behavioral).
- He does not have the muscle strength and coordination to hold and operate the scissors (biomechanical, developmental, motor control, neurodevelopmental).
- The room is too noisy, and Joey hates the way the metal scissors feel in his hand (sensory).

Data collected by the occupational therapist during the evaluation process indicate that Joey lacks a consistent hand preference and cannot smoothly open and close the scissors. The occupational therapist may use an if–then sequence to help develop intervention and the desired outcome. For example, *if* Joey developed a consistent hand preference for fine motor tasks and developed the ability to stabilize his hand with his ring and little fingers, *then* the ability to cut using scissors would emerge. Ongoing data collection and assessment of the intervention (e.g., formative evaluation) is essential to determine the effectiveness of interventions.

Learning Activity 5.10 provides a description of a preschooler who has some issues with his occupational performance. Readers are encouraged to consider various hypotheses for the child's performance and behaviors. Learning Activity 5.11 provides further information about using hypotheses in occupational therapy practice.

The occupational therapist analyzes the client's performance using formal observation, assessments, and procedures or some combination of those approaches. Knowledge and skills, theoretical principles of pediatric practice, evidence-based

Learning Activity 5.10. Developing a Hypothesis Using Frames of Reference

Directions: Andrew attends a local preschool for 4-year-olds. He does not sit in his chair during snacks; instead, he screams and runs away, disturbing the mealtime of others.

- What might be reasons for Andrew's behavior?
- Consider each of the following frames of reference, and write a hypothesis consistent with the frame.
- Which frame of reference seems to be the most plausible reason for the behavior?
- What data do you have or need to support your hypothesis?

Frame of Reference	Hypothesis
Behavioral	
Biomechanical	
Cognitive	
Coping	
Developmental	
Motor control/learning	
Neurodevelopmental	
Occupational	
Sensory integration	

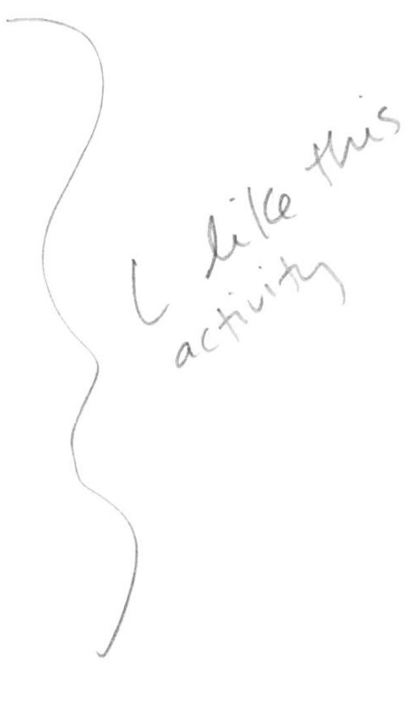

Learning Activity 5.11. Using Hypotheses

- Before beginning an evaluation, do you stop and reflect on several possible hypotheses for the reasons for referral and concerns presented?
- Do you vary evaluation strategies and processes for the young children who are referred for an occupational therapy evaluation? If so, how?
- Multiple frames of reference are used in early childhood occupational therapy practice. With your colleagues, investigate a frame of reference commonly used in early childhood occupational therapy, and present a short in-service about this frame of reference.

practices, and the experience of the occupational therapist all guide clinical reasoning for the therapist's selection and application of theories and frames of reference in the evaluation process (AOTA, 2008b). The evaluation allows the therapist in early intervention or early childhood practice to identify the client's strengths and needs, identify areas of instructional or environmental strengths and barriers, determine additional information that needs to be collected, and develop a hypothesis to explain the person's occupational performance concerns.

Learning Activity 5.12 provides readers with additional resources on frames of reference and decision making.

Choosing Assessments Tools for the Evaluation Process

With all the different assessment tools on the market, how do occupational therapists determine which assessment tool to use? First, the occupational therapist must determine the purpose of the tool. If the child is enrolled in a preschool program, a therapist may want to review the curriculum-based assessment being used by the program. These data may serve the purpose of evaluation for occupational therapy.

Second, if additional information is needed, remember that all tools published are not equal. Therapists should review the assessment manual to determine the technical adequacy of the tool. What is the stated purpose of this tool? Who were the participants used for data collection? How many participants were included in the data collection? Were children with disabilities included? What are the tool's reliability and validity? Is there a racial or cultural bias? For example, a tool that was developed from data gathered in Minnesota may not be appropriate for use in New Mexico because no data indicate that the early childhood population of the states are equivalent.

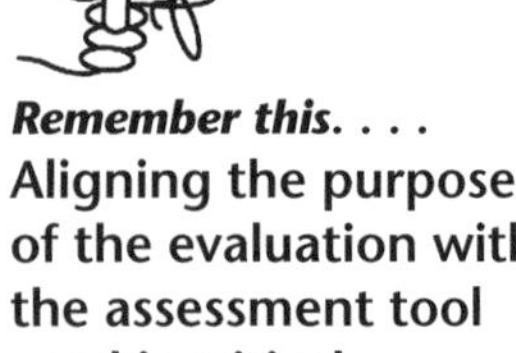

Remember this. . . .
Aligning the purpose of the evaluation with the assessment tool used is critical.

Third, therapists should be aware of the data provided by the test. If the test provides standard scores, but the therapist wants to identify functional skills that the child needs to learn, this test is a mismatch. Aligning the purpose of the evaluation with the assessment tool used is critical (see Table 5.1). Therapists may find authentic assessment methods to provide the data needed. Generally, tests with standard scores are used for determining diagnosis or eligibility. If the child has been determined to be eligible for a program, an occupational therapy evaluation would focus on identifying the child's strengths and needs related to participation in daily living skills and other functional tasks. A standardized measure would not provide this information.

As stated in Box 5.2 and in the previous section, decisions should not be made on a sole measure. Occupational therapists working in states where standardized

Learning Activity 5.12. Further Reading on Frames of Reference

- Read the *Occupational Therapy Practice Framework* (AOTA, 2008b).
- Read about common frames of reference used in early childhood occupational therapy:
  - Kramer, P., & Hinojosa, J. (1999). *Frames of reference for pediatric occupational therapy* (2nd ed.). Philadelphia: Lippincott Williams & Wilkins.
  - Candler, C., Clark, G., & Swinth, Y. (2008). School-based services: What does OT bring to the IFSP and IEP table? *Journal of Occupational Therapy, Schools, and Early Intervention, 1,* 17–23.
  - Handley-More, D., & Chandler, B. (2007). Occupational therapy decision making. In L. L. Jackson (Ed.), *Occupational therapy services for children and youth under IDEA* (3rd ed.). Bethesda, MD: AOTA Press.

scores determine a child's need for service should work with their administration to align this requirement with current practice. Table 5.6 provides a list of some of the more common assessment tools used in early childhood.

Determining Need for Occupational Therapy Intervention

On the basis of federal and state laws, teams determine which children are eligible and entitled to early intervention services (IDEA Part C) or special education (Part B). The decision for eligibility and entitlement rests on the IFSP or IEP team, as stated in IDEA. The team determines the child's (and family's, under Part C) needs, establishes goals and outcomes, and then determines the services necessary to meet those goals and outcomes. Occupational therapists do not evaluate children to "qualify" them for occupational therapy (Polichino et al., 2007); the occupational therapist's evaluation provides information for the team decision about entitlement and services needed for the child to benefit from the educational program.

The occupational therapy evaluation provides information to the team about the child's performance and functioning in the natural or least restrictive environment and about the child's participation in preschool activities. The team uses this information to develop the plan (e.g., the IFSP under Part C or the IEP under Part B). Occupational therapy services are added to the plan or program when the team determines that the expertise of the occupational therapist is necessary for the child to meet the identified outcomes or goals. Occupational therapists need to be familiar with their state practice act and perspectives of the state regulatory board regarding who is able within their state to make recommendation(s) for occupational therapy services and the frequency and duration of occupational therapy services. This information should be shared with all members of an IFSP or IEP team. The occupational therapist must be a part of this decision in some states and, as a matter of best practice, should participate in the decisions in all circumstances. Differences of opinion between the occupational therapist and the team, if not reconciled, should be brought to the attention of the program supervisors, agency administration and, if necessary, the state regulatory board.

After the child has been determined to need occupational therapy services, ongoing evaluation is important. "Ongoing assessment and documentation of progress towards identified goals makes therapists accountable for the right thing—improved performance in children's daily lives" (Linder & Clark, 2000, p. 137). Assessment and documentation answer such questions as, Is the child making progress?

Is this intervention strategy effective? If the child's rate of progress continues at this rate, will the goal or outcome be met? Formative evaluation and progress monitoring allow the therapist to change the intervention plan if the child's performance is not improving at the rate necessary for the child to meet the goal or outcome. The term *ongoing assessment* is used in education to indicate that student data are continually collected to make decisions. This information is necessary for decision making during the IFSP periodic review or the IEP annual meeting, in which the occupational therapist, as a member of the IFSP or IEP team, should participate.

Occupational therapists may evaluate children in multiple areas of development. Occupational engagement as the focus of occupational therapy fits well with the current focus in early childhood on functional abilities used in natural environments. The areas that are the focus of the evaluation are generally influenced by the agency, early childhood team, and therapist's knowledge and skills.

Role as a Team Evaluator

Often, agencies use the knowledge and skills of an occupational therapist and include him or her as a team evaluator of a child's development, including physical, adaptive, social–emotional, communication, cognitive, and sensory development. These agencies recognize that as health and human services professionals, occupational therapists are also knowledgeable about problems that can interfere with child development, such as social–emotional disorders, developmental delays, neurological impairments, genetic disorders, muscle disorders, and musculoskeletal problems. Occupational therapists may serve as members of an evaluation team to administer screenings and diagnostic assessments to determine eligibility. In this role of evaluator, the occupational therapist is bringing his or her knowledge to the team and would participate in the team report on the child. The results of the screening or evaluation may lead the team to recommend an occupational therapy evaluation to explore certain areas in more depth, and a specific occupational therapy report may be written, depending on the requirements of the state regulatory agency.

Some agencies use the occupational therapist as a multidisciplinary team member who administers various components of the evaluation and provides an occupational therapy evaluation, either during the initial eligibility evaluation, by virtue of what they address and evaluate, or as a separate evaluation after the IFSP is developed and an occupational therapy evaluation is identified as one of the services needed to support the desired outcome. For example, the early intervention team may be trained in administration of the Developmental Assessment of Young Children (Voress & Maddox, 1998). Various members of the team, including the family, will conduct the initial evaluation of the child to determine whether the child has a significant delay that entitles him or her to early intervention services in that state. The occupational therapist may be a part of that initial multidisciplinary team but may also provide further assessment of a specific area, such as feeding, in which the child is significantly delayed. This process may occur in states in which the same team members provide the evaluation and the services to children and families or states in which all evaluations are the responsibility of the ITD program and intervention services are provided by the provider network.

Some states have multidisciplinary teams that provide evaluations, write the IFSP, and then contract with various agencies (a provider network) to provide the identified services. Because the evaluation is completed, the therapist from the contracted agency should be able to begin services, collecting ongoing data as part of the service provision. Reevaluation should occur after several months unless a significant change or event occurs earlier.

Occupational therapists may serve as service coordinators for IFSP services or as case managers for families, depending on their agency procedures. In this arrangement, occupational therapists generally facilitate necessary evaluations but may also participate as evaluators, according to agency or state procedures. For example, as a service coordinator for a medically fragile infant, the occupational therapist may work with the hospital to determine the evaluations that have been conducted by that agency and then identify whether any additional ones need to be conducted before writing the IFSP. Considering evaluations from other agencies is effective and decreases the need to repeat tests.

Teams need to be clear on the occupational therapist's role. Occupational therapists should have established competency in any assessment method they will use as part of that role. Documentation of the results needs to indicate their role in the evaluation and their findings.

One issue that arises in relation to these practices is the billing of services, particularly in early intervention. For example, as part of a multidisciplinary team, occupational therapists, along with a second professional (perhaps a speech–language pathologist [SLP]), participate in the initial eligibility evaluation of an infant for the ITD program. The occupational therapist may bill Medicaid, if the child is Medicaid eligible, for an occupational therapy evaluation or an extended developmental assessment. The SLP could bill for a speech–language evaluation. These types of arrangements are usually detailed in the interagency agreements between state agencies that are part of the state early intervention application for federal funding under the Part C program.

Early Childhood Outcomes

How can early intervention and early childhood programs document effectiveness in helping a child achieve the desired outcomes and benefit to the family? In the 1990s, as the government moved toward a results-oriented and accountability approach, the importance of measuring outcomes at all levels emerged. Data from national studies on secondary students with disabilities showed outcomes indicating that special education services were not preparing students for independent living and work experiences (Wagner, Blackorby, Cometo, & Newman, 1993). The government became more results oriented in an attempt to determine the quality and effectiveness of services, so measures were developed to gather data on a regular and consistent manner across the nation.

In 2003, OSEP funded the Early Childhood Outcomes Center (ECO). The purpose of ECO "to promote the development and implementation of child and family outcome measures for infants, toddlers, and preschoolers with disabilities" (ECO, 2004, p. 2). This accountability system established outcomes for children and indicators for family benefits. States were required to report on child outcomes and family indicators beginning in 2005.

Parts B and C have three outcomes for children. For the child outcomes in Parts B and C, states had to determine the percentage of infants and toddlers with IFSPs or the percentage of preschoolers with IEPs (or IFSPs) who demonstrated improvements on the following three outcomes:

1. Positive social–emotional skills (including social relationships)
2. Acquisition and use of knowledge and skills (including early language, communication, and literacy)
3. Use of appropriate behaviors to meet their needs (including self-care skills and moving in environment).

Data can be collected in different ways, but most states use the Child Outcome Summary Form (COSF) developed by ECO (2009) to collect data on children with IFSPs and IEPs. This form is not an assessment; it requires those who have participated in evaluating the child to score the child's current functioning at a minimum of entry into the program and exit from the program. At least 6 months must elapse within these two points to complete the form. States may collect data more frequently than program entrance and exit (e.g., at 6-month IFSP review meetings) for their own purposes. The COSF allows teams to determine whether the child has shown progress toward the desired outcomes, has lost skills, or remains the same. In essence, the initial COSF can be thought of as a measure of baseline performance or current level of performance on entrance to the program. The exit COSF can be thought of as the status at program exit. To guide decision making, a decision tree was created using the COSF (Figure 5.1).

States also need to report on family outcomes for Parts B and C. States must report the percentage of families who believe that participating in Part C early intervention services has helped them

- Know their rights,
- Effectively communicate their children's needs, and
- Help their children develop and learn.

States must also report the percentage of parents with a preschool-age child with an IEP (Part B) who report that schools facilitated parent involvement. These data, generally collected by surveys, are a way to hold agencies and states accountable for providing services that families value and are in line with the law and parent safeguard procedures. For further information on ECO, including tutorial modules and crosswalks for various assessment tools, the reader is directed to the ECO Web site (www.fpg.unc.edu/~eco/index.cfm). The site is user friendly and contains maps about national collection methods and samples of forms used.

Role of Occupational Therapy in Promoting Early Literacy as an Outcome of Early Childhood Programs

One of the most important outcomes for early childhood programs is the development of early literacy. Early childhood is a critical time for developing the prerequisites for literacy. Occupational therapists working in early childhood have the ability to promote early literacy within their services. Making explicit that early

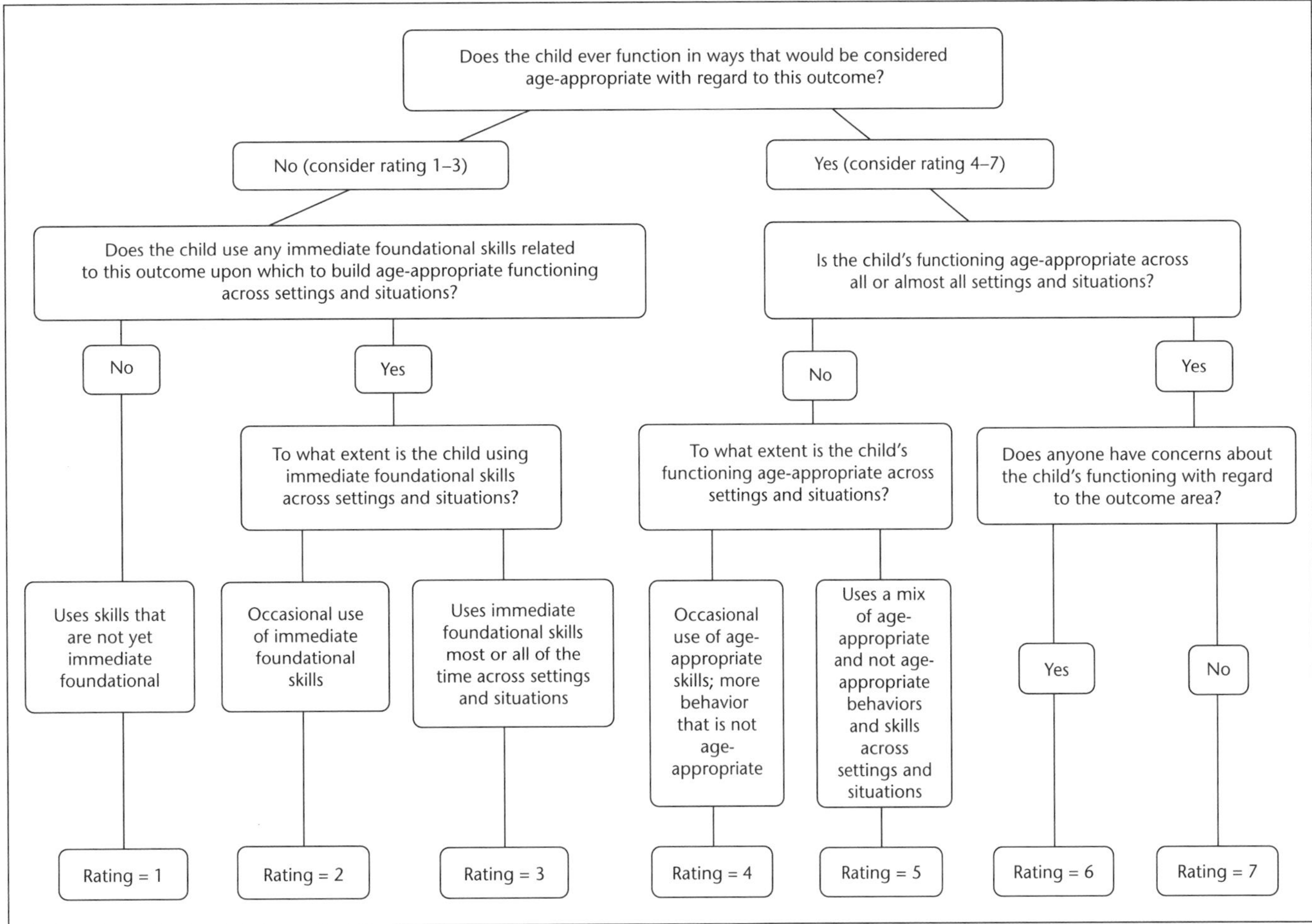

Figure 5.1. Decision tree for determining early childhood outcomes.

Source. Early Childhood Outcomes Center (2009). Used with permission.

childhood occupational therapy is relevant to literacy is critical in shaping the profession's role in literacy, especially reading and writing. Many of the interventions and activities that occupational therapists use enhance literacy skills (i.e., reading, writing, speaking, and listening). Occupational therapists use books, writing tools, alphabet toys, and assistive technology devices to enhance literacy skills. Research has shown that knowledge of the alphabet is the best predictor of reading success both during the first year of reading (Adams, 1990) and later (Honig, 2001). Research has also shown that the single most important activity to enhance literacy is shared book reading (Bus & van IJzendoorm, 1995; Dwyer & Neuman, 2008; Sulzby, 1985). Smith and Dickinson (2002) identified a study by Dickinson and Sprague (2001) in which "the quality of support for writing when children were 4 years of age was found to be related positively to their language and literacy growth at the end of kindergarten" (p. 269).

As providers of early services to children and families, occupational therapists may have a strong influence on the development of preliteracy skills in children from a very early age. Moustafa (1997) found that children who are from low-income families may begin kindergarten without having read a book; by contrast, children from middle-income homes have had approximately 6,000 books read to them.

Gettinger and Stoiber (2008) reported research by Whitehurst and Lonigan (2001): "Children who enter kindergarten with limited literacy and language skills rarely catch up and are at high risk of being referred for special education services" (p. 198).

Occupational therapists can work with programs to emphasize reading and writing readiness. Dickinson and Sprague (2001) collected data from programs with high accountability, such as Head Start. Reading was observed in only 65% of the classrooms. Consequently, even when teachers knew that they were being observed, researchers did not observe any reading in 35% of the early childhood settings (e.g., Head Start) over a 2-day period. In 58% of the classrooms, they did not observe any individual or small-group reading time. They also found that teachers in 72% of the rooms did not display efforts to support writing.

Marvin and Wright (1997) found that many parents of children with disabilities did not expect that their children would become literate. They also found that the parents and child care providers were less likely to encourage children with a speech–language disability to ask questions or answer the adult's questions during book reading than they were to encourage children without speech–language disabilities. Children with other disabilities were not as likely to point to pictures in the book. Opportunities for drawing and writing activities were even more discrepant than for typically developing peers. Many children were not exposed to early writing or reading materials by parents, day care providers, or even professionals working with them. The children with disabilities did not have the same opportunities to play with writing materials or have books read to them as frequently as their typically developing peers. Even the professional staff did not encourage age-appropriate preliteracy tasks for the children, possibly because the children were developmentally delayed.

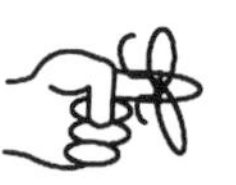

Remember this. . . .
Occupational therapists are in a unique role to encourage reading and writing activities through their knowledge of underlying visual–perceptual, visual–motor, fine motor coordination, and interaction skills.

Occupational therapists are in a unique role to encourage reading and writing activities through their knowledge of underlying visual–perceptual, visual–motor, fine motor coordination, and interaction skills. The Center for Early Learning Literacy (www.earlyliteracylearning.org/) has information for therapists and for families. Box 5.5 lists some of the activities that occupational therapists working in early childhood could encourage and facilitate with families and caregivers to promote literacy in reading, writing, speaking, and listening.

Case Studies

Many different models are used by occupational therapists across the United States to evaluate and serve children in early childhood. Occupational therapists may practice in homes, child care centers, community preschools, special education early childhood programs, or government-funded programs such as Early Head Start or Head Start. The case studies presented here may vary from your setting, but the processes of the *Framework* (AOTA, 2008b) should be woven into any practice area.

Early Intervention Evaluation

Zeva, an occupational therapist, is a member of the early intervention team. Other members include an early childhood teacher, social worker (who also functions as the service coordinator), physical therapist, and SLP. Their agency received a referral for a 6-month-old infant, Jonah. Jonah's pediatrician made the referral because

Box 5.5. Activities Occupational Therapists Use to Support Literacy in Early Childhood

The following activities encourage literacy in young children:

- Read aloud to a child.
- Have child find pictures (e.g., book, magazine, photo album, catalog).
- Have child identify colors (e.g., book, magazine, catalog).
- Have child use pointing a finger to identify pictures in a book.
- Have child make a choice regarding which book to read first.
- Have child turn pages of book.
- Have child point to letters of the alphabet that they know (usually letters in his or her name).
- Talk about the story (Why? What? Who?).
- Talk about the feelings of the people in the story.
- Recite rhymes.
- Perform finger plays.
- Scribble or draw on an easel (or paper on refrigerator).
- Use crayons or short pencils for drawing.
- Play with magnetic letters or small wooden letters.
- Use finger paints to form simple lines and shapes.
- Encourage the child to draw simple lines and shapes (e.g., imitate, copy).
- Copy letters of the child's name.
- Play with toys for drawing and writing such as Magna Doodle, Etch-a-Sketch.
- Use assistive technology (e.g., switches, computers, bent markers, adapted pencils).
- Position crayons or writing instruments in the child's hands.
- Use a light box to illuminate the child's work.
- Have child "sign" his or her name to the work.
- Have child "read" store signs or logos while riding in the car.

Jonah was not eating and was not gaining weight. Jonah lives with his mother, Maria, and his maternal grandmother, Jenna.

The agency has provided training to all the team members so that they are familiar with evaluations for eligibility. As the designated service coordinator, the agency social worker makes the initial contact with the families to orient them to the early intervention program and gather the family's concerns and priorities. Jonah does not have a known disability (e.g., no medical condition or diagnosis), so he will be evaluated to determine whether there is a developmental delay. The team will identify two people who will make the home visit and conduct the initial eligibility evaluation to determine whether Jonah is eligible as a child with a disability. (Jonah's state does not serve at-risk children in the ITD program.) Because Jonah has a feeding concern, Zeva and the early childhood teacher, Rosa, are identified as the team's primary evaluators.

Zeva called Jonah's mother, Maria, before the evaluation. They discussed Maria's concerns about Jonah's development and feeding. They reviewed Jonah's schedule and routines and identified the best time of day for the evaluation. They talked about the family's active role in the evaluation and who would be present for the assessment. Zeva and Maria discussed the assessment tool, and on the basis of Maria's concern about Jonah's nutrition, Zeva decided to include a screening tool for nutrition.

Zeva and Rosa arrived at Jonah's home during the predetermined time. They talked with Maria and Jenna about Jonah's birth, medical, and developmental history while Jonah warmed up to the visitors. Maria facilitated his participation in the evaluation, using his toys when necessary. Zeva and Rosa observed the interaction and scored Jonah's skills as he played with his mother. Jonah's cognitive, communication, physical, adaptive, and social–emotional development were documented by the occupational therapist and early childhood teacher during this natural interaction with the mother and grandmother. At times, they prompted Maria about items that were on the assessment tool. For example, Maria was given a mirror toy and asked whether Jonah would smile at his reflection

Because feeding was the primary area of concern, further information was gathered in that area. Zeva held Jonah while Maria prepared his bottle. While holding him, Zeva was able to check Jonah's postural tone, balance reactions, and reaction to other people's touch. While Maria fed Jonah, Zeva observed Jonah's feeding skills and his interactions with his parent and his self-regulation as he was eating. Zeva noted significant discrepancies in Jonah's sucking and swallowing skills. In addition to Zeva's role as a team evaluator to determine developmental performance and eligibility for services under Part C early intervention, she identified a need for a more in-depth occupational therapy evaluation of Jonah's feeding skills. Zeva interviewed Maria and Jenna to learn more about Jonah's strengths and needs in the area of feeding and eating.

Before leaving the home, Zeva and Rosa scored the assessment tool and provided Maria and Jenna with a general summary of Jonah's skills in the areas of cognitive, communication, physical, social–emotional, and adaptive skills. Because Jonah's evaluation was conducted as the mother facilitated Jonah's skills during play and the evaluators coached her, Maria felt she was a member of the team and that her concerns were being addressed. Together, Zeva and Maria set a time during the next week for Zeva to return for a second observation of Jonah's developmental skills and for a further occupational therapy evaluation of Jonah's oral–motor skills. (A second observation is often important with infants and young children because their performance can change or their initial performance may have been unreliable because of fear of strangers.) Zeva referred Maria to a dietitian on the basis of the results of the nutrition screening. Vision and hearing had already been addressed by the pediatrician.

Rosa explained to Maria and Jenna that a written summary report would be sent to them within 2 weeks. A date was scheduled within the next 3 weeks for a meeting to discuss Jonah's strengths and needs as well as any family needs identified during the family-directed assessment. An IFSP would be developed at that time and would contain outcomes that correspond to the family's initial concerns. Identified services will be provided to Jonah through the system used by his state.

Preschool Evaluation

Angel started child care at age 3 when her mother, LaDonna, returned to work. After 4 weeks of attending day care, Angel's child care provider was concerned that Angel was having difficulty with language skills, fine motor skills, and imitating motor actions. Angel's parents agreed to an evaluation by the local education agency and signed the consent form for a full and individual evaluation.

Reini is the occupational therapist who serves the school district in which Angel's child care is located. An occupational therapy evaluation was requested as part of the eligibility determination evaluation. Reini received the referral for Angel and contacted the child care center and Angel's parents to discuss their concerns (i.e., gathering information for the occupational profile). According to the parents, Angel had no history of medical, health, or developmental concerns. Reini asked the child care provider to identify the daily routines and activities at the day care and agreed to observe Angel during the small-group playtime and table time activities. Reini also scheduled a visit to the home during LaDonna's day off. LaDonna described the family routines and activities. They agreed that Reini should come in the afternoon when Angel awoke from her nap.

Reini arrived at the child care center at the agreed-on time and observed the child care provider, Angel, and other children. Watching Angel's performance during the natural routine and activities allowed Reini to analyze the activity demands, Angel's performance skills, and the child care provider's instructions. Reini was able to observe how the child care provider interacted with all the children and how behaviors were reinforced and promoted or discouraged and not allowed.

Because the child care center did not use a specific curriculum-based approach, Reini brought an assessment tool with her and was able to score most of the items during her 30-min observation. After the observation of Angel's performance skills during the natural activities, Reini spent some time with Angel and three same-age peers who were playing together. Reini used dynamic assessment principles during this interaction.

Dynamic assessment uses a test–teach–retest sequence to facilitate a child's skills in activities where difficulty is observed. For example, Angel had difficulty stringing the Cheerios on a piece of yarn during her day care tabletop activity. In the small group, Reini had Angel put Cheerios on a type of plastic lace called *spaghetti string*. Because this lace was stiffer, the task was easier, and Angel could put three Cheerios on the string. When the yarn was reintroduced, Angel could put one Cheerio on it. Initially, Angel had difficulty with this task, but when the task was reintroduced and taught with a modification, she could perform the new task. When the initial task was presented again, Angel was able to perform the task correctly at least once. Dynamic assessment allowed the evaluator to identify effective interventions as well as determine how quickly the child was able to respond to the instruction and intervention. Angel appeared to be a good candidate for intervention because she could modify her performance with minimal physical or verbal prompting. Modeling was an important strategy to use with Angel to enhance her performance.

Reini talked with the child care provider about Angel's performance and discussed the provider's initial concerns. The observations of Angel's performance skills were validated through this interview. Reini made suggestions to enhance Angel's fine motor and preliteracy skills (e.g., sit her next to a peer who can model the desired behavior; use short and chubby crayons to help her grasp them; encourage tearing, pushing, and squeezing with Play-Doh).

Reini met with LaDonna to observe Angel's skills in the home. (*Note.* Not all states will allow a portion of the evaluation in the home because preschool services are under Part B and are related to the child's academic and functional performance in connection with the curricular expectations of the educational environment.)

Although Angel demonstrated some delays at home, she was able to perform more skills independently in the home than in the child care environment, indicating that generalization of skills to other settings was not yet emerging.

LaDonna volunteered that she had been searching Web sites for information on developmental skills and was aware that Angel was delayed in her language, play, and fine motor skills. She was interested in suggestions to increase Angel's skills in those areas.

Reini shared her findings with LaDonna. Angel's current performance was significantly delayed, according to peers and developmental standards. She responded favorably to dynamic assessment, indicating that some of the skills could be facilitated using scaffolding methods (e.g., verbal prompts, modifications). Reini believed that Angel would demonstrate a positive response to interventions with an occupational therapist.

Reini completed her occupational therapy report, and this information was included in the multidisciplinary evaluation report. In her report, Reini followed the AOTA *Guidelines for Documentation of Occupational Therapy* (AOTA, 2008a) and IDEA requirements. The major headings that she used are listed in Appendix 5.A (Appendixes 5.B and 5.C are also provided as samples). Readers should refer to the documentation forms used by their agencies.

Reini met IDEA requirements by using multiple methods of evaluation (e.g., observation, interview, and testing). Reini followed the process identified in the *Framework* (AOTA, 2008b) by including data gathered during the occupational profile, analyzing Angel's occupational performance, and interpreting the data as they related to the initial concern. Reini followed her agency's guidelines by including information about the curriculum (e.g., what needs to be taught), instruction (e.g., strategies or interventions that would be appropriate to facilitate Angel's participation in her environment), and environmental modifications that would enhance Angel's performance. On the basis of the parent's and caregiver's concerns and Angel's performance, Reini outlined Angel's strengths and needs and suggested programming to increase Angel's skills in the areas of her needs.

Reini knew that if Angel was eligible for special education services, the IEP team would consider the occupational therapy report when making the final decision about Angel's services. She planned to attend the IEP meeting and would work with the team to develop functional, meaningful goals for Angel.

Conclusion

Occupational therapists evaluate and assess infants, toddlers, and preschoolers under early childhood services. Although services may vary according to the program setting, federal mandates, and state practice act regulations, the focus on promoting health and participation through engagement in occupations should be consistent throughout occupational therapy practice. Engaging the child in play, preliteracy activities, eating, dressing, and other activities and occupations of their daily routine are primary outcomes of occupational therapy services in early childhood programs. "All people need to be able or enabled to engage in occupations of their need and choice, to grow through what they do, and to experience independence or interdependence, equality, participation, security, health, and well-being" (Wilcock & Townsend, 2008, p. 198).

How Very Far We Have Come: Away From Home (1965–1968)

When Dan (as he now preferred to be called) was 15, he decided that he wanted to attend the state school for students with disabilities. He felt (and correctly so) that he had learned all he could from the "little school" that had been established by his mother and others. The Main Street School had grown to serve many children but still met in the church basement and, despite efforts, was not an accredited private school. Dan wanted to go to college, and he needed to graduate from an accredited school.

This year Congress had passed new legislation that for the first time authorized grants to state institutions and state-operated schools for children with disabilities. An infusion of federal money and federal oversight would strengthen the state school. Lydia was hesitant, but she could not deny Dan opportunities that she could not supply. When Dan was 6, she thought she could get him admitted to public school. Now, these many years later, she realized that this was the opportunity, even if it met Dan living away from home.

Annie and Mark didn't want Dan to go, either. Mark was now taller than either older twin, and he defended Dan vigorously whenever anyone made fun of him or attempted to belittle him. He was worried about Dan being bullied at the school. Dan reassured his siblings, quelled whatever fears he had, and attended the state residential school, which was 120 miles away.

At the state school, which had benefited from the new federal funding and new teachers, Dan discovered an affinity for math. He had always done well in math, but now he excelled and took special advanced correspondence courses that the math teacher arranged for him and monitored. His social world also expanded. Although he had always been included in family activities, not attending public school had always set him apart. Now, he socialized with teenagers from all over the state and realized, in many ways, how fortunate he had been to have a family such as his. Although federal legislation the next year established federal grant programs for local schools to serve students with disabilities, Dan decided to stay at the state school, where he knew the quality of the education offered and had made many friends.

Fraternal twins Dan and Annie graduated from high school in 1968, never having attended the same school.

Questions

1. How did the Elementary and Secondary Education Act Amendments of 1965 change the educational opportunities for children with disabilities?
2. In addition to providing grant funds to state schools to serve students with disabilities, the Elementary and Secondary Education Act Amendments of 1966 also established what other entities? Why is this important?
3. What other events occurred during this time frame that influenced how people with disabilities were thought of, considered, and treated?

References

Adams, M. J. (1990). *Beginning to read: Thinking and learning about print.* Cambridge, MA: MIT Press.

American Occupational Therapy Association. (1995). Clarification of the use of the terms assessment and evaluation. *American Journal of Occupational Therapy, 49,* 1072.

American Occupational Therapy Association. (2004). Occupational therapy services in early intervention and school-based programs. *American Journal of Occupational Therapy, 58,* 681–685.

American Occupational Therapy Association. (2005). Standards of practice for occupational therapy. *American Journal of Occupational Therapy, 59,* 663–665.

American Occupational Therapy Association. (2008a). Guidelines for documentation of occupational therapy. *American Journal of Occupational Therapy, 62,* 684–690.

American Occupational Therapy Association. (2008b). Occupational therapy practice framework: Domain and process (2nd ed.). *American Journal of Occupational Therapy, 62,* 625–683.

Anderson, S., Boigon, S., Davis, K., & deWaard, C. (2007). *Oregon Project for Preschool Children Who Are Blind or Visually Impaired* (6th ed.). Medford: Southern Oregon Education Service District.

Ayres, J. (1989). *Sensory Integration and Praxis Tests manual.* Los Angeles: Western Psychological Services.

Bagnato, S. (2006). Formalizing informed clinical opinion assessment procedures is more likely to yield accurate results. *Endpoints, 2*(3), 1–2. Retrieved September 16, 2009, from www.dec-sped.org/uploads/docs/conference/2008_handouts/ASM199%20W22_Research%20Foundations_CJ%20for%20EI%20Eligibility.pdf

Bagnato, S. (2007). *Authentic assessment for early childhood intervention.* New York: Guilford Press.

Bagnato, S., Neisworth, J., & Munson, S. (1997). *Linking assessment and early intervention: An authentic curriculum-based approach.* Baltimore: Brookes.

Bailey, D., McWilliam, R., Aytch Darkes, L., Hebbeler, K., Simeonsson, R., Spiker, D., et al. (1998). Family outcomes in early intervention: A framework for program evaluation an efficacy research. *Exceptional Child, 64*(3), 313–328.

Bayley, N. (2005). *Bayley Scales of Infant Development* (3rd ed). San Antonio, TX: Harcourt Assessment.

Beery, K., Buktenica, N., & Beery, N. (2006). *Beery VMI* (5th ed.). La Mesa, CA: Jerome M. Sattler.

Bricker, D. (2002). *Assessment, evaluation, and programming system for infants and children* (2nd ed.). Baltimore: Brookes.

Bus, A. G., & van IJzendoorn, M. H. (1995). Mothers reading to their three-year-olds: The role of mother–child attachment security in becoming literate. *Reading Research Quarterly, 40,* 998–1015.

Clark, G. F. (2008). The Infants and Toddlers With Disabilities Program (Part C of IDEA). *OT Practice, 13*(1), CE-1–CE-8.

Crepeau, E., Cohn, E., & Schell, B. (2003). *Willard and Spackman's occupational therapy.* Philadelphia: Lippincott Williams & Wilkins.

Dickinson, D. K., & Sprague, K. E. (2001). The nature and impact of early childhood care environments on the language and early literacy development of children from low-income families. In S. B. Neuman & D. K. Dickinson (Eds.), *Handbook of early literacy research* (pp. 263–280). New York: Guilford Press.

Dodge, D., Colker, L., & Heroman, C. (2002). *Creative Curriculum® for Preschool* (4th ed.). Washington, DC: Teaching Strategies.

Dodge, D., Rudick, S., & Berke, K. (2006). *The Creative Curriculum® for Infants, Toddlers, and Twos* (2nd ed.). Washington, DC: Teaching Strategies.

Dunn, W. (1999). *Sensory Profile: Users manual.* San Antonio, TX: Psychological Corporation.

Dunn, W. (2000). Best practice philosophy for community services for children and families. In W. Dunn (Ed.), *Best practice occupational therapy* (pp. 1–9). Thorofare, NJ: Slack.

Dunn, W. (2002). *Infant/Toddler Sensory Profile: Users manual.* San Antonio, TX: Psychological Corporation.

Dunn, W. (2006). *Sensory Profile School Companion.* San Antonio, TX: Harcourt Assessment.

Dunst, C., Bruder, M. B., Trivette, C., Hamby, D., Raab, M., & McLean, M. (2001). Characteristic and consequences of everyday natural learning opportunities. *Topics in Early Childhood Special Education, 21,* 68–92.

Dwyer, J., & Neuman, S. (2008). Selecting books for children birth through four: A developmental approach. *Early Childhood Education Journal, 35,* 489–494.

Early Childhood Outcomes Center. (2004). Considerations related to developing a system for measuring outcomes for young children with disabilities and their family. Retrieved April 21, 2010, from www.fpg.unc.edu/~eco/pages/papers.cfm#developingasystem

Early Childhood Outcomes Center. (2009). *Decision tree for summary rating discussions.* Retrieved July 14, 2009, from www.fpg.unc.edu/~eco/assets/pdfs/Decision_Tree.pdf

Elementary and Secondary Education Act Amendments of 1965, Pub. L. 89–313.

Elementary and Secondary Education Act Amendments of 1966, Pub. L. 89–750.

Fisher, A. (2005). *Assessment of motor and process skills.* Hampton Falls, NH: AMPS Project.

Folio, G., & Fewell, R. (2000). *Peabody Developmental Motor Scales* (2nd ed.). Austin, TX: Pro-Ed.

Frankenberg, W., Dodds, J., Archer, P., Bresnick, B., Maschka, P., Edelman, N., et al. (1990). *Denver II.* Denver, CO: Denver Developmental Materials.

Furuno, S., O'Reilly, K., Hosaka, C., Inatsuka, T., Allman, T., & Zeisloft, B. (2004). *Hawaii Early Learning Profile (HELP): Birth to 3.* Palo Alto, CA: VORT Corporation.

Gettinger, M., & Stoiber, K. C. (2008). Applying a response-to-intervention model for early literacy development among low-income children. *Topics in Early Childhood and Special Education, 27*(4), 198–213.

Giangreco, M., Cloninger, C., & Iverson, V. (1998). *Choosing outcomes and accommodations for children* (2nd ed.). Baltimore: Brookes.

Greenwood, C., Carta, J., Bagget, K., Buzhardt, J., Walker, D., & Terry, B. (2008). Best practices in integrating progress monitoring and response to intervention concepts into early childhood systems. In A. Thomas & J. Grimes (Eds.), *Best practices in school psychology V* (pp. 535–547). Bethesda, MD: National Association of School Psychologists.

Greenwood, C., Carta, J., Walker, D., Hughes, K., & Weathers, M. (2006). Preliminary investigations of the application of the early communication indicator (ECI) for infants and toddlers. *Journal of Early Intervention, 28,* 178–196.

Grisham-Brown, J., Hemmeter, M., & Pretti-Frontczak, K. (2005). *Blended practices for teaching young children in inclusive settings.* Baltimore: Brookes.

Haley, S., Coster, W., Ludlow, L., Haltiwanger, J., & Andrellos, P. (1992). *Pediatric Evaluation of Disability Inventory.* Boston: PEDI Research Group.

Hammill, D., Pearson, N., & Voress, J. (1993). *Developmental Test of Visual Perception* (2nd ed.). Austin, TX: Pro-Ed.

Handley-More, D., & Chandler, B. (2007). Occupational therapy decision making. In L. L. Jackson (Ed.), *Occupational therapy services for children and youth under IDEA* (3rd ed.). Bethesda, MD: AOTA Press.

Hardin, B., & Peisner-Feinberg, E. (2001). *Early Learning Accomplishment Profile examiner's manual (LAP–E).* Winston-Salem, NC: Kaplan Press.

Hardin, B., & Peisner-Feinberg, E. (2004). *Learning Accomplishment Profile (LAP–E).* Winston-Salem, NC: Kaplan Press.

Hinojosa, J., Sproat, C. T., Mankhetwit, S., & Anderson, J. (2002). Shifts in parent–therapist partnerships: Twelve years of change. *American Journal of Occupational Therapy, 56,* 556–563.

Honig, A. (2001). *Teaching our children to read.* Thousand Oaks, CA: Corwin Press.

Individuals With Disabilities Education Improvement Act of 2004, Pub. L. 108–446, 20 U.S.C. § 1400 *et seq.*

Jackson, L. (Ed.). (2007). *Occupational therapy services for children and youth under IDEA* (3rd ed.). Bethesda, MD: AOTA Press.

Johnson-Martin, N., Attermeier, S., & Hacker, B. (2004). *The Carolina curriculum for infants and toddlers with special needs* (2nd ed.). Baltimore: Brookes.

Johnson-Martin, N., Jens, K., Attermeier, S., & Hacker, B. (1990). *Carolina curriculum for preschoolers with special needs* (2nd ed.). Baltimore: Brookes.

Kaminski, R., & Good, R., III. (1996). *Dynamic indicators of basic literacy skills.* Eugene: University of Oregon.

Knox, S. (1997). Knox Preschool Play Scale. In L. D. Parham & L. S. Fazio (Eds.), *Play and occupational therapy for children* (pp. 35–51). St. Louis, MO: Mosby.

Kramer, P., & Hinojosa, J. (1999). *Frames of reference for pediatric occupational therapy* (2nd ed.). Philadelphia: Lippincott Williams & Wilkins

Linder, T. (1993). *Transdisciplinary play-based assessment: A functional approach to working with young children* (2nd ed.). Baltimore: Brookes.

Linder, J., & Clark, G. F. (2000). Best practices in documentation. In W. Dunn (Ed.), *Best practice occupational therapy* (pp. 135–146). Thorofare, NJ: Slack.

Losardo, A., & Notari-Syverson, A. (2001). *Alternative approaches to assessing young children.* Baltimore: Brookes.

Macy, M. G., Bricker, D. D., & Squires, J. K. (2005). Validity and reliability of a curriculum-based assessment approach to determine eligibility for Part C services. *Journal of Early Intervention, 28,* 1–16.

Martin, N. (2006). *Test of Visual–Perceptual Skills (TVPS–3).* Novato, CA: Academic Therapy Publications.

Marvin, C., & Wright, D. (1997). Literacy socialization in the homes of preschool children. *Language, Speech, and Hearing Services in Schools, 28,* 154–163.

McLean, M. (2005). Using curriculum-based assessment to determine eligibility: Time for a paradigm shift? *Journal of Early Intervention, 28,* 23–27.

McLean, M., & Crais, E. (2004). Procedural considerations in assessing infants and preschoolers with disabilities. In M. McLean, M. Wolery, & D. Bailey (Eds.), *Assessing infants and preschoolers with special needs* (pp. 45–70). Columbus, OH: Prentice Hall.

Miller, L. (2006). *Miller Function and Participation Scales.* San Antonio, TX: Harcourt Assessment.

Moustafa, M. (1997). *Beyond traditional phonics: Research discoveries and reading instruction.* Portsmouth, NH: Heinemann.

Moyers, P. A., & Dale, L. M. (2007). *The guide to occupational therapy practice* (2nd ed.). Bethesda, MD: AOTA Press.

National Association for the Education of Young Children, & National Association of Early Childhood Specialists in State Departments of Education. (2003). *Early childhood curriculum, assessment, and program evaluation: Building an effective, accountable system in programs for children birth through age 8.* New Brunswick, NJ: Authors.

Neisworth, J. T., & Bagnato, S. J. (2004). The mismeasure of young children: The authentic assessment alternative. *Infants and Young Children, 17,* 198–212.

Newborg, J. (2004). *Battelle Developmental Inventory* (2nd ed.). Scarborough, OH: Thomson Nelson.

Parks, S., Furuno, S., O'Reilly, K., Inatsuka, T., Hosaka, C., & Zeisloft-Falbey, B. (1994). *Hawaii Early Learning Profile (HELP).* Palo Alto, CA: VORT Corporation.

Peterson, N. (1987). *Early intervention for handicapped and at-risk children: An introduction to early childhood special education.* Denver, CO: Love.

Polichino, J. E., Clark, G. F., Swinth, Y., & Muhlenhaupt, M. (2007). Evaluating occupational performance in schools and early childhood settings. In L. Jackson (Ed.), *Occupational therapy services for children and youth under IDEA* (3rd ed., pp. 23–58). Bethesda, MD: AOTA Press.

Rous, B., & Townley, K. (Eds.). (2006). *Building a strong foundation for school success: Kentucky's early childhood continuous assessment guide.* Frankfort: Kentucky Department of Education.

Salvia, J., & Ysseldyke, J. (1995). *Assessment in special and remedial education* (6th ed.). Boston: Houghton Mifflin.

Schultz-Krohn, W. (1997). Early intervention: Meeting the unique needs of parent–child interaction. *Infants and Young Children, 10,* 47–60.

Schultz-Krohn, W., & Cara, E. (2000). Occupational therapy in early intervention: Applying concepts from infant mental health. *American Journal of Occupational Therapy, 54,* 550–554.

Shackelford, J. (2002). *Informed clinical opinion* (NECTAC Notes No. 10). Chapel Hill: University of North Carolina, FPG Child Development Institute, National Early Childhood Technical Assistance Center. Retrieved March 8, 2009, from www.nectac.org/~pdfs/pubs/nnotes10.pdf

Slentz, K., & Hyatt, K. (2008). Best practices in applying curriculum-based assessment in early childhood. In A. Thomas & J. Grimes (Eds.), *Best practices in school psychology V* (pp. 519–534). Bethesda, MD: National Association of School Psychologists.

Smith, M. W., & Dickinson, D. K. (2002). *Early language and literacy classroom observation toolkit.* Baltimore: Brookes.

Sparrow, S., Balla, D., & Cicchetti, D. (2007). *Vineland Adaptive Behavior Scales–II.* Bloomington, MN: Pearson Assessments.

Squires, J., Potter, L., & Bricker, D. (1997). *Ages and Stages Questionnaires: Social and emotional.* Baltimore: Brookes.

Squires, J., Potter, L., & Bricker, D. (1999). *Ages and Stages Questionnaires* (2nd ed.). Baltimore: Brookes.

Sulzby, E. (1985). Children's emergent reading of favorite storybooks: A developmental study. *Reading Research Quarterly, 20,* 458–481.

Ulrich, D. (2000). *Test of Gross Motor Development* (2nd ed.). Framingham, MA: Therapro.

Voress, J. K., & Maddox, T. (1998). *Developmental assessment of young children.* San Antonio, TX: Psychological Corporation.

VORT Corporation. (1995). *HELP for Preschoolers Checklist.* Palo Alto, CA: Author.

Wagner, M., Blackorby, J., Cameto, R., & Newman, L. (1993). *What makes a difference? Influences on postschool outcomes of youth with disabilities: The third comprehensive report from the National Longitudinal Transition Study of Special Education Students.* Menlo Park, CA: SRI International.

Wetherby, A., & Woods, J. (2006). Early social interaction project for children with autism spectrum disorders beginning in the second year of life. *Topics in Early Childhood Special Education, 26,* 67–82.

Whitehurst, G. J., & Lonigan, C. J. (2001). Emergent literacy: Development from prereaders to readers. In S. B. Neuman & D. K. Dickinson (Eds.), *Handbook of early literacy research* (pp. 11–29). New York: Guilford Press.

Wilcock, A., & Townsend, E. (2008). Occupational justice. In E. B. Crepeau, E. S. Cohn, & B. B. Schell (Eds.), *Willard and Spackman's occupational therapy* (11th ed., pp. 192–199). Baltimore: Lippincott Williams & Wilkins.

Woods, J., Kashinath, S., & Goldstein, H. (2004). Effects of embedding caregiver-implemented teaching strategies in daily routines on children's communication outcomes. *Journal of Early Intervention, 26,* 175–193.

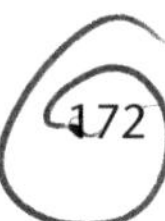

Appendix 5.A.
Sample Headings for Occupational Therapy Report for Infants and Toddlers

Demographic Information

- Child's name, date of birth, school district/early intervention agency, parents' name, parents' address.

Referral Information

- Date and source of referral, concerns for referral, diagnoses/conditions, pertinent medical history, precautions/contraindications.

Evaluation

- Occupational profile
  - Who is seeking occupational therapy service, why services are being sought (e.g., concerns and priorities), which areas of occupations are successful/problematic, where occupational performance is successful/problematic, outcomes
- Analysis of occupational performance
  - Each area of occupation is screened/evaluated to determine the child's strengths/needs in this area. Information is documented in this chart.

Area of Occupation	Brief Summary of Performance
Self-help skills	Include sleep, eating, bladder/bowel, ability to calm
Education	*Note.* May not be applicable if child is not in early intervention or child care program
Work	*Note.* May not be applicable for child's age; list if child has chores
Play and leisure skills	Visual attentiveness to mobile, reaching for toes
Social participation	Interactions with others

- Developmental performance
  - Specific evaluations conducted in areas of concern should be listed (see sample chart below). For a child with feeding concerns, for example, areas of concern could be broken into drinking, biting and chewing, and spoon and finger feeding. The child's current performance is then listed under strength or needs areas.

Area of Concern: Feeding
Sources of Data: Parent interview, observation, and medical reports
Date(s) of Evaluation: September 15, 2009

Area	Skills Present (Strengths)	Skills Not Mastered (Needs) based on peer/developmental or medical expectations
Drinking	• Drinks from a cup • Drinks milk and juice	Difficulty coordinating suck/swallow/breathe when drinking—has to stop after every sip to breathe
Finger feeding	• Attempts to pick up easily dissolvable foods • Can bring hands to mouth to suck on fingers	• Has difficulty grasping foods due to tightness (spasticity) in fingers • Attempts to bring hand to mouth with food but typically cannot release food into mouth

Summary

- Occupational performance
  - Describe the child's occupational performance as it relates to performance skills, performance patterns, context(s), activity demands, and client factors
  - Describe underlying factors causing the functional performance limitations in occupational performance.

Recommendations

- Provide specific skills child needs to learn. Describe why this child does or does not need the expertise of the occupational therapist.

Appendix 5.B.
Sample Headings for Early Childhood Team Report

Demographics

- Name, birth date, parents' names, addresses, parents' phone number

Team Members and Agency Staff

- List all team members, their roles, and their agencies. Include team members from other agencies who have sent a report.

Child's Strengths and Interests

- List characteristics about this child that were noted during the evaluation. Parent input can be included.

Concerns and Priorities

- List parents', caregivers', and other significant individuals' concerns and priorities for this child.

Child Assessments Used and Results

- Data may be entered into this chart for easy reading. List name, title, and agency affiliation of evaluator(s). Include medical reports, if applicable.

Health Status
Assessment/Date
Evaluator
Results

Vision
Assessment/Date
Evaluator
Results

Hearing
Assessment/Date
Evaluator
Results

Physical Development: Large Motor Skills
Assessment/Date
Evaluator
Results
Observations

Physical Development: Fine Motor Skills

Assessment/Date

Evaluator

Results

Observations

Cognitive Development

Assessment/Date

Evaluator

Results

Observations

Communication Development

Assessment/Date

Evaluator

Results

Observations

Social–Emotional Development

Assessment/Date

Evaluator

Results

Observations

Adaptive (Daily Living Skills) Development

Assessment/Date

Evaluator

Results

Observations

Family-Directed Assessment

- If the family participated in a family-directed assessment, summarize the information here. Link the family's concerns, priorities, and resources to build the family's capacity to meet the child's needs.

Summary

- Document whether the child meets eligibility for early intervention services and the criteria met (e.g., medical condition, developmental delay).
- Summarize developmental strengths and needs.

Service Recommendations

- State whether early intervention services are recommended.
- State the general areas of development that need to be addressed.

Appendix 5.C.
Headings for Occupational Therapy Report for Preschoolers

Demographic Information

- Child's name, date of birth, school district, parents' names, parents' address.

Referral Information

- Date and source of referral, concerns for referral, diagnoses/conditions, precautions/contraindications; significant medical history.

Evaluation

- Occupational profile
  - Who is seeking occupational therapy services, why services are being sought (e.g., concerns and priorities), which areas of occupations are successful/problematic, where occupational performance is successful/problematic, outcomes
- Analysis of occupational performance
  - Each area of occupation is screened/evaluated to determine child's strengths/needs in this area. Information documented in the following chart.

Area of Occupation	Brief Summary of Performance Within the Educational Program and Activities
Activities of Daily Living (self-help and living skills)	
Education	
Work	
Play and Leisure	
Social Participation	

- Specific evaluations conducted in areas of concern are listed in the following chart. Data are used to compare the child's performance with the expected performance and document the discrepancy noted.

Data Source	Date	Child's Performance	Expected Performance	Discrepancy

Summary

- Occupational performance
  - Describe the student's occupational performance as it relates to performance skills, performance patterns, context(s), activity demands, and client factors.
  - Describe underlying factors causing the functional performance limitations in occupational performance.
- Educational needs: Describe needs required for the child to receive an appropriate education.
  - *Instruction:* What types of instruction appear most helpful for this child to learn?
  - *Curriculum:* What are the specific skills and concepts the child must learn?
  - *Environment:* What adaptations, modifications, positioning, and assistive technology are needed for student to be successful.

Recommendations

Using the previously mentioned data, describe why this child does or does not need the expertise of the occupational therapist.

CHAPTER 6

Working Where Life Is Lived: Promoting and Using the Rhythms of Daily Life

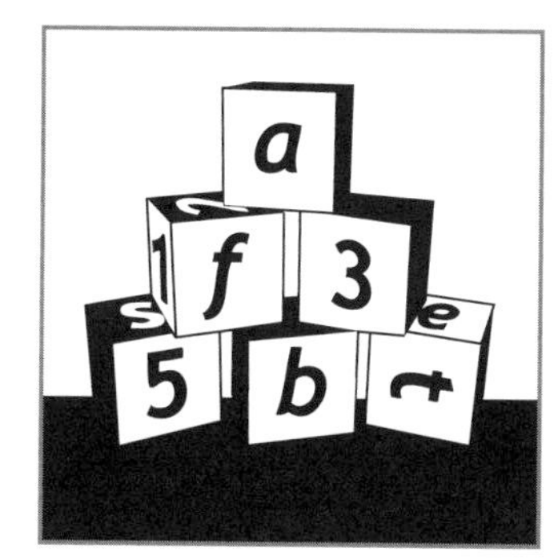

Amy Russell Yun, MS, OTD, OTR/L, and
Barbara E. Chandler, PhD, OTR/L, FAOTA

Learning Objectives

After reading this material and completing the examination, readers will be able to

- Identify the development and attributes of routines;
- Identify routines of daily living and their importance in the lives of young children and their families;
- Delineate what encompasses the natural environment in practice serving young children;
- Delineate relationships among biology, behavior, and occupation in families with young children;
- Identify evidence supporting occupational therapy intervention in practice settings serving the needs of young children;
- Delineate the skill set necessary for working in natural environments, especially as a home visitor;
- Recognize co-occupations and the importance and use of this concept in working with families.

> The whole of human organization has its shape in a kind of rhythm. It is not enough that our hearts should beat in a useful rhythm, always kept up to a standard at which it can meet rest as wholesome *strain* without upset. There are many other rhythms which we must be attuned to: the *larger rhythms* of night and day, of sleep and waking hours, of hunger and its gratification and finally the big four—work and play and rest and sleep, which our organism must be able to balance even under difficulty. The only way to attain balance in all this is actual doing, actual practice, a program of wholesome living as the *basis* of wholesome feeling and thinking and fancy and interests. (Meyer, 1922, cited in Cottrell, 2005, p. 27)

These words of wisdom from one of the founders of occupational therapy are as true now as they were almost 100 years ago. They speak to the power of routines in influencing both mental and physical health. They speak to the power of "doing" as a way of organizing our experiences and, in some ways, of making meaning of them and of our lives.

There are few places in which our routines are as ingrained as in our own homes, where, generally, we are able to create and exert control over the rhythms of our lives. Tenets long held in occupational therapy are emerging as basic concepts in many programs for young children. The use of naturally occurring activities present in daily routines in natural environments is now the mantra of early childhood programs. How shall we enfold others into this perspective while maintaining that which is unique about occupational therapy?

This chapter discusses routines as naturally occurring and evolving phenomena, the various purposes they serve, their complexity, and how they are proposed to be used in early childhood services. Environments of intervention, which are federally mandated to be "in natural environments, including the home, and community settings in which children without disabilities participate" (20 U.S.C. § 1432(4)(G)), and the justification of any intervention not provided in the natural environment are discussed along with the history of home visiting and the skills sets needed for this practice environment. A brief discussion of early brain development and how it is influenced by experience is included. The chapter concludes with ways to foster child and family functioning to support a child's unique needs using the rhythms of a child's and family's day and from a strengths-based perspective.

Routines

Since the founding days of our profession, occupational therapists have been cautioned not to overlook the value of routines:

> [I]t is important that things should move on a regular schedule in order that everything should work smoothly and that there be no confusion. This becomes so much a matter of habit to us that we may fail to realize how beneficial this regular life may be to patients . . . a regular life has much to do with improvement or recovery. (Dunton, 1921, pp. 34, 35)

Indeed, "a regular life" has much to do with the rhythm and flow of a person's day, with meeting instrumental needs, and with reciprocal interactions with others. When a person becomes a parent, this regular life changes dramatically and necessitates a reconstruction of daily life to account for the new roles, expectations, and 24-hr-a-day responsibilities of caring for a small helpless human being—one who speaks a different language of sighs and cries and eyes.

The wisdom of mothers says, "There is a rhythm to this." Slightly used parents (whose children are 6 months old or older) often speak to new parents of "the cycle." They say things like, "Give yourself some things that you have to do every day, but give yourself some breathing room, too" or "There is a rhythm to this. Feed, diaper, sleep, do what you need to do for yourself, *but fast,* diaper, play, feed, diaper, then you can go out if you need to, but it won't be for as long as it used to be, and it won't be as easy with your new traveling partner and his regalia" or "Don't get used to it, you just get into a routine that works for everyone, and then your child grows and develops or needs a new routine." Welcome to parenthood.

In the occupational therapy literature, *routines* have been defined as follows:

> Patterns of behavior that are observable, regular, repetitive, and that provide structure for daily life. They can be satisfying, promoting, or damaging. Routines require momentary time commitment and are embedded in cultural and ecological contexts. (American Occupational Therapy Association [AOTA], 2008, p. 643)

Routines have also been described as "habitual, repeatable, and predictable ways of acting" (Corbin, 1999, cited in Clark, 2000, p. 127s) that "provide a structure that serves to organize and maintain individual lives" (Christiansen & Townsend, 2004, p. 4).

Routines consist of sequential steps, have a temporal aspect, and may or may not have an interactive effect or intersection with the routines of others. Routines usually provide a comforting rhythm to daily life. The patterns of our daily lives in many ways define us. They provide order and may help us feel organized (Fiese et al., 2002). For example, a mother completing her morning routine of shower; dress; drink coffee; apply makeup; and gather briefcase, keys, and purse desires her routine to temporally intersect with her teenage son's morning routine (wake at the last minute, don clothes from yesterday, pick up backpack from floor, and meet Mom at front door). If the sequencing and timing works right, another routine or coroutine then follows, that of the drive to school and then office. "Routines typically involve instrumental communication conveying that 'this needs to be done'" (Fiese et al., 2002, p. 382). If "this" is not done—either in sequence or with a step omitted—the disruption may be minor or may require an alteration in what would have been a subsequent routine. Teenage son forgot glasses, which disrupts the drive to school or office and necessitates a return trip to the house. This disruption is minor and can be seen as a hassle. A major deviation in a routine may have dire consequences, as when a parent who does not usually take the baby to child care encounters traffic, takes an unfamiliar route and, in the haste to get to work on time, forgets the sleeping child in the car seat in the back seat, only remembering when a colleague says, "So how was it doing the morning day care run?"

Routines develop in contexts, exist as long as they serve a purpose, and are altered because of a variety of variables. Self-care, work, leisure, and rest make up the usual mix of daily routines. Caregiving for or of others may be a significant part of a daily routine at different points in people's lives. Routines may also be perceived as boring and, at times, overwhelming, even when acknowledged as necessary to get things done. Who hasn't thought he or she just couldn't bear to stop the car and pick up that gallon of milk on the way home after a long, hard day at work?

Routines involve a level of *automaticity;* that is, they are done automatically, having developed over time to meet a need (Bargh, 1997). This automaticity may mask other aspects of an experience that are important. For example, a parent may have developed a diapering routine with the first child, who was easygoing as an infant and toddler and responded to the sequencing of the routine and the mother's talking while being diapered. A second child may find the positional and sensory aspects of diapering unpleasant and may be overwhelmed by Mom's chattering and thus try to "escape" by wiggling or crying excessively. In this situation, the routine may meet an instrumental need, but other needs are unmet.

Routines can be maladaptive and potentially destructive. Excessive gambling after work, drinking each evening, or watching excessive amounts of television a day are routines that have a high potential of interfering with other, more productive activities, such as paying attention to children in the family.

Because the practice of occupational therapy is concerned with the daily occupations of people, the role of routines in occupational engagement is of great interest. The construction, deconstruction, or alteration of routines or use of existing routines as a means or conduit of intervention are common practices in occupational therapy. For occupational therapists working in early childhood, routines will almost always involve the child and another person, usually a parent but sometimes a sibling, grandparent, or other caregiver. Occupations that involve two or more people are termed *co-occupations* (Zemke & Clark, 1996). Moreover, co-occupations are occupations that "by their very nature, require more than one person's involvement . . . active agency of the participant is requisite; that is both people must be seen as actors to define their activity as co-occupation" (Zemke & Clark, 1996, p. 213). Co-occupations involve social interactions that are reciprocal, are interactive, and may consist of *nested activities,* which are activities that are dependent on one another (Dunlea, 1996; Esdaile & Olson, 2004).

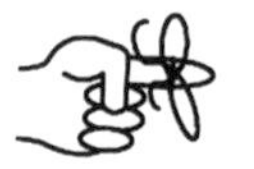

Remember this. . . .
Routines play a role in the construction of the self (Clark 2000, p. 132s).

Co-occupations are extremely important to acknowledge and understand when working with young children and their families and when considering the family routines that unfold daily and that provide rich opportunity for learning and growth. The *Occupational Therapy Practice Framework: Domain and Process* (2nd ed.; AOTA, 2008) advocates that occupational therapists consider co-occupations in an integrated view of the client's engagement in relationships with significant others within the client's context. It is easy to see how this concept applies to practice with infants and young children. According to Dunlea (1996), many occupations in which mothers and young children engage center on "the repertoire of social interactive routines that evolve within the mother–infant dyad" (p. 228). These occupations are reciprocal; the behavior of one partner responds to something previously done by the other partner (Dunlea, 1996; Esdaile & Olson, 2004). This lens should also be applied by occupational therapists working in center-based settings. The way in which teachers or day care providers engage in their occupations shapes the way in which children in their care may participate in their own occupations. Done well, it is like a beautifully orchestrated dance, without the music.

Learning Activity 6.1 provides an opportunity to analyze and apply the concept of co-occupation in a real-life example.

Many studies remind occupational therapists working from a family-centered perspective to consider family routines and rituals (Humphry, 2002; Kellegrew, 2000; Segal, 2004). Increasing evidence has shown this emphasis to be beneficial. Family routines and rituals have been reported as having positive effects on family members' health (Fiese et al., 2002) and promoting family identity and resilience (Schuck & Bucy, 1997). Evans and Rodger (2008) found that families with young children use mealtime and bedtime routines to organize the activity, teach children about social engagement, and facilitate the achievement of daily demands.

en Table Dance

ge 5 stays very busy, engaging in many co-occupations with her
engaging in the occupation of feeding the children, they may
or eating. The way the mother *scaffolds,* or structures,
n it, which in turn shapes what the mother does.
ing different food textures by making green
or she may cajole, gently threaten, dupe,
calling them "egg pudding." The
's participation and performance in

which she and her children

are them with one or more colleagues who have done
your responses and approaches, and identify co-occupations in
which you have participated or currently participate.

1. How do you evaluate performance within co-occupations?
2. How do you consider caregiver components within co-occupations?
3. Identify tools that can assist you with the evaluation process when viewing or considering co-occupations.
4. How *may* or *do* you structure your interventions to address co-occupations of infants and toddlers and their caregivers?

Routines and Rituals: Providing Structure and Meaning to Life

When occupational therapists consider routines, they must consider several issues. What are the form, function, and meaning of the routines for all involved clients? When (the temporal aspects) do clients engage in specific occupations, activities, or tasks? In what order (the sequence of parts of a routine or the sequence of routines) do clients engage in these occupations or activities? Is there a meaning or a purpose to the way clients organize their routines? We must also consider co-occupations embedded within the routine and consider whether the routines are effective for all involved clients. Clark (2000) described routines as playing a role in the construction of the self.

Remember this. . . . **Routines are the activities we use to get things done in our lives. They ebb and flow with our natural patterns, shaping what gets done and when it happens.**

Routines are the activities we use to get things done in our lives. They ebb and flow with our natural patterns, shaping what gets done and when it happens. Routines involve instrumental communication, which conveys information about "what needs to be done." Children learn over time that a weekday routine has certain expectations, that their parents are all about business and there is no fooling around in the morning. Routines require an episodic time commitment in which people give little afterthought to activities after their completion. Routines involve repeating activities over time so that there is continuity in the way they are done and people behave.

Routines are not the same as rituals, although a routine may become a ritual. The *Occupational Therapy Practice Framework* defines a *ritual* as "symbolic actions with spiritual, cultural, or social meaning, contributing to the client's identity and reinforcing values and beliefs. Rituals have a strong affective component and represent a collection of events" (AOTA, 2008, p. 643). Fiese et al. (2002) differentiated between family routines and family rituals in three ways: communication, commitment, and continuity. Rituals involve symbolic communication and may convey a sense of family (group) identity and cohesion. They involve a strong affective component for members of the group and provide continuity in meaning across generations (Fiese et al., 2002). Although specific routines may be forgotten after their completion, routines that turn into rituals often live in the mind of the participants (Fiese et al., 2002). Often there is overlap between routines and rituals, which is illustrated by the example in Box 6.1.

Much of what we know about routines comes from qualitative research designed to gain insight into the lived experience. Anthropologists and sociologists have been studying the development and purposes of routines for a long time. Recent publications in other disciplines have investigated routines in families by applying an ecocultural approach. *Ecocultural theory,* based on the ecological systems perspective (Bronfenbrenner, 1976), proposes that families accommodate or adjust their daily occupations in response to environmental variables and cultural influences (Bernheimer, Gallimore, & Weisner, 1990; Kellegrew, 2000).

Routines may serve protective functions for people, such as helping them cope with pain or illness (Frare, Axia, & Battistella, 2002), maintain health (Denham, 2003; Fiese, 2007), cope with stress or anxiety (Markson & Fiese, 2000), ease burdens associated with disruptions to other routines (Fiese, 2007), and provide a sense of connectedness (Gilis, 1996). Research has suggested relationships between routines and sleep–wake cycles (Sprunger, Boyce, & Gaines, 1985). Routines may serve to protect or buffer children from harmful stress (Fiese & Wamboldt, 2001; Kliewer & Kung, 1998). Routines and rituals provide a familiar structure for the family. Lack of routines or physical disorganization in the environment often leads to temporal and affective disorganization and increased stress levels as more energy and time are spent "getting things done."

Routines develop out of a transactional and reciprocal process of interactions. In considering family routines, those transactions involve a child or children and

Box 6.1. Remembering Dad's Mornings

Jennifer (a friend of the authors) recalled the impact her childhood morning routine had on her. Both of her parents worked. Her father would return each morning from his night-shift job, making sure to send his wife off to her job with a kiss. He would then wake the children, assist them in getting cleaned up and ready for school (often taking time to review homework), fix breakfast for them, and send them off to school. Jennifer could not remember what was specifically involved with the routine. What she did recall was how her father set the mood for the day. She clearly recounted the kiss and that her father played classical music during breakfast every day. She thinks the routine must have involved activities of daily living (e.g., waking, toileting, bathing, dressing, eating, feeding, grooming) and instrumental activities of daily living (e.g., care of others, meal preparation, home management) because "they need to get done." She referred to play being incorporated at times, but other than referencing a few incidents could not describe it on a daily basis or address when shifts occurred. Now in her 30s, Jennifer reflected on the meaning that this "routine turned to ritual" holds for her, leaving her feeling valued and loved. She reproduces aspects of this routine-become-ritual with her own family, hoping to have a similar impact.

an adult, usually a parent. In some cases, an older sibling fills the adult role. It is hypothesized (and accepted by many grandmothers worldwide) that predictable routines contribute to positive outcomes for family functioning. Research has shown that predictable routines help parents feel that they are, indeed, good parents because they are competent in taking care of their children (Brody & Flor, 1997; Seaton & Taylor, 2003). Predictable routines enable parents to keep track of information relevant to their children, whether it is an immunization appointment for an infant or "Meet the Teachers" day at high school. Monitoring of child activities contributes to the sense of competence in the parent role. Participation in ongoing and predictable routines also serves as a bonding mechanism for parents and children (Spagnola & Fiese, 2007). Routines assist children in developing and adapting to their environment. Bellagamba and Tomasello (1999) suggested that young children are more inclined to imitate activities that appear to have purpose.

Caregivers use daily routines to create temporal patterns of action punctuated by outcomes as the context for infants to learn about occupation (Humphry, 2002). Occupations (and routines) are *scaffolded,* or actively structured, by parents so children can participate in them as independently as possible (Primeau, 1998). As the child combines intrinsic capacities into a pattern that meets a need or responds to expectations of others, behavior is said to emerge (Humphry & Wakeford, 2008). Parents foster their children's competence as adults by orchestrating and scaffolding their child's engagement in occupations. This "dance" relies on the interactions of parent and child and the active participation of both. The decisions as to what objects will be available to both parent and child are part of this dance.

> By deciding what objects and people a child can access, in promoting some and limiting other activities, and through organization of daily routines, caregivers create their own socio-cultural niches for children. . . . In this way, caregiving creates a unique ecology for each child and ensures that childhood occupations reflect the cultural characteristics of the group. (Humphry, 2002, p. 175)

An example of scaffolding or active structuring is presented in Box 6.2.

Box 6.2. Scaffolding With Bananas

Unlike the "dreaded squishy scrambled eggs," homemade banana bread is eagerly anticipated and consumed in the family with three children under age 5 described earlier. The children "let" their mother help them. While she turns on the oven and adjusts the oven shelves (a "mommy-only" job), they get the plastic baking pans, bowls, and measuring cups from the bottom cabinets. This recipe, adjusted by mom, amazingly requires one level cup of each of the dry ingredients! Mom gets the ingredients, which are located in higher places, and fills the cups to slightly overflowing. The children "measure" the ingredients by scraping extra sugar and flour into a container to ensure a level measure and empty the cups into the bowl. Mom "opens" the bananas and the 2-year-old peels the fruit (what fun!) and then smashes it with a masher. While she does that, the 4-year-old sifts the dry ingredients into a bowl. Mom deals with the raw eggs. It is a lot more work for Mom to allow some activities and objects and limit others, but the children are learning and feel proud of their accomplishments at the end. Plus, there is banana bread!

Routines With Children

What of the families whose every day involves caring for and raising a child with a disability? Werner-DeGrace's (2004) article on everyday occupations of families with children with autism provides an illuminating perspective: "I began experiencing a sense of shame for not taking the time previously to understand the challenges these families faced at creating, engaging in, and sharing meaning in their families' occupations" (p. 549). The use of naturally occurring routines as the venue for intervention in the homes of infants and toddlers with disabilities through early intervention programs is identified as the preferred means of intervention in almost all early childhood literature (Pretti-Frontczak, Barr, Macy, & Carter, 2003).

A routine is not simply a time of day during which something is done. To identify a routine as simply a time of day does not begin to describe the complexities involved in these seemingly simple acts or the potential for use as a venue of intervention. Although the professional in early childhood may advocate using routines, what does that mean to families? Is it perceived as the best way to help their child? Is it seen as an intrusion in a carefully (or not so carefully) constructed daily life?

"The organizational features of routines . . . linked with other mechanisms of developmental processes" (Spagnola & Fiese, 2007, p. 284) influence child behavior and family functioning. How does intervention focusing on daily routines in the natural environment to address infant and toddler developmental needs intersect with the daily routines of the family? Routines construct order and meaning throughout the day. "Acts as simple as encouraging children to hang up their clothing or put away their toys even when it is a struggle can make the difference between independence (doing) and learned helplessness (having things done for)" (Chandler, Schoonover, Frolek Clark, & Jackson, 2008, p. 1). Routines are the "magnificent mundane" of daily life.

How Do Occupational Therapists Use Routines and Rituals?

Routines and rituals provide occupational therapists with information about a family's group process, cultural and ecological contexts, and interactions among members (Fiese et al., 2002). By appreciating that "learning takes place in the context of relationships," we recognize the needs of infants and toddlers with disabilities to receive "services that enhance rather than disrupt the typical activities unique to each family" (Pilkington, 2006). As such, understanding family routines is a critical aspect of working with families, particularly those with infants or young children.

The early childhood literature suggests that approaches provided within the context of natural environments, which include parents, are effective (Childress, 2004). In a study on reducing challenging behaviors in children with autism, considering family context improved goodness of fit and both the stability and the durability of the interventions (Moes & Frea, 2002). Macy and Bricker (2007) used a single-subject design with three students with disabilities and found that embedding goals into classroom routines improved the social skills of preschool students with disabilities. Embedding is readily accepted by many adults working in early childhood programs as a process of including a facilitating activity into the time and place in which it most naturally fits and enhances specific aspects of that activity or experience of the child (Pretti-Frontczak & Bricker, 2001). Others, especially Dunst (2006); Dunst, Bruder, Trivette, and Hamby (2006); and Dunst et al. (2001), have held that embedding disrupts that which naturally occurs and only that which is already occurring should be used as a venue of intervention. This perspective raises the question of why intervention is necessary if a child's daily routines are already providing everything that is needed for growth and development. Although the first two studies likely provide affirmation for the many occupational therapists who already deliver contextually driven services, note that (1) delivering services in this manner is complex and involves many challenges and that (2) sadly, neither study was done by occupational therapists.

Places of Occupational Engagement

Early intervention services, as a system of service provision, were included in the Education of the Handicapped Act Amendments of 1986 for the first time in a way other than demonstration and pilot projects. Since then, providing early intervention services within settings that include typically developing peers has been emphasized. In 1991, Congress added the language of "natural environments" as part of the definition of early intervention services and required them as a component of the individualized family service plan (IFSP). The Individuals With Disabilities Education Improvement Act of 2004 (IDEA 2004) states that services for infants and toddlers

> to the maximum extent appropriate, are provided in natural environments, including the home, and community settings in which children without disabilities participate. (20 U.S.C. § 1432(I)(4)(G) *et seq.*)

The implementing regulations further define *natural environments* as follows:

> To the maximum extent appropriate to the needs of the child, early intervention services must be provided in natural environments, including the home and community settings in which children without disabilities participate. (34 C.F.R. Part 303.12(b))

IDEA was reauthorized in 2004, but the proposed implementing regulations for Part C of the law, which governs early intervention, have never been approved and were withdrawn in January 2009. Until new regulations are promulgated, states must adhere to the current federal regulations addressing Part C, which were amended in 1999 and reflect the 1997 version of IDEA.

The current implementing regulations require that states have

> (c) Policies and procedures to ensure that—
>
> (1) To the maximum extent appropriate, early intervention services are provided in natural environments; and
>
> (2) The provision of early intervention services for any infant or toddler occurs in a setting other than a natural environment only if early intervention cannot be achieved satisfactorily for the infant or toddler in a natural environment. (34 C.F.R. § 303.167(c)(1)(2))

What does it mean to provide early intervention in a child's home, child care center, or other place where young children and their caregivers or families engage in occupations? What is the meaning or influence of place? Occupational engagement is inextricably bound up with place:

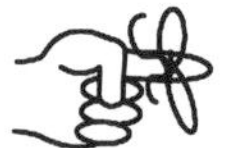

Remember this. . . .
"[T]he link between person, place, and occupation is so strong that one cannot consider occupations without considering that they involve people in places" (Hamilton, 2004, p. 174).

> The contribution of place is an important and necessary element of occupation . . . all occupational situations have three components: places, people (with their attributes, thoughts, feelings, and memories), and the occupations in which people are engaged. Thus, the link between person, place, and occupation is so strong that one cannot consider occupations without considering that they involve people in places. (Hamilton, 2004, p. 174)

Spivack (1973) identified 13 "archetype" places, which elicit and support behaviors that meet basic human needs. The 13 archetype places, in terms of the behavior they support, are those that support the need to sleep, mate, groom, feed, excrete, store, play, route, meet, compete, and work; the need for territory; and the need for shelter. Although not all of these behaviors primarily take place at home, many do, particularly for the family unit.

The home provides another aspect essential for human mental health—the need for privacy. This need is inherent in the territorial approach (Sack, 1992), in which people want private or personal spaces to be safe, nonthreatening, and secure as well spaces over which they have control (Ralph, 1976). When needs are met by the behaviors occurring in context, occupational functioning occurs, and a person has a feeling of satisfaction. When the place or environment does not allow for these needs to be met (too noisy for sleep, too crowded for privacy), needs are unmet and dissatisfaction occurs.

Sociologists use the term *life-world* to denote "the routine patterns and interactions of everyday life" (Hamilton, 2004, p. 180). What is the life-world within each house or home?

> Just as the person brings abilities and capacities and desires mastery and competence in a setting, the place makes occupational performance demands on the individual that can change within the same setting during the course of a day. The demands that a place makes on everyday occupations can vary according to difficulty, complexity, familiarity, intricacy, speed, effort, integration, exertion, responsiveness, timing, span, and scope. (Hamilton, 2004, p. 183)

It is clear that the environment is not a constant state even within what we would like to think of as the safe confines of home. The term *environmental press* was coined to describe the environmental aspects or forces (human and nonhuman) of a place that influence behavior (Murray, 1938). Environments afford opportunities and demand certain patterns of behavior. Environments can organize behavior or can contribute to disorganization. When we speak of using routines in natural environments as the venue of intervention, we presuppose that (1) a routine exists and (2) the routine is facilitative. Common sense and our experiences tell us that this is not always the case. As early childhood occupational therapists, we must then recognize routines that facilitate the growth and development of the child in the context of the family and recognize those routines that do not. We must know how to go about assisting in such a way that intervention fits with the family life, a process that may involve facilitating the development of routines and modifications to the place or space. Indeed, if the family's daily routines wholly supported the child in his or her development, would there be a need for early childhood intervention?

When we provide intervention in the natural environment, primarily the home, do we understand, comprehend, and give credence to what it means to enter someone's home? *Ontological security* is a stable mental state derived from a sense of continuity and order with regard to the events and experiences in one's life (Dupuis & Thorns, 1998). A sense that people and things and, sometimes, places are reliable and will not change contributes to ontological security. Home is one of the most important sources of ontological security; it is "where people feel in control of the environment, free from surveillance, free to be themselves and at ease, in the deepest psychological sense, in a world that might at times be experienced as threatening and uncontrollable" (Kearns, Hiscock, Ellaway, & Macintyre, 2000, p. 361). Home should provide constancy in the social and material environment. It is a space that becomes a place through the daily routines of living that occur there and imbue it with meaning and is a secure base around which identities (e.g., mother, father, daughter, son, sister, brother, cousin) are constructed. Early childhood intervention may occur in other naturally occurring places where children and families go, but most early intervention services are provided in the home.

Home Visiting: Who Are These Strangers at the Door?

Professionals working in early intervention might think they are pioneers on the frontiers of working in the home. That is far from true. Early intervention practitioners are simply the latest in a long line of people who have viewed the natural environment as the logical and most efficacious place or space to influence health and development.

Who Has Been Here Before?

Home visiting to offer aid, guidance, or support has a long history, starting with religious groups visiting the ill as part of their mission in the third and fourth centuries. Much health care throughout history has been provided outside of institutions; one of the main reasons was that the institutions were seen as the source of many ills.

In medieval England, *outdoor relief* meant any health or poverty assistance provided outside of an institution. Some "pauper relief," usually in the form of food or clothing, was brought to the home. In the early days of the United States, in-home care was provided to some children in poverty, but eventually almshouses replaced the home visiting. In the mid-1800s, around the time of the Civil War, there was a shift back to providing support in the home, especially as it related to the effects of poverty.

Religious orders were some of the earliest providers of home care service (Kunstaetter, 1987). The Sisters of Mercy, founded in Ireland in 1831, worked with families in their homes in Ireland and then the United States and continue to do so today. The Congregation of the Sisters of Bon Secours, founded in Paris in 1824, opened hospitals in France, Ireland, and England before coming to the United States and opening a hospital in Baltimore in 1919. This hospital had an outreach mission: Staff went into homes and into the community to help reduce the prevalence of disease, poverty, and unsanitary conditions. Many occupational therapists practicing today were trained at or continue to work in one of the many Bon Secours hospitals or home care facilities currently operating in this country.

Home care was part of the Settlement House efforts of the late 19th and early 20th centuries. In response to rapid urbanization, industrialization, and immigration, settlement houses were established in major cities to provide hygiene, nutrition, health, education, and acculturation information and services to immigrants. Often staffed by upper-class, educated women, to whom gainful employment was denied, the services offered by settlement houses focused on the family and, often, the mother and her children. Occupational therapy traces one of its roots to the settlement houses.

In the early part of the 20th century, public health agencies focused on community needs related to clean water, street sanitation, food safety, and the like. No public agencies, other than hospitals, were addressing the individual needs of citizens. In 1910, the Visiting Nurse Association (VNA) of New York City was established to meet those needs. VNAs were soon replicated across the country in urban areas. Rural areas seldom had accessible health care, and health care for women and children was particularly poor.

Since the 1920s, home care (home health) agencies have employed nurses and therapists to make home visits to those who are homebound (AOTA, 1981). Although most services are to elderly people, who are more likely to be homebound, services to mothers, infants, and children also occur. The focus of home health care for children and their mothers is to promote the daily occupations that occur in a home (Box 6.3).

The legislation that authorized the Infants and Toddlers With Disabilities program stressed providing services in natural environments because it is a well-established way of providing health and developmental knowledge and care, which is the focus of the program. In the 1970s, home visits were made by occupational therapists and others working under the Handicapped Children's Early Education Assistance Act of 1968, one of the roots of IDEA. IDEA reflected the advocacy that had occurred to bring the legislation to passage (e.g., Part C of IDEA is a result of advocacy for "family-centered, community-based, coordinated care"). Part C is based, in part, on the following needs:

Box 6.3. Personal Vignette

I made home visits on Level II fieldwork in 1975, visiting young children and their families as part of an early intervention program (*early intervention* at that time referred to services for children birth to age 5) funded under the Handicapped Children's Early Education Assistance Act. In the 1980s, I and many other occupational, physical, and speech therapists worked in rural and urban health care with children and their families in their homes. The goal then, as now, was to promote health and development through family competency and capacity to meet the needs of the young child.

—Barbara Chandler

Sec. 631. FINDINGS AND POLICY.

(a) FINDINGS.—

Congress finds that there is an urgent and substantial need—

(1) to enhance the development of infants and toddlers with disabilities, to minimize their potential for developmental delay, and to recognize the significant brain development that occurs during a child's first 3 years of life;

. . . .

(4) to enhance the capacity of families to meet the special needs of their infants and toddlers with disabilities; and

(5) to enhance the capacity of State and local agencies and service providers to identify, evaluate, and meet the needs of all children, particularly minority, low-income, inner city, and rural children, and infants and toddlers in foster care. (20 U.S.C. § 1431)

Learning Activity 6.2 asks you to consider how policy and practice are interrelated.

What Skills Make a Welcomed and Effective Home Visitor?

The simple act of entering a client's natural environment adds a dimension of involvement encountered in few other areas of practice. Through the seemingly simple act of entering the client's space, the therapist has already altered the client's place. Often, the act of being observed changes the behavior of clients. Many interventionists, particularly early in working with a client, have arrived at a client's home and found it obvious that the home was not in its "typical" state.

Working in different environments affords occupational therapists different opportunities and challenges and contributes to a different perspective on occupational therapy practice. Home visiting allows us to see where daily occupations

Learning Activity 6.2. Policy and Practice

To care for the child, you must care for the entire family.

—Mary Breckinridge (Frontier Nursing Service, n.d.)

Mary Breckinridge founded the Frontier Nursing Service (FNS) in Kentucky in 1925 after completing a "needs assessment" that consisted of interviewing families and lay midwives in four eastern Kentucky counties, riding more than 700 miles on horseback. Almost 90 years later, the FNS still serves as a model for rural health care. Although not all care is provided in the home now, home care services and home visiting are still essential services (FNS, n.d.).

Questions

One of the purposes of IDEA is to support rural family capacity.

1. What does it mean to be a home visitor, whether you are doing home health or early intervention with young children?
2. How do Mary Breckinridge's words resonate in the language of IDEA related to working with families in their natural environments to enhance their ability to care for their child with special needs?
3. What are the special challenges of working in a rural environment?

are carried out. Although some clinical or center-based programs integrate an occasional visit to families' homes (usually to ensure that the home environment is safe and has the supports that the client needs to be able to return home) in anticipation of discharge to the home environment, single visits differ from programs in which home visiting is the typical mode of service provision. Practice in settings in which home visiting is the primary mode of intervention, such as home health or early intervention, is different. Although the first few visits may offer the therapist the vantage point of "guest," this perspective shifts over time. The number of visits it takes for this transformation to happen varies, but it is clear that there is a point at which guest status evaporates. The client no longer views the visit as a special occasion, and the therapist is integrated into the family's routine for that particular day or time of day.

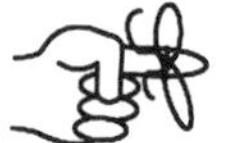

Remember this. . . .
"To care for the child, you must care for the entire family" (Breckinridge, cited in Frontier Nursing Service, n.d.).

What does an occupational therapist need to do to be welcomed and effective as a home visitor? First, recognize that the visitor does not control the environment. The therapist is visiting someone's home. The people who live there control the environment and may be amenable or resistant to modifications. Therefore, the use of environmental or routine modification must be carefully presented. Flexibility is essential in responding to unfolding circumstances. Using a holistic perspective, scanning the environment for potential, and recognizing the possibilities for taking action are essential. The ability to think, reflect, and synthesize quickly is essential for the problem solving that must occur in the environment. Therapists must recognize supports—perceived, embedded and, most important, enacted—to foster growth and competence leading to occupational engagement. Therapists must be comfortable trying assistive technology and hypothesizing what will work. Organization, both of time and the therapist's space within the setting, is needed to work in the natural environment.

Perhaps what is most important is the ongoing clinical reasoning process and therapeutic use of self. Home visiting quickly shows what works and what does not, thereby allowing the therapist's clinical reasoning process to continue to find other solutions to problems. Many of the practices promoted today closely resemble practices advocated more than 100 years ago. Mary Richmond (1899), in *Friendly Visiting Among the Poor,* stated six rules for home visiting, including looking beyond present need to future needs, providing adequate levels and types of help, matching intervention to the particular need, and requiring "maximum feasible participation" from those who are helped. Sound familiar?

Evidence for Practice

Occupational therapists are also faced with the challenge of finding and using evidence to support interventions in situations in which services are mandated to be individualized and contextual. Many fields of study are looking at these same issues, and some of the challenge arises from the need to keep up with current evidence in related fields, such as psychology, education, and neuroscience. Many of the disciplines involved in early childhood practice use criteria to determine whether a practice is evidence based or scientifically based that differ significantly from the criteria used in most of health and medicine, which are based on epidemiology. Buysse and Wesley (2006) defined *evidence-based practice* in the early childhood field as "a decision-making process that integrates the best available research evidence with family and professional wisdom and values" (p. xiv).

Occupational therapists may find themselves discussing evidence-based practice with their colleagues from other professions in early childhood and hear of a practice termed "evidence based" when there is one research article supporting it. What does "best available research" mean? Occupational therapists must understand how colleagues are defining *evidence*. We must also participate in research activities and understand how to evaluate research articles and their conclusions. Learning Activity 6.3 provides some suggestions and resources for locating and evaluating evidence in practice.

Brains of Babies

In 2000, the National Research Council and the Institute of Medicine published *From Neurons to Neighborhoods: The Science of Early Childhood Development* (Shonkoff & Phillips, 2000), which synthesized and updated knowledge from the behavioral,

Learning Activity 6.3. Finding and Using the Evidence

Analyze how you access and use evidence-based information to guide your practice.

Write your responses so that you may refer to them.

1. **How** do you use evidence within practice?
2. **Where** can you access this information (subscriptions, Internet, library)?
3. **What** specific sources do you use?
4. Are there **additional types** of information you should explore?
5. **How** can you obtain this information?

Accessing evidence can be challenging for occupational therapists, particularly those working in smaller, rural areas or in community-based pediatric settings. With the emphasis on evidence-based practice, occupational therapists need to use creativity in solving this challenge. Wise practitioners explore several options.

1. *Form a journal club* with other occupational therapists, and pool your resources to gain access to additional resources. Just like social support can help you with your exercise routine, forming a group is a great way to keep up the motivation for keeping current or finding that answer.
2. *Write a critically appraised topic (CAT) or critically appraised paper (CAP), and investigate.* If several people have similar interests, you could even consider writing a CAT or CAP together. The National Board for Certification in Occupational Therapy (NBCOT) allows practitioners to participate in professional study groups and online study groups designed to advance knowledge through active participation (see www.nbcot.org).
3. *Access state libraries.* Many states provide state employees access to the state library, which is often linked to all the public university libraries in the state. Many local libraries also now offer access to databases in a variety of fields.
4. *Find information on the Internet.* Below is a list of places from which occupational therapists can access relevant evidence.
   - *AOTA:* www.aota.org/Educate/Research.aspx (members only)
   - *Campbell Collaboration:* www.campbellcollaboration.org
   - *CanChild Centre:* www.canchild.ca/
   - *Cochrane Collaboration:* www.cochrane.org
   - *OT CATS:* www.otcats.com/
   - *OT Search/Wilma West Library:* www.aotf.org/html/otsearch.shtml (members only)
   - *OT Seeker:* www.otseeker.com.

social, and neurological sciences related to early childhood development. This study had several key findings:

- Early experiences affect the development of the brain and lay the foundation for intelligence, emotional health, and moral development, but the focus on the period from zero to three is too narrow.
- Healthy early development depends on nurturing and dependable relationships.
- How young children feel is as important as how they think, particularly with regard to school readiness.
- "Society is changing, and the needs of young children are not being met in the process" (Shonkoff & Phillips, 2000, p. 8).

Occupations, Routines, Neuroscience, and Development

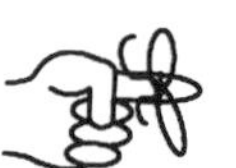

Remember this. . . . **Environmental experience is "recognized to be critical to the differentiation of brain tissue itself. . . . Nature's potential can be realized only as it is enabled by nurture" (Cicchetti & Tucker, 1994, p. 538).**

Recent developments in the neurosciences are pertinent to the discussion of routines in working with young children and their families. All occupational therapists study the structure and function of the nervous system in their professional preparation programs, but because our understanding of the nervous system progresses daily, a review of recent developments in the understanding of the nervous system is in order. Although many experienced therapists may recall the nurture–nature debate, we now know that the debate has essentially been declared a draw (McEwen, 2003; Shonkoff & Phillips, 2000). Environmental experience is "recognized to be critical to the differentiation of brain tissue itself. . . . Nature's potential can be realized only as it is enabled by nurture" (Cicchetti & Tucker, 1994, p. 538). The human central nervous system (CNS) reacts to and modifies itself in relation to the environment (Schore, 2001). A contextual perspective, as suggested by Humphry and Wakeford (2006), allows occupational therapists to understand the maturation of the infant's brain in relation to the environment and to keep in mind that there is a transactional relationship between biological variables, environment, and behavior (Stoff & Cairns, 1996).

We have long known that the infant, toddler, and early preschool years represent an important period for the emergence of self-regulation (Kopp, 1982). Advances in neuroscience are revealing how. Development and brain organization are viewed as "a process of transaction between (1) genetically coded programs for the formation of structures and connections among structures and (2) environmental influence" (Fox, Calkins, & Bell, 1994, p. 681). Understanding the timing of how neurodevelopment typically unfolds is crucial for occupational therapists. Although this section highlights particular information, it is strongly recommended that readers review this process in a recent neuroscience text.

Critical or Sensitive Periods of Development

A *critical period* is a temporally circumscribed period of postnatal development during which specific input is required to establish a particular behavior, presumably because the input plays a central role in establishing the neural system that supports the behavior (Knudson, 2005; Stiles, 2008). Although this concept emerged from animal studies (Harlow, Dodsworth, & Harlow, 1965), it has also been applied to human development, specifically attachment behaviors (Bowlby, 1969) and language. Initially, critical periods were viewed as rigidly adhering to a time window determined by intrinsic factors. More recent research has suggested that development is more plastic, prompting researchers to refer to these periods as *sensitive periods* and suggesting that timing is not the only essential factor contributing to development. Evidence has suggested that the first few years of life are sensitive periods for socioemotional development (Schore, 1994, 2001; Schore & Schore, 2008; Shonkoff & Phillips, 2000).

Genetically, during the third trimester, the human brain is programmed to undergo a growth spurt, which continues through the first 24 months of life (Dobbing & Sands, 1973). Human babies generate significantly more neurons and form more synaptic connections than are actually needed (Schore, 2001). Environmental experiences enable or constrain the structure and function of the developing brain through experience-dependent "pruning." This process, called *competitive interaction,* is environmentally driven. The brain selects connections that are most effective in relaying information (Schore, 1994) and prunes the excess neurons and synapses. As a result, neural circuits used by the CNS remain intact, and unused neural circuits die off (Chechik, Meilijson, & Ruppin, 1999).

Rinaman, Levitt, and Card (2000) suggested that the late prenatal period and early postnatal periods are crucial for limbic–autonomic circuit development. During this period, significant shaping of synapses involved with autonomic nervous system (ANS) functioning, including the subcortical sympathetic and parasympathetic branches and cortical (limbic) components of the CNS, takes place. This development is particularly prominent in the right hemisphere (Chiron et al., 1997; Schore, 1994), which matures earlier than the left hemisphere. Again, understanding that maturation is experience dependent (Schore, 1996, 2000), events that influence ANS–limbic circuit development are embedded in the infant's ongoing experiences, particularly those that involve affect-regulating attachment transactions (Schore, 2001). In other words, the experiences infants and young children have every day contribute to the formation of their nervous systems and therefore have long-lasting effects on their lives (Schore, 1997). Maturation of regulatory systems that support ANS functioning and control emotions manifests behaviorally as emergence of self-regulation skills during the first few years of life (Schore, 1994, 2000).

A main task of infants and young children, particularly those born early, is to maintain homeostasis in the face of a changing environment (Als et al., 2004; Clark, Woodward, Horwood, & Moor, 2008). The ability to survive depends in part on the ability of an organism to maintain homeostasis in the face of constant challenge by intrinsic or extrinsic forces or stressors (Weinstock, 1997). These challenges can be conceptualized as stress: Stressful stimuli cause disruptions in an organism's physiology, whether the threat or stress is real or perceived. The physiological response is consistent with the degree of stress (McEwen & Stellar, 1993).

"Subtle differences in maternal behavior affect infant attachment, development, and physical well-being" (Champoux, Byrne, DeLizio, & Suomi, 1992, p. 254). The interactive regulatory transactions that cocreate a secure attachment bond also influence the development and expansion of the regulatory systems involved in the infant's appraisal of and coping with stress (Schore, 2001). Schore (2001) proposed a psychoneurological model of early development that posits that infant mental health or healthy stable social–emotional development is dependent on biological structural systems, primarily in the brain, that organize during the early months of infancy, in part in response to experienced environmental conditions and events.

Brazelton and Cramer (1990) noted that in critical phases of development, "by learning the baby's 'language,' as reflected by autonomic, state, motor, and attentional behaviors, parents can synchronize their own states of attention and inattention to the baby's" (p. 121). Schore (2001) asserted that direct links exist between secure attachment, development of efficient right brain regulatory functions, and adaptive infant mental health; conversely, traumatic attachment is associated with inefficient right brain regulatory functions and maladaptive infant mental health. In Schore's model, the first few years of life are critical periods for the development of self-regulation: "[S]pecific critical conditions or stimuli are necessary for development and can influence development only during that period" (Erzurumlu & Killackey, 1982, p. 207).

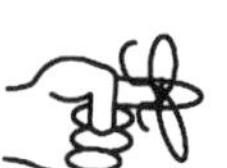

Remember this. . . .
The extent to which parents are responsive and sensitive to the needs of their child is an important predictor of regulatory competence.

Supplee, Shaw, Hailstones, and Hartman (2004) suggested that the extent to which parents are responsive and sensitive to the needs of their child is an important predictor of regulatory competence. They asserted that parent and child factors interact in a bidirectional fashion. Parents of extremely preterm children had more difficulties scaffolding the interactions around cues from their children and providing well-timed support. Preterm children who have difficulties regulating arousal and affect may require more facilitation of soothing and calming from caregivers, but they are likely to send ambiguous signals. Caregivers are likely to react by becoming more intrusive to get their child to respond, which in turn may overstimulate the child. Supplee et al. stated that this overstimulation may set up an aversive social interaction between parties, is likely to have ongoing effects on the development of the mutually rewarding relationship between parent and child, and may become more pronounced over time as challenges to self-regulation increase (Dunn, 2007). Studies such as Supplee et al.'s support the need to address the needs, perceptions, and skills of caregivers in intervention approaches.

Evidence emerging during the past 20 years has advocated the need to focus on the social and emotional needs of infants and young children (Schore, 2001; Schore & Schore, 2008; Shonkoff & Phillips, 2000). This research has led to recommendations to expand early intervention services in ways that build the capacities of families who have children with disabilities and professionals who work with young children. Parents, siblings, extended family members, caregivers, day care providers, therapists, teachers, and early education professionals are all recognized as having profound influences on children's development (Brazelton & Cramer, 1990). These recommendations were reflected in policy changes during the reauthorization of IDEA in 2004.

Using the *Occupational Therapy Practice Framework* to Guide Practice

The *Occupational Therapy Practice Framework* (AOTA, 2008) describes *occupational therapy* as "facilitating interactions among the client, the environments or contexts, and the activities or occupations in order to help the client reach the desired outcomes that support health and participation in life" (p. 647). This approach is congruent with the recommendations from the National Research Council and Institute of Medicine (Shonkoff & Phillips, 2000) and is congruent with the infant mental health approach. Responsive relationships with consistent primary caregivers build positive attachments that support healthy social–emotional development and form the foundation of mental health for infants, toddlers, and preschoolers (Schore, 2001). Landry, Smith, and Swank (2006) discussed contingent responding as a way to provide infants with emotional–affective support. They described such interactions as being characterized by caregivers demonstrating the following behaviors:

- Conveying sensitivity and warmth in voice when talking to the infant
- Supporting the young child's focus, interests, needs, and attention through adult behaviors
- Being attentive to and responsive to the infant's signals and actions
- Verbal encouragement.

Contingent responses do not focus on redirecting the child or restricting interests, nor do they involve physical intrusiveness or harshness toward the child.

The concept of co-occupation is important in working with families on contingent responses (Dunlea, 1996). Occupational therapists help parents and other care providers respond contingently to children within co-occupations. This process profoundly influences the development of children. Co-occupation is not exclusively the verbal messages or the relationships one has with a child. It is the whole picture. Occupational therapy interventions focus on modifying the environment or contexts and activity demands or patterns, promoting health, establishing or restoring and maintaining occupational performance, and preventing further disability and occupational performance problems (AOTA, 2008). The way in which care providers arrange and maintain the physical and social environments, the way in which they select activities, the objects they use and the manner in which they use them, and the timing of activities, as well as the relationships, all influence the trajectory of the child and the care provider's development, health, and well-being.

> Parents and other regular caregivers in children's lives are "active ingredients" of environmental influence during the early childhood period. Children grow and thrive in the context of close and dependable relationships that provide love and nurturance, security, responsive interaction, and encouragement for exploration. Without at least one such relationship, development is disrupted and the consequences can be severe and long lasting. If provided or restored, however, a sensitive care giving relationship can foster remarkable recovery. (Shonkoff & Phillips, 2000, p. 7)

People, Places, and Practices

What is the "whole" of working with parents and children in their home using naturally occurring routines to foster "parent-mediated everyday childhood learning opportunities" (Dunst, 2006, p. 1)? The whole is supporting occupational engagement in context, or putting it all together. Campbell (2004) and Humphry and

Wakeford (2006) reiterated the importance of framing development through a contextual perspective. They suggested that the contextual perspective is valuable for occupational therapy because it emphasizes viewing the elements of the change process—such as the person engaged in occupations, societal efforts, context, cultural practices, and social interactions—as inseparable and interdependent. It can be argued that this perspective is one of dynamic systems—multiple systems interacting and influencing each other. The occupational therapy literature recognizes and emphasizes this interaction and the importance of context and environment as not only contributing to selection of particular occupations but also making profound contributions to the manner in which people engage (Clark et al., 1991; Primeau, 1998).

Building Rapport: Who Is the Client?

The profession of occupational therapy considers clients to be "(1) individuals and other persons relevant to the individual's life, including family, caregivers, teachers, employers, and others who also may help or be served indirectly; (2) organizations such as business, industries, or agencies; and (3) populations within a community" (AOTA, 2008, p. 669). Understanding the perspective of the caregiver is essential in providing family-centered care. Caring for a child with a disability often places increased demands on families (McGuire, Crowe, Law, & Van Leit, 2004; Werner-DeGrace, 2004). Additionally, occupational therapists may be called to provide services for at-risk families, who experience disruptions in parenting capacity through factors such as maternal depression or abuse and neglect. Occupational therapists may work with families who are involved with other state and private agencies, such as social services, departments of behavioral health and developmental services, substance abuse treatment services, and housing support agencies providing services for adult care providers. An organizational client may be the regional Head Start agency with whom the occupational therapist consults related to enrollment of and enhancement of services for young children with disabilities in the Early Head Start, Head Start, preschool, or child care programs.

Pilkington and Malinowski (2002) suggested that occupational therapists discover and use what already exists rather than impose all things new. Developing an occupational profile, followed by an analysis of occupational performance (AOTA, 2008), provides the occupational therapist with the essential information to develop an intervention plan that is individualized, family centered, and contextually driven. When working with young children, the child may be the initial client who brings the occupational therapist to the family, but the parents or other caregivers become clients as well as they participate in and eventually complete any change process.

Mattingly and Fleming (1994) described occupational *storytelling* (describing what has happened) and *story making* (describing what we hope will happen) as strategies used to elicit therapeutic changes. In occupational storytelling and story making, the therapist attempts to elicit a picture of the client as an occupational being (Lawlor & Mattingly, 1998). This process may be used to learn the family's perspective of who the child is and who the family is. It may help the occupational

Learning Activity 6.4. Listen to Our Story . . .

If you were asked whether babies develop in isolation, how would you respond? Most likely, you would laugh. Now, consider how you practice:

- How does the way in which you practice reflect your knowledge of and skills in working with young children in their complex, multilayered environments and contexts?
- Provide several specific examples of how you enact your beliefs about how babies develop and how families incorporate a new baby into their "story."
- Articulate how your evaluations and interventions address the multiple contextual layers and capture information about the child's and family's story.

therapist to identify the child's abilities and how the family scaffolds the child's engagement in occupations. Storytelling and story making also help families explore potential futures for the child and assist in goal development.

Clinical reasoning studies of occupational therapy practice in multiple and diverse settings demonstrated that the client's or patient's story was revealed through the assessment process and then was used to guide the intervention process (Larson, 2000, 2006; Mattingly & Fleming, 1994). Bernheimer and Weisner (2007) suggested that storytelling is more natural for parents, less intrusive, and better than asking parents to complete a form that reduces their and their child's actions to a number or "some of the time."

Learning Activity 6.4 asks you to reflect on how you use story making and storytelling when getting to know and working with families with young children,

Context and Environment

The natural environment may include the child's home, daycare, playgrounds, and the like (Chandler, 2009; Hanft & Pilkington, 2000). When discussing environment and context, the *Framework* suggests that occupational therapists consider "the wide variety of interrelated conditions both external and internal to the client that influence performance" (AOTA, 2008, p. 645). As occupational therapists, we understand that it is not just what one does that matters but that the way in which one engages within specific chosen occupations is also important (Wilcock, 1998). We also understand that "central to the practice of occupational therapy is the way in which therapists conceptualize development of everyday activities" (Humphry & Wakeford, 2008). The activity is not a means to an end—it is the end. It is a valued and meaningful occupation in and of itself.

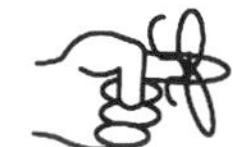

Remember this. . . .
The activity is not a means to an end—it is the end. It is a valued and meaningful occupation in and of itself.

The *Framework* uses the term *environment* to refer to "the external physical and social environments that surround the client and in which the client's daily life occupations occur" (AOTA, 2008, p. 645). The *physical environment* is the "natural and built nonhuman environment and the objects in them" (AOTA, 2008, p. 645). In early intervention, this environment may include the home or child care center and the terrain that surrounds them. Physical aspects such as steps, landings, flooring, toys, and furniture all need to be considered because they may enhance or detract from occupational performance or safety within performance. Experienced

Learning Activity 6.5. Slip Sliding Away . . . or Not

Bella is ready to find out what is on the other side of the living room! It looks like a toy that would be wonderful to pick up and mouth. Which surfaces might facilitate Bella's effort to pivot in prone and get over there?

- Is it a thick shag carpet that challenges movement by providing increased resistance in the form of friction?
- Is it a slick wood floor that may allow Bella to move easily or, possibly, not provide enough traction?
- Or is it a linoleum floor that has seen too many footsteps and is uneven and is potentially hazardous to Bella?

In what way are you explicit about the importance of environmental factors when you educate families so that they are empowered to make good decisions?

---

occupational therapists probably automatically consider these and a multitude of other physical factors. Many therapists are tuned into the influence that sensations in environments have on the ability of infants and young children to self-regulate (Williamson & Anzalone, 2001).

Learning Activity 6.5 asks you to ponder the effects of different environments on occupational performance.

Winnicott (1987) asserted, "There is no such thing as a baby; there is a baby and someone" (p. 88). Social environments are constructed by the presence, relationships, and expectations of people, groups, and organizations with whom the client has contact (AOTA, 2008). It is difficult to discuss the social environment without addressing context. The *Framework* defines *context* as "a variety of interrelated conditions that are within and surrounding the client that influence performance" (AOTA, 2008, p. 645), including cultural, personal, temporal, virtual, physical, and social conditions. The *Framework* reflects the transactional nature of people, occupation, and environments; it is understood that one component cannot be viewed in the absence of the others. As cultural contexts influence how occupations are chosen, prioritized, and organized, occupational therapists need to gain insight into how the client frames issues affecting performance.

Activity Demands

The concept of using activities in particular ways dates back to the beginning of the profession of occupational therapy and, indeed, farther back to roots in moral treatment. In an early text related to occupational therapy, Dunton (1919) cited Robert Chase as follows:

> No feature in the treatment (of the insane) is more highly valued than occupation, systematically applied and judiciously carried out. Work is a law of our nature which demands expression. . . . To understand this one has only to reflect on the depressing effect of inaction, then turn to the satisfaction and strength that result from the agreeable use of one's mental and physical powers. (p. 14)

The *Framework* uses the term *activity demands* to refer to "the specific features of an activity that influence the type and amount of effort required to perform the activity" (AOTA, 2008, p. 634). When analyzing activity demands, occupational therapists consider the following elements:

- Specific objects (and their properties) used in the activity (e.g., soft toy bunny, plastic giraffe)
- Physical space required by the activity (e.g., open floor, playpen)
- Social demands (e.g., ask for "more," use "inside" voice)
- Sequence and timing (e.g., put into container, then put lid on)
- Actions or skills needed to perform the activity (e.g., grip spoon, recognize front and back of shirt)
- How body functions and how body structures are used during the performance of the activity (e.g., bowel and bladder control for toilet training, opposition of thumb for precise grip of crayon).

Activity demands are specific to the way in which an activity is conducted; altering one feature of an activity may change demand in other features. Although occupational therapists have attended to how people engage within occupations, activities, and tasks for almost a century (Dunton, 1921), it appears that this idea is now supported in findings from other disciplines such as biomechanics (Bhat & Galloway, 2007; Lee, Liu, & Newell, 2006), psychology (Als et al., 2004; Fonagy, Gergely, & Target, 2007; Spencer, Vereijken, Diedrich, & Thelen, 2000), education (Brown, Fox, & Brady, 1987), and neuroscience (Schore, 2001).

Dunton (1921), in the previously mentioned quote, referred to the systematic application and judicious carrying out of occupations. Today, occupational therapists refer to this concept as the "just-right challenge" (Ayres, 1973). Activities are provided in a systematic manner that challenges the client in ways that promote therapeutic growth or change but is not so difficult as to frustrate him or her. We achieve this balance by closely observing the client as he or she engages within the occupation or activity, and we modify the activity according to the client's needs. Occupational therapists refer to these processes as *grading* and *adapting* activities.

Grading and adaptation serve different functions in occupational therapy. Occupational therapists *grade,* or incrementally and sequentially increase or decrease, the demands of an activity in ways that stimulate the client's functioning (Crepeau & Boyt-Schell, 2008). This approach is consistent with the establish–restore intervention approach (AOTA, 2008) because its goal is to improve the client's underlying capacities and skills. An occupational therapist might grade drinking from a straw by using a lip block to help pediatric clients establish isolated lip movements while drinking.

Adaptations change demands of an occupation or activity so that they are congruent with the client's ability level and allow him or her to participate in a valued occupation or meaningful activity (Crepeau & Boyt Schell, 2008). An occupational therapist might select a spoon with a shallow bowl to enable a child who has difficulty isolating lip movements to remove food from the spoon to participate in eating. Not only is whether a person engages in occupations, activities, or tasks important, but how one engages within these occupations, activities, or tasks influences health, well-being, and development (Wilcock, 1998).

Learning Activity 6.6. NO MORE Toy Bags on the Floor!

An occupational therapist who works in early intervention is frustrated because her supervisor has informed her that she is not allowed to use "special therapy toys" as part of her intervention. According to her supervisor, the items are not part of the child's natural environment because these toys were not already in the home and thus were inappropriate in early intervention or early special education settings. The occupational therapist's counterargument is that the toys are assistive technology that enable the child to explore his environments in ways that typically developing children do.

Review IDEA 2004, and analyze this issue from both sides of the argument.

- Whose interpretation is most accurate, given what you know about working in natural environments?
- If you had to articulate a rationale to your supervisor, how would you construct it?
- What evidence are you using to support your assertions?

Refer to Chapter 8 for perspectives on use of assistive technology.

Learning Activity 6.6 presents a dilemma that many occupational therapists face related to designing interventions and fostering competence. What would you do?

Occupational orchestration is one way in which environment and context influence the child's development (Pierce, 2000; Primeau, 1998). Clark et al. (1991) described *orchestration* as the way people consciously

> make decisions, every day, about what to do and what not to do . . . they configure activities within time that can be chunked and correspondingly labeled . . . each day, the person creates his or her daily experiences through planning, orchestrating, and participating in occupations. (p. 301)

With children, particularly with younger children, "someone besides the child selects and orchestrates many other childhood occupations, assuming the child will participate" (Humphry, 2002, p. 172). Parents make choices about where and when a child may play; they include or exclude play objects on the basis of their own beliefs and values, thereby actively shaping their children (Pierce, 2000). Often these decisions take into account the needs of other family members and are made in relation to the context in which the family lives. In this way, young children's development is influenced by others who are close to the child.

A child's disability, delay, and temperament "indirectly [affect] a child through the parent–child relationship, which, in turn, holds a reciprocal association with the child's development" (Humphry, 1989, p. 738). Following a parent's lead, always finding something positive to say about the child and the parent, "interpreting" the child to the parent, and facilitating parent interaction were all identified by occupational therapists as ways that they facilitate or foster parent–child interaction (Mayer, White, Ward, & Barnaby, 2002). Some parents and caregivers of children in early childhood programs have disabilities, chronic illness, or other challenges of their own, and occupational therapists may be called in to help them engage in the occupation of caregiving to the children in their care. Box 6.4 suggests resources for parents and caregivers with disabilities that may help them to carry out their parent or caregiver role.

Box 6.4. Resources for Working With Parents Who Have a Disability or Chronic Illness or Condition

Caregivers may have specific challenges of their own, and occupational therapists may be called in to help them engage in the occupation of caring for the children in their care. The following resources may be helpful when working with parent(s) who have a disability or chronic illness or condition:

- Abledata. Resource Center for Parents With Disabilities (www.abledata.com/abledata.cfm?pageid=113573&top=16046§ionid=19326).
- Center for Independent Living Toronto (www.cilt.ca/parenting.aspx). Resources include the Parenting With a Disability Network.
- Developmental Disability.org (www.developmentaldisability.org/ChallengesFacingParents.htm).
- Esdaile, S. A., & Olson, J. A. (2004). *Mothering occupations: Challenge, agency, and participation.* Philadelphia: F. A. Davis.
- Nicholson, J., Biebel, K., Hinden, B., Henry, A., & Stier, L. (2001). *Critical issues for parents with mental illness and their families.* Rockville, MD: Substance Abuse and Mental Health Services Administration. Retrieved from http://mentalhealth.samhsa.gov/publications/allpubs/KEN-01–0109/default.asp
- Parents With Disabilities Online (www.disabledparents.net/).
- Through the Looking Glass center (http://lookingglass.org/index.php). Adaptive baby care equipment and book are available for purchase.

Performance Patterns and Skills

To reiterate, *routines* are "patterns of behavior that are observable, regular, repetitive, and that provide structure for daily life. They can be satisfying, promoting, or damaging. Routines require momentary time commitment and are embedded in cultural and ecological contexts" (AOTA, 2008, p. 643). Routines are designated performance patterns. Routines and other performance patterns influence and are influenced by client factors, activity demands, performance skills, and contexts and environments. The way in which these components interact influences the client's occupational performance. Performance patterns have always been—and always will be—essential to occupational therapy practice.

It is easy to understand that families make changes in response to family events such as the addition of a new family member or a family member's illness. Some evidence suggests that families of children who have disabilities, such as autism, experience disruptions to their routines (Werner-DeGrace, 2004) and that mothers may adapt in ways that jeopardize their own well-being (McGuire et al., 2004). Bernheimer and Weisner (2007) also found that families with children with disabilities make *accommodations,* or intentional adjustments, to sustain their daily routines. The accommodations were made in response to mundane circumstances of everyday life, as opposed to simply being responses to stress. Accommodations occurred in response to high rates of "child hassle," or the effects that a child's problems had on the family's routines. Bernheimer and Weisner (2007) identified six types of impact:

1. Behavioral (e.g., frequent tantrums)
2. Medical (e.g., unusual care demands)
3. Communication skills (e.g., nonverbal)
4. Social appropriacy (e.g., tiresome overtures)
5. Activity rate (e.g., extremely active)
6. Responsiveness. (p. 195)

Kellegrew (2000) found that the way mothers orchestrated daily routines "appeared to be a blended process between accommodation to everyday events and anticipation of future needs" (p. 258). Children's performance skills emerge in this way.

Occupational therapists can educate first-time parents about the use of routines to promote positive behaviors in young children. Routines may be structured as opportunities to help the young child practice and develop skills (Kellegrew, 2000), and they may be modified to incorporate sensory experiences to prepare a child for the main activity, such as feeding (Dunn, 2007). For example, a therapist could work with a family to establish a routine to enable a young child diagnosed with autism to make transitions from one activity to the next. A child in potty training might be able to maintain continence by incorporating a toileting routine into a day care setting. An occupational therapist could help prevent injuries to a child whose parent has a developmental delay by incorporating a prebath safety check routine.

Even though it is common for intervention approaches to focus on routines, Segal (2004) cautioned, "It is not uncommon for families to not follow their [occupational therapists'] suggestions and recommendations" (p. 507). Segal (2004) and Fiese et al. (2002) noted that when families do not follow through with suggestions, the therapist should consider whether he or she has inadvertently suggested altering an important, symbolic family ritual that is important to the family's sense of identity rather than a mundane, instrumental routine, or whether other reasons might explain the resistance. Therapists should also consider the family's dynamics to ensure that parents are not being neglectful of parental duties because of other contextual factors, such as drug abuse or severe depression.

Research on routines has suggested that time constraints are a major consideration for most families (Brotherson & Goldstein, 1992; Kellegrew, 2000). This problem may be even more true for families in which a child has a disability, given that the caregiving demands are higher (McGuire et al., 2004). Kellegrew (2000) found that "children who were less competent in self-care skills were less likely to be given opportunities for self-care independence when time was limited" (p. 258). Occupational therapists need to work with families to assist them in finding times that will work and need to be respectful of families' time constraints. Doing so may positively influence the development of self-care in children with disabilities who require additional practice proficiency. Occupational therapists also need to examine the influence that performance patterns have on the stress levels of young children and the people who care for them.

Areas of Occupation

Occupational therapists in early childhood encounter many occupations in their work in homes, child care centers, preschools, and other environments. Occupations are complex sets of behaviors that have meaning and purpose for a person and include underlying elements that build on one another and interact and involve context, including spatial and temporal dimensions. Children's occupations are "culturally valued, coherent patterns of actions that emerge through transactions between the child and environment and as activities the child either wants to do or is expected to perform" (Humphry, 2002, p. 172).

Occupational therapists must consider many types of occupations in which clients might engage. *Areas of occupation* are categories into which activities or occupations can be sorted and include activities of daily living, instrumental activities of daily living, rest and sleep, education, work, play, leisure, and social participation (AOTA, 2008). It is helpful to remember these categories, their functions, usual location, and ways in which they are demonstrated when working with clients to facilitate health, development, and learning.

Automaticity, Intentionality, and Mindfulness in Occupational Therapy

Automaticity refers to mental operations, including aspects of thinking, feeling, and doing (Bargh, 1997), that, once learned, can be performed with little awareness or conscious effort (Schneider & Shiffrin, 1977). These mental operations and the corresponding performance of tasks take decreased time and effort (Eggen & Kauchak, 1997). The example of driving a car is often cited. Initially, learning to drive takes significant mental energy. Once learned, people can often do the task and other things such as listen to the radio, converse with passengers, and mentally process the day. Automaticity serves a purpose because it allows people to conserve mental energy and multitask.

Intentionality can be defined as the cognitive ability to represent goals beyond the here and now of perception (Rochat, 2007). *Mindfulness* involves intentionally bringing one's attention to the internal and external experiences occurring in the moment (Baer, 2003; Dumas, 2005). In other words, mindfulness involves thinking about how one thinks and feels during a particular situation and considering why one thinks or feels that way. Some evidence has suggested that practicing mindfulness allows people to have a clear, calm mind that is focused on the present moment in a nonjudgmental way (Singh et al., 2006). By examining how one thinks and feels, this approach allows people to see alternative ways of perceiving and responding to events, creating the possibility for implementing those alternatives (Kabat-Zinn, 1994). How intentional are parents as they orchestrate their children's occupations?

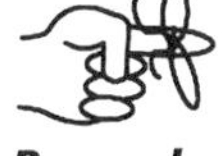

Remember this. . . .
Occupational therapists discover and use what is rather than impose all things new (Pilkington & Malinowski, 2002).

Humphry (1996) reminds us that families are open systems, influenced by outside forces but each having its own boundaries, often acting as a unit, and striving for homeostasis. Pilkington (2006) suggested that occupational therapists "have a clinical plan in mind (and a 'kit bag' of natural learning strategies) to explore with a family" as a strategy that enables therapists to be adaptive in natural environments. She noted that although the occupational therapist may have ideas about how to address the client's occupational performance, rather than use preconceived, "canned" plans, the occupational therapist needs to collaborate with the family and sort through strategies to determine which ones align with the family's needs and "druthers."

As stated earlier, routines are crucial conditions for development in many areas, including influencing the child's CNS. Applying terms from psychoneurobiology (Schore, 1994), routines may be considered *growth facilitating* or *growth inhibiting*. Consider the contextual perspective as applied to our understanding of neuroscience, stress response, self-regulation, and occupation.

Implications of Research on Routines for Occupational Therapy Intervention

Although routines have long been recognized within occupational therapy practice as being important, reviewing how occupational therapists actually use them in intervention is important. Of particular importance is how occupational therapists recognize how performance patterns, such as routines, interact with and influence other aspects of occupational engagement.

Routines, Self-Regulation, and the Reflective Occupational Therapist

Occupational therapists often educate and coach family members to enhance their abilities to read their children's behavioral cues. Occupational therapists should be able to read autonomic signs of stress. This skill is essential in early intervention and early childhood practice because the child client usually does not have sufficient language in his or her communication repertoire and will use nonverbal signals (behavior) to communicate. Preschool-age children, who—one hopes—have more verbal skills, communicate through behavior as well. All behavior is communication (Mims & Chandler, 1992).

Accurately understanding these cues enables caregivers to more effectively communicate with their children and gain insight into their physiological or emotional needs. The occupational therapist may then collaborate with family members to identify the child's habits so that consistent routines can be identified or constructed. The routines enable young children to anticipate what happens next. Through repeated engagement in routines, the child learns and is better able to attain and maintain homeostasis, leading to development of a sense of control over the body and emotions and a sense of mastery. In addition, the child may feel more secure in the relationship and begin to trust the primary caregivers. This trust forms the basis of a secure attachment, which in turn allows the child to engage in the occupations of exploring the environment and play. From the caregivers' perspective, the child behaves more positively, which allows the child and the caregiver to view their relationship more positively.

For example, an occupational therapist is talking with the mother of a young boy with autism about the importance of the physical environment in providing structure. The mother reveals that she is frustrated with trying to teach her son to dress himself: "I know he can do it, but he won't." The mother and occupational therapist examine how the room is set up in relation to the task the boy is being asked to do. Recommendations and problem solving include adding visual cues to help him identify where specific items of clothing can be found. Sorting the clothing to reflect the sequencing or temporal aspect of putting them on was the second suggestion (underwear in the first bin, shirts in the second, pants in the third, socks in the fourth, and shoes in the last bin). As the boy grows taller, the bins can be replaced by furniture (e.g., a dresser). The mother later reports that her son is proud of his ability to dress himself because he knows the "rules" of dressing.

Routines Teach Social Skills

Interventionists first use two classroomwide interventions—developmentally appropriate practices in inclusive early childhood programs and affective interventions—

to influence children's attitudes. When needed, it is also recommended that early childhood occupational therapists use four individualized interventions:

1. *Incidental teaching of social behavior:* Reinforce positive behavior as it is shown (e.g., "I like how you shared with Nora"), and redirect negative behavior and tell child why ("We don't hit").
2. *Friendship activities:* Pair child with another who shares similar interests; adult stays to initially foster interaction.
3. *Social integration activities:* Provide group activities structured around turn taking ("Now you are leader," etc.).
4. *Explicit teaching of social skills* (e.g., "We say 'thank you' when someone gives us a toy," "We wipe our noses with a tissue and then throw it in the trash can").

When a particular intervention is not effective, early childhood practitioners should proceed to another, perhaps more intensive, intervention that might involve additional teacher planning and preparation time and relatively straightforward classroom changes.

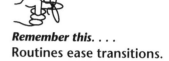

Remember this. . . .
Routines ease transitions.

As babies grow, they experience contact with more people and learn expectations and patterns for social interaction. Greeting routines and caregiving routines help children learn important socialization skills and build communication skills. As the child ages, routines become more complex and provide opportunities to engage in more intricate social interactions. What may initially start off as imitation, in terms of waving "bye-bye," will later evolve into play involving sharing, taking turns, and symbolic communication. The regulation of affect and emotion during regular gatherings will be tempered by the meanings ascribed to repetitive events and the communication of feelings (Fiese, 2007, p. 46).

Routines Ease Transitions

Transitions involve moving from one activity, person, or place to the next and are a fact of life. Most people who live and work with young children know that transitions are often a challenge, particularly when the transition involves leaving a preferred activity for a less preferred one. Introducing a transition routine can help children understand and anticipate the next step.

Intentionally planning or designing transitions is a skill that has huge potential benefits for supporting children's participation and performance in home environments, schools, and other group settings. Although the first step always involves observing the situation to gain information on the child (client factors) and context (to help children anticipate the transition), many professionals use preparatory cues, such as a 2-minute warning, to introduce the idea of a transition in advance of the actual transition. This approach gives the child time to adjust to the idea of changing activities. Using special activities such as transition songs (Table 6.1) or transition games may create a bridge from one activity or caregiver to the next, enabling the child to successfully transition. Consistently using a particular song or activity at a particular time of day may also assist the child. For example, using a book or toy during diaper changing to engage the child's interest may allow him or her to remain still for the duration of the task.

Table 6.1. Songs to Ease Transitions

Clean-Up Songs	Purpose	Tune
Twinkle, twinkle little star, Time to clean up where you are, Put a (fill in the blank—toy, book, etc.) back in its place, Put a smile on your face, Twinkle, twinkle little star Time to clean up where you are	Cleaning up toys	Twinkle, Twinkle Little Star
Clean up, clean up! Everybody, everywhere! Clean up, clean up! Everybody do your share!	Cleaning up toys	Unknown
I see something, I see something Out of place, out of place It does not belong there It does not belong there Where does it go? Where does it go?	Putting things where they belong	Frére Jacques/Where Is Thumbkin?
This is the way we pick up our toys, Pick up our toys, Pick up our toys, This is the way we pick up our toys, Before we go out to play (Fill in the blank with next step; four or five syllables work best.)	Putting things where they belong • May also be used for transitions (e.g., "This is the way we go to lunch. . . ."). • Have children march, clap hands while walking, etc.	This Is the Way We . . .
To make up your own tune, select a familiar children's song. Make sure it involves repetition. Use simple language to phrase your request. Also, be sure your song has the same number of syllables in each line as the original. Be creative and have fun!		

Learning Activity 6.7 provides an opportunity to combine, compare, and contrast current perspectives on early childhood and what constitutes best practice to meet the needs of young children and their families. The reader is referred to Odom and Wolery (2003) for a detailed review of resources related to foundational theories and practices in early childhood programs for children with special needs.

Directions for Research on Routines in Early Childhood

We still have much to learn about the role of routines in terms of supporting child development. Howe (2002) suggested that professionals need to know more about how family routines develop, stabilize, and reorganize over time. More information is needed on how families adapt to major life transitions, such as the addition of a new child or in response to learning that a child has a disabling condition. There is also a need to understand how family routines affect developmental outcomes. Kellegrew (2000) suggested further exploration of the relationship between maternal understanding of the child's present and future occupational potential and home routines to learn which routines promote development. Research should also explore the temporal factors of routines and how they affect performance. Understanding the protective aspects of family routines and how they relate to adaptation and coping could have important implications for health promotion or interventions. Learning Activity 6.8 describes a perspective and a way of thinking that has implications for occupational therapy's role in early childhood programs now and in the future.

Learning Activity 6.7. From Many Perspectives

Review the occupational therapy process from the *Occupational Therapy Practice Framework: Domain and Process, 2nd Edition* (AOTA, 2008).

- Describe ways in which you address the needs of the child and his or her caregivers within their context(s).
- Describe ways in which you promote the capacities of the child and caregivers (parents, guardians, paid care providers).

From Neurons to Neighborhoods (Shonkoff & Phillips, 2000) includes several recommendations from the National Research Council and the Institute of Medicine regarding the provision of services for young children:

- Increase resources allocated to the social and emotional needs of young children.
- Create more well-designed early intervention programs for children at risk.
- Make early intervention services more accessible for working parents.
- Design early intervention programs that deal with the full range of problems that families face, including substance abuse, domestic violence, mental health issues.
- Increase collaboration between disciplines to determine relationships between environmental and bio-genetic factors.

It has been nearly a decade since *From Neurons to Neighborhoods* was published. Reflect on your practice, and describe how your practice reflects or does not reflect the report's recommendations.

Learning Activity 6.8. Facing the Challenges in Early Childhood Practice

Read the following story, and relate it to the future of occupational therapy in early childhood programs and evidence-based practice.

Changing the Water (*Author unknown*)

> A young couple were experiencing difficulties. In a new town, with a new job, no support, money tight, and a new crying baby, they argued frequently.
>
> The maternal grandmother visited the family to see her new granddaughter and witnessed the turmoil. After curt words between the young parents and a slammed door, the grandmother put two pots of water to heat on the stove. She added noodles to one pot, eggs to the other and used the rest to make coffee. She poured two cups. She then gently fished the noodles out into one bowl and the eggs into another.
>
> With the two bowls in front of her daughter, she asked calmly, "What do you see?" "An odd lunch, served much too early," the daughter replied.
>
> "Think again—touch the noodles," said the grandmother.
>
> "Ick, they're limp and sticky!" exclaimed the daughter.
>
> "Now peel the egg." Of course, it was hard boiled.
>
> "OK, Mom, I am not going to talk about what just happened." Her mother simply said, "I want to talk about what I cooked. Each of these objects faced the boiling water, the same adversity so to speak, but each reacted differently, right? The noodles were strong, hard, and unbending. The boiling water changed them, made them, as you said, limp and sticky. The eggs only had their thin shells for protection. They looked the same until you peeled them and found them, of course, to be hardened and dried out from being in the boiling water. And the coffee beans? Same adversity, same boiling water, but they responded uniquely, they changed the water."
>
> "I chose how I respond to adversity," said the grandmother. "I chose to change the water."

- How will we, as occupational therapists, respond to the changes in early childhood services? Will we lead or will we follow?
- How will we "change the water?"

Conclusion

The importance of early childhood in a person's life is gaining greater and greater importance as we understand more about what happens in the first years. If we are to reduce the burden of care and, more important, encourage human potential, we must not be shy about what we bring to these efforts. We understand how to use the rhythm of life through daily occupations to foster health, growth, and development. And we know we should start at the beginning.

How Very Far We Have Come: Annie and Grace (1968–1979)

Annie attended the state university on scholarship and majored in education. She had decided early in life that she wanted to teach. The summer after graduation, she married Coleman, whom she had met in third grade. Coleman had served two tours in Vietnam, had been wounded once, and was happy to be home and married to Annie. While she started her first teaching job, he attended the local community college.

In 1975, their daughter Grace was born. Grace had a cleft palate and, as they would discover over time, several other congenital anomalies. It would be years before the link would be made between these and Coleman's exposure to Agent Orange while in Vietnam. Annie resigned her teaching position when it became clear that Grace's needs were great and Annie's health coverage would not assist. (The insurance company called Grace's condition "preexisting" because she had been born with it.) Coleman quit school and found a steady job with an income greater than what Annie had been making teaching, but money was still tight.

The family was able to get some help for Grace through a mix of charitable institutions, but they also incurred enormous medical bills for several surgeries that Grace required. She was an engaging little girl, and Coleman and Annie wanted the best for her. Annie had an opportunity to substitute teach some days, but no preschool was interested in enrolling Grace because of her special needs. Maggie's daughter, Annie's cousin Corinne, was working at the local Head Start program. Although she taught 4-year-olds, she told Annie that Head Start had to have at least 10% of their enrollment consisting of children with disabilities and that the class for 3-year-olds had openings. Annie was not sure that they were eligible for Head Start, but with all the medical bills, they were. In fact, Grace had just recently been deemed eligible for Medicaid. Annie immediately called Head Start, and Grace was enrolled. While at Head Start, Grace also worked with speech and occupational therapists, who showed the teachers activities that would be helpful for Grace and that could be done every day.

Questions

1. What needs and advocacy led to the establishment of Head Start?
2. When and why did Head Start set aside 10% of its enrollment for children with special needs?
3. How is the development of the Head Start program reflective of the Great Society aspirations of the 1960s?

References

Als, H., Duffy, F. H., McAnulty, G. B., Rivkin, M. J., Vajapeyam, S., Mulkern, R. V., et al. (2004). Early experience alters brain function and structure. *Pediatrics, 113*(4), 846–857.

American Occupational Therapy Association. (1981). The role of the occupational therapist in home health care. *American Journal of Occupational Therapy, 35,* 809–810.

American Occupational Therapy Association. (2008). Occupational therapy practice framework: Domain and process (2nd ed.). *American Journal of Occupational Therapy, 62,* 625–683.

Ayres, J. (1973). *Sensory integration and learning disorders.* Los Angeles: Western Psychological Services.

Baer, R. A. (2003). Mindfulness training as a clinical intervention: A conceptual and empirical review. *Clinical Psychology: Science and Practice, 10*(2), 125–143.

Bargh, J. A. (1997). The automaticity of everyday life. In R. S. Wyer, Jr. (Ed.), *The automaticity of everyday life: Advances in social cognition* (Vol. 10, pp. 1–61). Mahwah, NJ: Lawrence Erlbaum.

Bellagamba, F., & Tomasello, M. (1999). Re-enacting intended acts: Comparing 12- and 18-month-olds. *Infant Behavior and Development, 22*(2), 277–282.

Bernheimer, L., Gallimore, P., & Weisner, T. (1990). Ecocultural theory as a context for the individualized family service plan. *Journal of Early Intervention, 14,* 219–233.

Bernheimer, L., & Weisner, T. (2007). "Let me just tell you what I do all day." The family story at the center of intervention research and practice. *Infants and Young Children, 20,* 192–201.

Bhat, A. N., & Galloway, J. C. (2007). Toy-oriented changes in early arm movements III: Constraints on joint kinematics. *Infant Behavior and Development, 30,* 515–522.

Bowlby, J. (1969). *Attachment and loss: Vol. 1. Attachment.* New York: Basic Books.

Brazelton, T. B., & Cramer, B. G. (1990). *The earliest relationship: Parents, infants, and the drama of early attachment.* Reading, PA: Addison-Wesley.

Brody, G., & Flor, J. (1997). Maternal psychological functioning, family processes, and child adjustment in rural, single-parent, African American families. *Developmental Psychology, 33*(6), 1000–1011.

Bronfenbrenner, U. (1976). *The ecology of human development: Experiments by nature and human design.* Cambridge, MA: Harvard University Press.

Brotherson, M., & Goldstein, B. (1992). Time as a resource and constraint for parents of young children with disabilities: Implications for early intervention. *Topics in Early Childhood Special Education, 12*(4), 508–527.

Brown, W., Fox, J., & Brady, M. (1987). Effects of spatial density on 3- and 4-year-old children's socially directed behavior during freeplay: An investigation of a setting factor. *Education and Treatment of Children, 10*(3), 247–258.

Buysse, V., & Wesley, P. (Eds.). (2006). *Evidence-based practice in the early childhood field.* Washington, DC: Zero to Three.

Campbell, P. (2004), Participation-based services: Promoting children's participation in natural settings. *Young Exceptional Children, 8,* 20–29.

Champoux, M., Byrne, E., DeLizio, R., & Suomi, S. J. (1992). Motherless mothers revisited: Rhesus maternal behavior and rearing history. *Primates, 33,* 251–255.

Chandler, B. (2009). Working where life is really lived. *ADVANCE for Occupational Therapy Practitioners, 25*(6), 8.

Chandler, B. E., Schoonover, J., Frolek Clark, G., & Jackson, L. L. (2008). The magnificent mundane. *School System Special Interest Section Quarterly, 15*(1), 1–4.

Chechik, G., Meilijson, I., & Ruppin, E. (1999). Neuronal regulation: A mechanism for synaptic pruning during brain maturation. *Neural Computation, 11*(8), 2061–2080.

Childress, D. C. (2004). Special instruction and natural environments: Best practices in early intervention. *Infants and Young Children, 17*(2), 162–170.

Chiron, C., Jambaque, I., Nabbout, R., Lounes, R., Syrota, A., & Dulac, O. (1997). The right brain is dominant in human infants. *Brain, 120,* 1057–1065.

Christiansen, C., & Townsend, E. (2004). *Introduction to occupation: The art and science of living.* Upper Saddle River, NJ: Prentice Hall.

Cicchetti, D., & Tucker, D. (1994). Development and self-regulatory structures of the mind. *Development and Psychopathology, 6,* 533–549.

Clark, C. A. C., Woodward, L. J., Horwood, L. J., & Moor, S. (2008). Development of emotional and behavioral regulation in children born extremely preterm and very preterm: Biological and social influences. *Child Development, 79*(5), 1444–1462.

Clark, F. A. (2000). The concept of habit and routine: A preliminary theoretical synthesis. *OTJR: Occupation, Participation and Health, 20*(Suppl.), 123s–137s.

Clark, F. A., Parham, D., Carlson, M. E., Frank, G., Jackson, J., Pierce, D., et al. (1991). Occupational science: Academic innovation in the service of occupational therapy's future. *American Journal of Occupational Therapy, 45,* 300–310.

Corbin, J. M. (1999, January). *The role of habits in everyday life* [Abstract]. Paper presented at A Synthesis of Knowledge Regarding the Concept of Habit, a research conference of the American Occupational Therapy Association, Pacific Grove, CA.

Cottrell, R. (2005). *Perspectives for occupation-based practice: Foundation and future of occupational therapy* (2nd ed.). Bethesda, MD: AOTA Press.

Crepeau, E. B., & Boyt-Schell, B. A. (2008). Analyzing occupations and activity. In E. B. Crepeau, E. S. Cohn, & B. A. Schell (Eds.), *Willard and Spackman's occupational therapy* (11th ed., 359–374). Baltimore: Lippincott Williams & Wilkins.

Denham, S. A. (2003). Relationships between family rituals, family routines, and health. *Journal of Family Nursing, 9*(3), 305–330.

Dobbing, J., & Sands, J. (1973). Quantitative growth and development of human brain. *Archives of Disease in Childhood, 48,* 757–767.

Dr. Seuss (Geisel, T. S.). (1960). *Green eggs and ham.* New York: Random House.

Dumas, J. E. (2005). Mindfulness-based parent training: Strategies to lessen the grip of automaticity in families with disruptive children. *Journal of Child and Adolescent Psychology, 34*(4), 779–791.

Dunlea, A. (1996). An opportunity for co-adaptation: The experience of mothers and their infants who are blind. In R. Zemke & F. Clark (Eds.), *Occupational science: The evolving discipline* (pp. 227–342). Philadelphia: F. A. Davis.

Dunn, W. (2007). Supporting children to participate successfully in everyday life by using sensory processing knowledge. *Infants and Young Children, 20*(2), 84–101.

Dunst, C. (2006). Parent-mediated everyday childhood learning opportunities: I. Foundations and operationalization. *CASEinPoint, 2*(2), 1–10.

Dunst, C., Bruder, M., Trivette, C., & Hamby, D. (2006). Everyday activity settings, natural learning environments, and early intervention practices. *Journal of Policy and Practice in Developmental Disabilities, 3,* 3–10.

Dunst, C., Bruder, M., Trivette, C., Hamby, D., Raab, M., & McLean, M. (2001). Characteristics and consequences of everyday natural learning opportunities. *Topics in Early Childhood Special Education, 21,* 68–92.

Dunton, W. R. (1919). *Reconstruction therapy.* Philadelphia: W. B. Saunders.

Dunton, W. R. (1921). *Occupation therapy: A manual for nurses.* Philadelphia: W. B. Saunders.

Dupuis, A., & Thorns, D. (1998). Home, home ownership, and the search for ontological security. *Sociological Review, 46*(1), 24–47.

Education of the Handicapped Act Amendments of 1986, Pub. L. 99–457, 20 U.S.C. § 1401, Part H, Section 677.

Erzurumlu, R., & Killackey, H. (1982). *Defining critical and sensitive periods in neurobiology.* In R. K. Hunt (Ed.), *Current topics in developmental biology. Neural development, Part III* (Vol. 17, pp. 207–240). New York: Academic Press.

Esdaile, S. A., & Olson J. A. (2004). *Mothering occupations: Challenge, agency, and participation.* Philadelphia: F. A. Davis.

Evans, J., & Rodger, S. (2008). Mealtimes and bedtimes: Windows to family routines and rituals. *Journal of Occupational Science, 15*(2), 98–104.

Fiese, B. (2007). Routines and rituals: Opportunities for participation in family health. *OTJR: Occupation, Participation and Health, 27*(Suppl.), 41s–49s.

Fiese, B., Tomcho, T. J., Douglas, M., Josephs, K., Poltrock, S., & Baker, T. (2002). A review of 50 years of research on naturally occurring family routines and rituals: Cause for celebration? *Journal of Family Psychology, 16*(4), 381–390.

Fiese, B., & Wamboldt, F. (2001). Family routines, rituals, and asthma management: A proposal for family-based strategies to increase treatment adherence. *Families, Systems, and Health, 18,* 405–418.

Fonagy, P., Gergely, G., & Target, M. (2007). The parent–infant dyad and the construction of the subjective self. *Journal of Child Psychology and Psychiatry, 48*(3/4), 288–328.

Fox, N., Calkins, S., & Bell, M. (1994). Development and neural plasticity: Behavioral and cognitive outcomes. *Development and Psychopathology, 6,* 677–696.

Frare, M., Axia, G., & Battistella, P. A. (2002). Quality of life, coping strategies, and family routines in children with headache. *Headache: The Journal of Head and Face Pain, 42*(10), 953–962.

Frontier Nursing Service. (n.d.). *How FNS began.* Retrieved October 11, 2009, from www.frontiernursing.org/History/HowFNSbegan.shtm

Gilis, J. (1996). Making time for family: The invention of family time(s) and the reinvention of family history. *Journal of Family History, 21,* 4–21.

Hamilton, T. (2004). Occupations and places. In C. Christiansen & E. Townsend (Eds.), *Introduction to occupation: The art and science of living* (173–196). Upper Saddle River, NJ: Prentice Hall.

Handicapped Children's Early Education Assistance Act of 1968, Pub. L. 90–538.

Hanft, B. E., & Pilkington, K. O. (2000). Therapy in natural environments: The means or end goal for early intervention? *Infants and Young Children, 12*(4), 1–13.

Harlow, H., Dodsworth, R., & Harlow, M. (1965). Total social isolation in monkeys. *Proceedings of the National Academy of Science of the United States of America, 54*(1), 90–97.

Howe, G. (2002). Integrating family routines and rituals with other family research paradigms: Comment on the special section. *Journal of Family Psychology, 16*(4), 437–440.

Humphry, R. (1989). Early intervention and the influence of the occupational therapist on the parent–child relationship. *American Journal of Occupational Therapy, 43,* 738–742.

Humphry, R. (2002). Young children's occupations: Explicating the dynamics of developmental processes. *American Journal of Occupational Therapy, 56,* 171–179.

Humphry, R., & Case-Smith, J. (1996). Working with families. In J. Case-Smith (Ed.), *Occupational therapy for children* (3rd ed., pp. 67–94). St. Louis, MO: Mosby.

Humphry, R., & Wakeford, L. (2006). An occupation-centered discussion of development and implications for practice. *American Journal of Occupational Therapy, 60,* 258–267.

Humphry, R., & Wakeford, L. (2008). Development of everyday activities: A model for occupation-centered practice. *Infants and Young Children, 21*(3), 230–240.

Individuals With Disabilities Education Act of 1997, Pub. L. 105–117.

Individuals With Disabilities Education Improvement Act of 2004, Pub. L. 108–446, 20 U.S.C. § 1400 *et seq.*

Kabat-Zinn, J. (1994). Foreword. In M. Lerner (Ed.), *Choices in healing* (pp. xi–xvii). Cambridge, MA: MIT Press.

Kearns, A., Hiscock, R., Ellaway, A., & Macintyre, S. (2000). Beyond four walls: The psycho-social benefits of home: Evidence from West Central Scotland. *Housing Studies, 15*(3), 387–410.

Kellegrew, D. H. (2000). Constructing daily routines: A qualitative examination of mothers with young children with disabilities. *American Journal of Occupational Therapy, 54,* 252–259.

Kliewer, W., & Kung, E. (1998). Family moderators of the relation between hassles and behavior problems in inner-city youth. *Journal of Clinical Child Psychology, 27,* 278–292.

Kopp, C. B. (1982). Antecedents of self-regulation—A developmental perspective. *Developmental Psychology, 18,* 199–214.

Knudson, A. (2005). A personal sixty-year tour of genetics and medicine. *Annual Review of Genomics and Human Genetics, 6,* 1–14.

Kunstaetter, R. (1987). Intelligent physiologic modeling: An application of knowledge-based systems technology to medical education. *Computer Methods and Programs in Biomedicine, 24,* 213–225.

Landry, S. H., Smith, K. E., & Swank, P. (2006). Responsive parenting: Establishing early foundations for social, communication, and independent problem-solving skills. *Developmental Psychology, 42,* 627–642.

Larson, E. A. (2000). The orchestration of occupation: The dance of mothers. *American Journal of Occupational Therapy, 54,* 269–280.

Larson, F. (2006). Care giving and autism: How does children's propensity for routinization influence participation in family activities? *OTJR: Occupation, Participation and Health, 26*(2), 69–79.

Lawlor, M., & Mattingly, C. (1998). The complexities embedded in family-centered care. *American Journal of Occupational Therapy, 52,* 259–267.

Lee, M., Liu, Y., & Newell, K. (2006). Longitudinal expressions of infant's prehension as a function of object properties. *Infant Behavior and Development, 29,* 481–493.

Macy, M., & Bricker, D. (2007). Embedding individualized social goals into routine activities in inclusive early childhood classrooms. *Early Child Development and Care, 177*(2), 107–120.

Markson, S., & Fiese, B. (2000). Family rituals as a protective factor for children with asthma. *Journal of Pediatric Psychology, 25*(7), 471–479.

Mattingly, C., & Fleming, M. (1994). *Clinical reasoning: Forms of inquiry in a therapeutic practice.* Philadelphia: F. A. Davis.

Mayer, M., White, B., Ward, J., & Barnaby, E. (2002). Therapists' perceptions about making a difference in parent–child relationships in early intervention occupational therapy services. *American Journal of Occupational Therapy, 56,* 411–421.

McEwen, B. S. (2003). Early life influences on life-long patterns of behavior and health. *Mental Retardation and Developmental Disabilities Research Reviews, 9,* 149–154.

McEwen, B., & Stellar, E. (1993). Stress and the individual: Mechanisms leading to disease. *Archives of Internal Medicine, 153,* 2093–2101.

McGuire, B. K., Crowe, T. K., Law, M., & Van Leit, B. (2004). Mothers of children with disabilities: Occupational concerns and solutions. *OTJR: Occupation, Participation and Health, 24*(2), 54–63.

Meyer, A. (1922). The philosophy of occupational therapy. *Archives of Occupational Therapy, 1,* 1–10.

Mims, S., & Chandler, B. (1992). Communication and behavior in the classroom. In C. Royeen (Ed.), *Classroom applications for school-based practice* (pp. 1–40). Bethesda, MD: American Occupational Therapy Association.

Moes, D. R., & Frea, W. D. (2002). Contextualized behavioral support in early intervention for children with autism and their families. *Journal of Autism and Developmental Disorders, 32*(6), 519–533.

Murray, H. A. (1938). *Explorations in personality.* New York: Oxford University Press.

Odom, S. L., & Wolery, M. (2003). A unified theory of practice in early intervention/early childhood special education: Evidence-based practice. *Journal of Special Education, 37*(3), 164–173.

Pierce, D. (2000). Maternal management of the home as a developmental play space for infants and toddlers. *American Journal of Occupational Therapy, 53,* 290–299.

Pilkington, K. (2006). Side by side: Transdisciplinary early intervention in natural settings. *OT Practice, 11*(6), 12–17. Retrieved January 8, 2010, from www.aota.org/Pubs/OTP/1997-2007/Features/2006/f-040306.aspx

Pilkington, K. O., & Malinowski, M. (2002). The natural environment II: Uncovering deeper responsibilities within relationship-based services. *Infants and Young Children, 15*(2), 78–84.

Pretti-Frontczak, K., Barr, D., Macy, M., & Carter, A. (2003). Research and resources related to activity-based intervention, embedded learning opportunities, and routines-based instruction: An annotated bibliography. *TECSE, 23*(1), 29–39.

Pretti-Frontczak, K., & Bricker, D. (2001). Use of the embedding strategy by early childhood education and early childhood special education teachers. *Infant and Toddler Intervention: The Transdisciplinary Journal, 11,* 111–128.

Primeau, L. (1998). Orchestration of work and play within families. *American Journal of Occupational Therapy, 52,* 188–195.

Ralph, E. (1976). *Place and placelessness.* London: Pion.

Richmond, M. (1899). *Friendly visiting among the poor.* New York: Macmillan.

Rinaman, L., Levitt, P., & Card, J. P. (2000). Progressive postnatal assembly of limbic–autonomic circuits revealed by central transneuronal transport of pseudorabies virus. *Journal of Neuroscience, 20*(7), 2731–2741.

Rochat, P. (2007). Intentional action arises from early reciprocal exchange. *Acta Psychologica, 124,* 8–25.

Sack, R. (1992). *Place, modernity, and the consumer's world.* Baltimore: Johns Hopkins University Press.

Schneider, W., & Shiffrin, R. M. (1977). Controlled and automatic human information processing: I. Detection, search, and attention. *Psychological Review, 84*(1), 1–66.

Schore, A. N. (1994). *Affect regulation and the origin of the self: The neurobiology of emotional development.* Mahwah, NJ: Lawrence Erlbaum.

Schore, A. N. (1996). The experience-dependent maturation of a regulatory system in the orbital prefrontal cortex and the origin of developmental psychopathology. *Development and Psychopathology, 8,* 59–87.

Schore, A. N. (1997). Early organization of the nonlinear right brain and development of a predisposition to psychiatric disorders. *Development and Psychopathology, 9,* 595–631.

Schore, A. N. (2000). Attachment and the regulation of the right brain. *Attachment and Human Development, 2,* 23–47.

Schore, A. N. (2001). Effects of a secure attachment relationship on right brain development, affect regulation, and infant mental health. *Infant Mental Health Journal, 22*(1–2), 7–66.

Schore, A. N., & Schore, J. R. (2008). Modern Attachment Theory: The central role of affect regulation in development and treatment. *Clinical Social Work Journal, 36*(1), 9–20.

Schuck, L., & Bucy, J. (1997). Family rituals: Implications for early intervention. *Topics in Early Childhood Special Education, 17*(4), 477–493.

Seaton, E., & Taylor, R. (2003). Exploring familial processes in urban low-income African American families. *Journal of Family Issues, 24,* 627–644.

Segal, R. (2004). Family routines and rituals: A context for occupational therapy interventions. *American Journal of Occupational Therapy, 58,* 499–508.

Shonkoff, J. P., & Phillips, D. A. (Eds.). (2000). *From neurons to neighborhoods: The science of early childhood development.* Washington, DC: National Academies Press.

Singh, N. N., Lancioni, G. E., Winton, A. S. W., Fisher, B. C., Wahler, R. G., McAleavey, K., et al. (2006). Mindful parenting decreases aggression, noncompliance, and self-injury in children with autism. *Journal of Emotional and Behavioral Disorders, 14,* 169–177.

Spagnola, M., & Fiese, B. (2007). Family routines and rituals: A context for development in the lives of young children. *Infants and Young Children, 20*(4), 284–299.

Spencer, J. P., Vereijken, B., Diedrich, F. J., & Thelen, E. (2000). Posture and the emergence of manual skills. *Developmental Science, 3*(2), 216–233.

Spivack, M. (1973, October). Archetypal place. *Architectural Forum,* 44–49.

Sprunger, L., Boyce, W., & Gaines, J. (1985). Family infant congruence: Routines and rhythmicity in family adaptations to a young infant. *Child Development, 56,* 564–572.

Stiles, J. (2008). *The fundamentals of brain development: Integrating nature and nurture.* Boston: Harvard University Press.

Stoff, D. M., & Cairns, R. B. (1996). *Aggression and violence.* Mahwah, NJ: Lawrence Erlbaum.

Supplee, L. H., Shaw, D. S., Hailstones, K., & Hartman, K. (2004). Family and child influences on early academic and emotion regulatory behaviors. *Journal of School Psychology, 42,* 221–242.

U.S. Department of Education. (1999). Part II. Assistance to states for the education of children with disabilities and the early intervention program for infants and toddlers with disabilities; Final Regulations. 64 FR 12406. 34 CFR §§ 300, 303.

Weinstock, M. (1997). Does prenatal stress impair coping and regulation of hypothalamic–pituitary–adrenal axis? *Neuroscience and Biobehavioral Reviews, 21*(1), 1–10.

Werner-DeGrace, B. (2004). The everyday occupations of families with children with autism. *American Journal of Occupational Therapy, 58,* 543–550.

Wilcock, A. (1998). *An occupational perspective of health.* Thorofare, NJ: Slack.

Williamson, G., & Anzalone, M. (2001). *Sensory integration and self-regulation in infants and toddlers: Helping very young children interact with their environment.* Washington, DC: Zero to Three.

Winnicott, D. W. (1987). *The child, the family, and the outside world.* Reading, MA: Addison-Wesley.

Zemke, R., & Clark, F. (Eds.). (1996). *Occupational science: The evolving discipline.* Philadelphia: F. A. Davis.

CHAPTER 7

Play in Early Childhood

Rebecca E. Argabrite Grove, MS, OTR/L, and
Frances A. Davis, MA, LPA

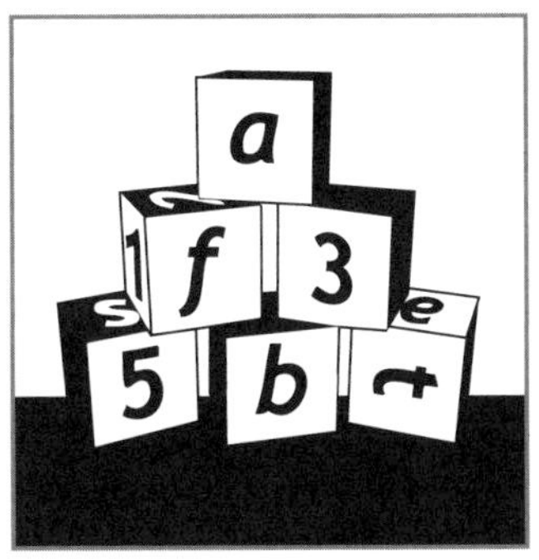

Learning Objectives

After reading this material and completing the examination, readers will be able to

- Delineate the characteristics and purpose of play within the context of infants', toddlers', and preschoolers' daily life;
- Delineate the opportunities, purpose, supports for, and value of play as a developmental intervention across multiple environments, including educational, of preschoolers', infants', and toddlers' daily life;
- Identify play assessments, goal selection, and the value of occupational therapist and parent partnerships in assessment and intervention;
- Delineate the application of the occupational therapy process related to play;
- Recognize how to design and modify supportive play environments for active engagement; and
- Recognize how to select and adapt toys, learning materials, and activities for individual or group participation.

> *Playing is fun. It's about interaction . . . playing with things and interacting with other people and kids. Kids like to have fun.*
>
> —Maia B. Grove, age 6

Play is a primary and quintessential occupation of early childhood, lending itself toward exploration and mastery of the environment and its tangible tools. Through play, children are motivated to interact with material objects and peers to bolster self-esteem and independence as derived through the successful repetition of fun. It is the innate sense of fun provided by the just-right challenge (Csikszentmihalyi, 1990) of play that compels a child to create his or her own space in the world.

Play, as defined by Wolfberg (1999), is an activity that is pleasurable, intrinsically motivated, flexible, nonliteral, and voluntary and involves active engagement. Similarly, play is described as having intrinsic motivation, pleasure, flexibility, and imagination (Berretta & Privette, 1990), while being free, having a joyous quality, being separated within the limits of time and space, having an unproductive and uncertain outcome, and governed by rules within the realm of make-believe (Caillois, 1961). The common characteristics associated with play, as described professionally over time, cross gender, age, and cultural differences to allow for a child's immersion in the fundamental human experience.

Play has been studied and documented professionally for many decades. Although difficult to define objectively for the purposes of scientific exploration, Alessandrini (1949) clearly articulated that

> [p]lay is a child's way of learning and an outlet for his innate need of activity. For each child it is a serious undertaking not to be confused with diversion or idle use of time. Play is not folly. It is purposeful activity. (p. 9)

The concept of play can be examined as a mélange of purposes all directed toward the development of a dynamic interaction between a child and his or her environment:

> Play develops language, say the linguists. Play develops the body, say the doctors and therapists. Play develops the mind, say the educators. Play allows children to work out their psychic challenges, say the psychologists. Mastery of the environment is the role of play, say the developmentalists. Play is a reflection of the child's culture, offer the anthropologists. Play keeps children occupied and out of the way while I fix dinner, says the parent . . . and on and on. (Chandler, 1997, p. iii)

Play is an excellent medium for supporting a child's learning and development. It can support acquisition, practice, mastery, and integration of learning (Barnett, 1990; Widerstrom, 2005) across developmental domains. By interacting with the environment and the objects and materials therein, children develop a sense of physical knowledge through categorization, seriation, and conservation. Manipulation of objects of various sizes and textures, as well as rough-and-tumble and outdoor active play, facilitate fine and gross motor skills. *Symbolic,* or pretend, play is the foundation for later use of symbols in the development of spoken and written language. As children become more skilled at using symbols, language and communication begin to blossom from gestures to single words and phrases and, eventually, to drawing and writing (Widerstrom, 2005).

Play is also an effective way to enhance social and emotional development. Children learn to share, resolve differences, practice manners, and cooperate with one another. As children develop a mastery of skills through play, self-esteem is enhanced and independence is supported. Gender roles and separation from parents are also developed within the context of play. Play is a fundamental support to child development in all domains, and it assists children with organizing and integrating life experiences (Cook, Tessier, & Klein, 2000; Frank, 1955).

Play, as the primary occupation of childhood, can be used not only as an indicator of development but also as an intervention. It provides value and quality to children's lives, and the occupational science literature has suggested that it should be considered and studied in its most naturalistic forms (Knox & Mailloux, 1997; Parham, 1996, 2008; Pollock, Stewart, Law, Sahagian-Whalen, & Toal, 1997).

Play and its inherent choices can be affected by many variables, of which age, gender, ability, and environment are just a few considerations. Miller and Kuhaneck (2008) found that play activities that are perceived as fun are more likely to be repeated because of the positive emotions associated with them. Repetition, in turn, creates patterns and preferences, which foster continued engagement in play, thereby contributing to mastery. Whether play activities are naturally occurring or prescribed as an intervention, consideration must be made for both a child's preferences and the importance of fun.

What Is Infant and Toddler Play, and Why Is It Important?

Newborn infants will change their pattern of sucking to listen to a familiar voice or story, turn their heads to locate a new sound, and lock gazes with their mother and imitate facial expressions (Brazelton & Cramer, 1990; DeCasper & Fifer, 1980; Meltzoff & Moore, 1983). By the age of 3 months, infants are capable of repeating the cooing sounds and facial expressions made by their parent and remembering which mobile moves when they kick (Marakova & Legerstee, 2008; Rovee-Collier, 1987). From birth, infants are actively expressing their interest in and using their capabilities to explore and act on their environment. In addition, infants' interactions with their environment can be selective on the basis of their previous experiences, current capabilities, and interests. D'Eugenio (1997) observed, "Play does not occur when there is uncertainty or fear" (p. 66).

Remember this. . . .
"Play does not occur when there is uncertainty or fear" (D'Eugenio, 1997, p. 66).

Descriptions or models of play vary according to the capabilities of the player, the social context, and the proposed purpose of the activity (Greenspan & Lewis, 1999; Parham & Fazio, 1997; Piaget & Inhelder, 1966, 1969). Consistent across definitions, however, are characterizations that denote play as enjoyable, exploratory, self-sustaining, activity based, and interest based or as involving social interaction (Burke, 1998; Parham & Fazio, 1997; Piaget & Inhelder, 1966, 1969; Raab, 2005; Vygotsky, 1978). Given these characterizations, it appears clear that from birth, children can engage in playful activities.

Infant and toddler play activities share many characteristics and experiences associated with models of development and evidence-based changes in children's neurological, motor, cognitive, linguistic, and social–emotional capabilities (Brazelton & Cramer, 1990; Bruner, 1972; Greenspan & Lewis, 1999). Consider the two processes of assimilation and accommodation seen as infants move from mouthing all objects to classifying objects into different groups on the basis of their properties and function (Piaget & Inhelder, 1966/1969). Across all stages described in Piaget's model of development, self-motivation and active participation and engagement with the objects and people in a child's environment are required for the development of the sensorimotor and cognitive capabilities through which children acquire and organize knowledge (Piaget & Inhelder, 1966/1969).

Vygotsky (1978), in his model of cultural learning, and Bandura (1992), in his discussion of delayed imitation, both described how infants and toddlers acquire new communicative and social capabilities through the recapitulation of guided facilitation and modeling observed activity. Vygostsky (1978) reported that development progressed when play activity began at the level of the child's capability or within their zone of proximal development and included the more complex capabilities of an experienced playmate. Bandura (1992) observed that play provides a context within which children can observe, practice, and learn socially appropriate behaviors, roles, and rules of engagement.

Remember this. . . .
Play provides a context within which children can observe, practice, and learn socially appropriate behaviors, roles, and rules of engagement (Bandura, 1992).

Consistent, contingent, parent–child play interactions are strongly associated with the development of social–emotional, cognitive, and motor competencies for infants and toddlers (Ainsworth, 1969; Zeanah, Larrieu, Heller, & Valliere, 2000). The building blocks of successful social interactions and emotional expression begin in infancy with the bidirectional communications and establishment of turn taking between parents and the newborn infant. Parents attend to the infant's continued and pleasant visual attention and calm awake state as a signal to provide new information about objects or new sounds and will continue until the infant disengages his or her attention from the person or object (Stern, 2002). At approximately 4 to 5 months, this pattern changes, and the infant becomes the initiator of social interaction, with infants recognizing the parent as an important person who enhances play experiences and provides interesting stimulation. The infant recognizes he or she can control the attention of parents and access parents with the use of certain kinds of gestures, sounds, and actions (Brazelton & Cramer, 1990).

The establishment of social–interactive play routines is informative for both the child's development and the parents' understanding of their role in that process. Infants and toddlers seek experiences and interactions in which they can be active and learn that adults can provide and help them maintain play activities. Allowing a child to take the lead not only ensures the engagement of infant–toddler interests and motivations but also promotes the development of self-concept and mastery over emotional regulation and expression. In successful play interactions, parents experience enhanced parenting self-efficacy (Brazelton & Cramer, 1990).

Finally, during the first 3 to 4 years of life, the child's brain undergoes rapid changes in the proliferation, establishment, and organization of neural connections that correlate with the recognition of patterns of sensory information, initiation and mastery of locomotion and manipulation, recognition and mastery of emotional and verbal communication, initiation and maintenance of social interaction, establishment of self-concept, and the acquisition of basic problem-solving strategies and concepts. The acquisition of capabilities that are important for the infant and toddler's day-to-day play activity and function and later socialization and academic success is sensitive to the developmental experiences of the child (Greenspan & Lewis, 1999). For better or worse, the day-to-day life of infants and toddlers provides the information and experiences that culminate in a typical 3-year-old child being capable of complex sentence construction, supported recall of the characters and the sequence of events in a story, riding a tricycle, drawing a simple representation of himself or herself, and providing empathy and assistance for others.

Role of Play in Infant and Toddler Development and Intervention

Appreciating the role of play in infant and toddler development and as a milieu for early intervention requires the joint consideration of child characteristics, play activity characteristics, and environmental context as a process through which development is expressed (Burke, 1998; Sameroff & Fiese, 2000; Schaaf & Burke, 1997). Consider the play activity of a 12-month-old infant sitting in a high chair in the kitchen who takes toys in and out of a large bowl while her mother cooks dinner. In this one activity, the child engages sensorimotor, visual–perceptive, and cognitive capabilities required to manipulate the toys in and out of the bowl. Most likely, there are pauses in play for verbal exchanges between the mother and child regarding both the child's play activity and the mother's activity. The mother says "take the toys out," the child responds with "ow, ow, ow" and the mother says "out, out, out."

Later, when the mother replaces the toys with a dish of food and the family begins eating dinner, the child may begin putting food in and taking it out of her dish until the mother says "time to eat." At this signal, the child observes the family eating and begins taking food out of the dish and putting it into her mouth. The mother smiles, and the child smiles back.

The child engages similar capabilities and experiences responsive supports from her mother in both activities but with different developmental outcomes. In the beginning of this routine activity of daily living (ADL), the child is engaged in independent sensorimotor and cognitive problem-solving play, whereas at the end of the activity, her interests changed to eating, social interactions, and family routines.

Play activities not only provide infants and toddlers a variety of experiences and opportunities to engage multiple capabilities but also promote new capabilities. For example, in the same scenario, the mother introduces a child-sized spoon during the play activity that the child initially places in and out of the bowl during independent play. She later begins to play at putting food on it, imitating her family members. After a few attempts, the child puts the spoon down, and her mother picks it up and finishes feeding the child with the spoon. At successive dinners, however, the mother continues to introduce the spoon until eventually the child uses the spoon to feed herself independently.

Within any play activity, the child's level of engagement and interest, present ability to perform the activity, materials available, and responses of other participants influence the process through which the infant's and toddler's development progresses. In addition, the context of available materials and support of parents influence the development of new competencies through the opportunities for new experiences they afford. Dunst (2006) referred to the combination of these contexts and interchanges, which have been occurring since the dawn of time, as *parent-mediated child learning*. For instance, the next step for the infant in the high chair putting her food in and taking it out of a bowl became feeding herself with a spoon out of a dish, because the mother introduced the spoon to the play activity and supported the child keeping the spoon during dinner.

The sensitivity and plasticity of the relationship between brain development and infant and toddler experiences in cognitive, social–emotional, language, and sensorimotor play activities also mean that effective intervention can alter the course of early childhood development (Shonkoff & Phillips, 2000). Play is a particularly rich medium for early intervention for several reasons:

- Infants and toddlers are self-directed and actively engaged with a variety of tasks, objects, and participants during play activities.
- Infants and toddlers are more likely to demonstrate their interests and current capabilities during play (Meisels, 1996).
- Play is a natural activity of infants and toddlers; therefore, it offers many daily opportunities for intervention.
- Parents are the first attachment figure and most common playmate for infants and toddlers. When offered opportunities to participate in intervention, they are more likely to continue to support intervention strategies.
- The Individuals With Disabilities Education Improvement Act (IDEA 2004) Part C: Infants and Toddlers With Disabilities requires that early intervention services be provided in natural environments, which include home and community settings and involve the interests, goals, and participation of the family (U.S. Department of Education, 2004).

> ***Remember this. . . .***
> **The sensitivity and plasticity of the relationship between brain development and infant and toddler experiences in cognitive, social–emotional, language, and sensorimotor play activities also mean that effective intervention can alter the course of early childhood development (Shonkoff & Phillips, 2000).**

Chai, Zhang, and Bisberg (2006) proposed three critical elements of natural environment practices: *naturalistic specialized instruction, natural settings,* and *parent–child interactions in daily routines and activities.* Infant and toddler play activities, when viewed as a developmental process, encompass all of these elements. Play is the most common natural learning activity for infants and toddlers, and parents are most often the principal play partner and supportive agent for child learning opportunities. Even though infants and toddlers can engage in play across a variety of settings, the family home is the most natural setting and affords the use of frequently occurring daily routines and play activities and familiar objects as opportunities to promote infants' and toddlers' development. The same three elements are important for the evaluation process when considering infant and toddler play as the activity setting or context of early intervention.

Infant and Toddler Play Evaluation

Typically, evaluation takes place for two reasons: (1) to determine eligibility for participation in a program or to receive intervention supports and (2) to inform and guide the intervention process. Eligibility determination often requires, in part, comparing a child's task performance or skills against that of a normative sample through the use of a structured protocol and standardized materials presented by an often unfamiliar adult. The demonstration of specific skills in a directed format, however, is not consistent with the characteristics of infant and toddler play activity, and the idiosyncratic nature of infant and toddler play choices. As a result, evaluation in infant and toddler programs requires use of more than one instrument or process to identify specific developmental needs. Observation of the infant or toddler at play in his or her home with familiar toys and people yields a great deal of specific information about play and learning through play. (See Chapter 5 for more information about evaluation in early childhood programs.)

Aside from eligibility, evaluation and intervention are not mutually exclusive; that is, the planned context and the strategies used during intervention guide both the selection of the assessment tool and the evaluation process (Macy & Bricker, 2006). For example, criterion-referenced and curriculum-based assessments, such as the Infant–Toddler Developmental Assessment (Erikson, 1996), which incorporates play activities into tasks based on developmental levels of skill mastery, provide information about conditions for child success and can provide evaluators and parents with useful information for identifying individualized goals and objectives (called *outcomes* on the individualized family service plan [IFSP]) and to review progress. The Assessment, Evaluation, and Programming System (Macy & Bricker, 2006) is a curriculum-based assessment that combines evaluation with a daily routine–based curriculum and can provide the practitioner and parent with guidance on where and when to implement a play-based intervention within the context of the family's daily routines (Macy & Bricker, 2006). Even more specific to an individual infant's or toddler's developmental status, interests, and play activities are performance assessments and interviews. Performance assessments involve observing the knowledge, skills, and emotional disposition children demonstrate in familiar settings as they explore and act on objects in their environment and interact with familiar people (Meisels, 1996). Performance assessments and interviews regarding play present an opportunity for parents to participate as valued members of the intervention team through the contribution of their knowledge of their child and the activities in which the child most often demonstrates the full range of his or her capabilities (Greenspan & Meisels, 1996). Being a member of the intervention team that values parent information and participation engages parents in a manner that builds their confidence to promote their child's development (Dempsey & Dunst, 2004; Rocco, 1996).

One form of performance assessment is nonstructured play observation, which establishes an alliance with the parents and includes their views on the child's strengths, challenges, and issues to be explored during the evaluation (Greenspan & Meisels, 1996; Segal & Webber, 1996). Segal and Webber (1996) described three primary components necessary to nonstructured play observations as (1) selecting the observer, (2) gathering background information, and (3) identifying the focus of observation.

Selection of the observer should be guided by the expertise of the observer and the focus of the observation. Nonstructured observations that involve observations of the child with his or her parent and observations of the child with the early intervention occupational therapist offer the opportunity for parents and occupational therapists to begin sharing their respective expertise and maintain such conversations during intervention.

Background information may include formal testing, medical information, previous intervention and child care provider reports, and parent experiences with the infant or toddler. When play is the chosen context of intervention, background information can be gathered with an interview and should include information about infants' and toddlers' preferred favorite play interests, activities, and play partners and the access the child has to them in daily experience.

The focus of a nonstructured play assessment differs according to the family-identified interests and expertise, the occupational therapist's expertise, and the intervention approach. For example, when the occupational therapist is the observer, the focus may be on the environmental context in which the play occurs; the interactions with parents or siblings; the range and functional use of the child's motor competencies; the child's regulatory responses or reactivity to new stimuli; change and interruption (Hirshberg, 1996); or the communication signals the parent responds to as he or she begins, supports, and ends play activities. Conversely, when the parent is the observer, the focus may be on the positional or sensory strategies the occupational therapist uses to support the child's activity. Nonstructured assessment can also provide opportunities for the occupational therapist and parents to attempt strategies for stimulating the child's use of new competencies (Dunst, 2006).

Interview assessments can provide both background information and guidance for intervention. Burke (1998) suggested using a descriptive interview in which parents describe the child's interactions with favorite activities and toys. Parent and child interaction during play activities can provide the occupational therapist with information regarding child abilities, emotional regulation and limitations, parent knowledge, and emotional status. One example is the Asset-Based Context Matrix (ABC Matrix; Wilson, Mott, & Batman, 2004), "a contextually based assessment tool that uses children's assets (personal interests and abilities) as factors promoting their participation in everyday natural learning environments" (Wilson & Mott, 2006, p. 1). As an interview assessment tool, it is specifically designed to provide intervention in the natural learning environment of infants', toddlers', and families' daily life.

The information gathered through discussions with the parents is organized according to characteristics of child behavior (interests, capabilities, and function) and the opportunities for the child to participate in play that engages his or her interests in three learning contexts: (1) family activities settings, (2) community activity settings, and (3) early childhood activities. Questions useful for exploring the child's interests in activities and that can be used to promote child development might include the following (Raab, 2005):

- What things catch and maintain the child's attention?
- What things encourage the child to work hard?
- What does the child do best?
- When is the child likely to try new things?
- When does the child appear especially excited or interested?

The ABC Matrix goes one step further than the previously discussed play assessments by providing a format for using the information gathered to plan and incorporate intervention activities into the child's and family's everyday life and culture (Wilson et al., 2004). The matrix may be helpful when working with people who may not be as familiar as occupational therapists with how to provide intervention supports within the context of already occurring, interest-based child and family activities. The therapist builds on, extends, supports, and enhances what the child is already doing in typical routines. The occupational therapy literature has always referred to this process as "embedding" intervention, but the early childhood literature does not use this term. Finally, the ABC Matrix allows the parent to document ongoing intervention success and change, thereby providing both the occupational therapist and the parent with information that sustains or alters the goals of intervention (Meisels, 1996).

Determining Play-Related Goals for Infants and Toddlers

Burke (1998) considered information on the quality of social, sensory, motor, cognitive, and language competencies to be important because the child uses those skills in daily family activities; they are the starting place for the occupational therapist and family when determining goals (outcomes). Infant and toddler behaviors, activities, goals, and motivations associated with play, however, are specific to individual child interests and the current context setting. As the child develops new and more complex capabilities, the combinations of capabilities the child engages to participate in play activities changes as well. Because children's choices in play activities are determined by the meaningful actions they can engage in pursuit of their interests (Raab, 2005), new competencies are then the next step for the child, not necessarily the next step in skill development or the next step for parents.

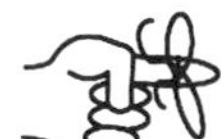

Remember this. . . .
As the child develops new and more complex capabilities, the combinations of capabilities the child engages to participate in play activities changes as well.

In addition, the focus and efforts of infants and toddlers may change quickly within a single play activity. Consider the 2-year-old pretending to diaper and feed his favorite stuffed bear. Initially he is focused on the perceptual–motor capabilities required to place and tape the diaper on the bear, but during feeding, the child becomes more focused on the conversation he is having with the bear about eating his dinner. Intervention that refocuses (interrupts) the child's attention to the motor capabilities he is using to feed the bear disrupts the child's current focus of language and social capabilities. For this reason, how the chosen intervention approach supports the child's lead and interests needs to be considered when determining the approach or strategies used with an individual child at a specific time.

Home-based early intervention often occurs weekly and lasts approximately 1 hr. The therapist works with the family member (usually the mother) to identify when opportunities for intervention occur naturally and to facilitate and implement other intervention activities and supports with the child. Infants and toddlers engage in many play activities throughout their day, and this process is then repeated (without the therapist) with the parent as the primary facilitator of opportunity and support. When family environment, parents' interests, and opportunity to participate in the chosen play intervention activities are considered, family capacity to support the child is built (Dunst, Hamby, Trivette, Raab, & Bruder, 2000; Lawlor & Mattingly, 1998; Rocco, 1996).

Planning and Implementing Intervention

Two promising approaches to planning and implementing intervention are consistent with the philosophy of occupational therapy and how occupational therapy services are provided in natural environments and are consistent with play as a developmental process: (1) activity-based instruction (Macy & Bricker, 2007) and (2) parent-mediated child learning (Dunst, 2006). Both approaches can be used in infants' and toddlers' home settings and include the participation of the parent.

Activity-based instruction embeds targeted child goals and behaviors into routine ADLs and may be complementary to curriculum-based assessments, such as the Assessment, Evaluation, and Programming System (Macy & Bricker, 2006). This approach is familiar to occupational therapists. Intervention is focused on modifying and expanding child capabilities in a manner that is meaningful or functional for the infant or toddler (Pretti-Frontczak & Bricker, 2004). An example of this approach would be placing favorite toys on the couch to encourage standing. Standing is not the primary interest or activity for the child but is instigated by the occupational therapist; it becomes a necessary activity for the child to pursue his or her interest in the toys on the couch.

A single learning capability can be embedded into several routine activities, an approach that increases the amount of practice and the likelihood that the child will continue practicing the new capability in the absence of the occupational therapist. Embedding new actions, behaviors, and toys or other play objects into routine ADLs facilitates the child's opportunities and abilities to "become actively involved or occupied with the environment, both in mind and in body . . . and an opportunity for children to learn how to engage in and elaborate play with objects" (Burke, 1998, p. 190).

Parent-mediated child learning (Dunst, 2006) is an early childhood, interest-based, learning intervention model that draws upon the natural interaction of the parent and the child. It promotes parents as the primary interventionist for their child and focuses on the context of everyday family and community activities as natural learning opportunities. Interest-based learning is based on the unsurprising fact that children's play reflects that in which they are interested and that they are active learners when they are thus engaged. The child's capabilities are promoted during interaction and participation in the activity (Raab, 2005).

The parent is supported by the occupational therapist to (1) identify child interests and the everyday activities that provide opportunities for interest-based child learning and (2) use responsive teaching strategies that enhance, increase, and encourage child capabilities and participation in different activity settings. Although similar to activity-based instruction, this approach influences infant and toddler development through play activities but is even more likely to promote the parent's confidence and competence to promote their child's development. Engaging parents in planning, intervening, and reflecting regarding the success of their efforts strengthens parents' self-efficacy beliefs, which in turn increases their competence and participation (Coleman & Karraker, 2003; Coleman et al., 2002; Teti & Gelfand, 1991).

As toddlers acquire more complex capabilities, they are able to engage and participate in more complex and extended ADLs. For the preschooler, the role of play continues to be a primary developmental process and environment for early learning. The increasing complexity of the preschooler's integrated capabilities and opportunities for participation in more complex social activities again reflect the combined influence of child characteristics, play activity characteristics, and environmental context and is a process through which development is expressed (Burke, 1998; Sameroff & Fiese, 2000).

Most infant and toddler play activities that occur in the home or community use objects and materials that can be found within those environments. It is recognized that some homes do not have toys, materials, or spaces that are appropriate or safe for child play and that other strategies will be necessary in those situations. When home-based and family-owned materials are used in play activities, it increases the likelihood that the child and parent will continue to use them in play activities between visits from the occupational therapist. Developmental supports can typically be provided by ensuring that infants and toddlers have opportunities to move about in and explore a variety of rooms, floors, and safe household objects. Box 7.1 lists common activities and materials found in many family homes that support play-based development for infants and toddlers.

Role and Purpose of Play in Preschool

Much empirical evidence supports play as facilitating the development of problem-solving and abstract reasoning skills, social communication, and anxiety management (Barnett, 1990). By allowing children to move, solve problems, relate to others, and cope with their own feelings, play initiates the process of occupational development and promotes competence, achievement, and acquisition of roles that transform into the necessary habits and roles of learning and subsequent adult daily life (Bryze, 2008).

Not only are there multiple definitions of play, but an elusiveness surrounds its purpose. Lieberman (1965) identified *playfulness* using criteria such as physical, social, and cognitive spontaneity; manifest joy; and a sense of humor, whereas Dattner (1969) emphasized the process of play in lieu of the product. Bundy (1993) purported that play serves three purposes: (1) as an activity in which humans engage, (2) as a primary medium for intervention, and (3) as a style used to approach problems and situations with flexibility (playfulness). Nonetheless, play allows children to walk (or tumble) through the process of discovery regarding self and the world around them through experimental, manipulative, physical, interactive, and imitative activities (Henry, 2008).

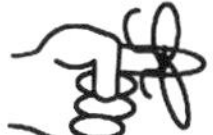

Remember this. . . .
Not only are there multiple definitions of *play,* but an elusiveness surrounds its purpose.

Play has a long cultural history within the confines of educational philosophy and curriculum. It was recognized by Plato and Aristotle in ancient Greece (Spariosu, 1991; Widerstrom, 2005) as producing relaxation as a remedy for pain from exertion (as related to occupation, defined therein as *work*), a definition necessitating that play have an element of pleasure. In ancient Greece, play, occupation (work), and leisure were viewed as three distinct but interdependent entities.

In 18th-century France, Rousseau believed that children learned through play. He was an influence on Pestalozzi in Switzerland, who developed a method of early education for orphans that was based on play and learning by discovery (Pestalozzi, 1799/1890). Friedrich Wilhelm Froebel, borrowing ideas from Rousseau and Pestalozzi, opened the first kindergarten in Germany that was based on the principles of play, natural development, and active participation (Widerstrom, 2005). The kindergarten movement quickly spread to England and the United States, where John Dewey (1902, 1938) predicated a child-centered curriculum based on the intrinsic motivation to learn.

One of the most well-known and influential educational leaders, Maria Montessori, who was a physician, began her work in the early 1900s in Italy with children who were orphaned or abandoned. Much like Piaget (Piaget & Inhelder, 1969), she believed in learning through sensory and motor experiences to take advantage of children's natural curiosity. The *Montessori method,* as it has come to be known, uses

Box 7.1. Selection and Adaptation of Infant–Toddler and Home-Based Activities, Learning Materials, and Toys

Activities:

- Cuddling or rocking with adult
- Dancing or moving to music
- Brushing teeth
- Washing hands and face
- Doing laundry
- Dressing and undressing
- Meal preparation
- Eating meals or snacks
- Going for a walk at home, in town, or at a park
- Chase and hiding games
- Feeding ducks at the park or pond
- Finger painting with pudding
- Playing with bubbles
- Going grocery shopping
- Helping with household chores (e.g., dishwashing)
- Picking up toys
- Playing finger games
- Playing in a wading pool
- Playing in the garden and sand outside
- Playing in kitchen cupboards
- Playing lap games (e.g., peek-a-boo, so big)
- Playing on park/playground equipment
- Playing with/taking care of pets
- Rough housing/playing tickle games.

Locations:

- Clear safe spaces in the living room, kitchen, or other family areas for crawling, walking, running, and ball play
- Safe outside gardens, yard, and neighborhood parks
- Stable, safe low tables, ottomans, couches, and chairs for pulling up, cruising, standing, and climbing.

Materials:

- Plastic bowls, cups, and spoons for imaginative and manipulative play
- Plastic food containers in a variety of sizes or empty cereal and food boxes for manipulative play
- Socks, gloves, and hats of different sizes for manipulative play
- Towels, washcloths, dishcloths, or small blankets
- Cardboard boxes and packing cases for motor exploration and imaginative play
- Magazines or newspaper store ads for manipulative play.

In addition, families may purchase interest-based, inexpensive, cause-and-effect toys for infants and manipulatives for toddlers such as

- Mobiles
- Large, bright cardboard books and pictures
- Medium-sized blocks, balls, and pop-beads
- Larger crayons and markers
- Playhouse toys
- Push–pull toys
- Teething toys and rattles
- Bubbles.

Learning Activity 7.1. All I Need to Know I Learned Through Play

The developmental roots of competence lie in the human capacity for play.

—M. Brewster Smith (1974)

- Reflect on your own personal experiences as a young child ages 3 to 5. Look at old photographs. If possible, ask your parent(s) or siblings about your play. What were your play environments?
- Define competence on the basis of your memories of the occupation of play at this age.

---

natural materials and ADLs such as sweeping, pouring, folding, and caring for plants and animals to foster development (Montessori, 1912).

Learning Activity 7.1 asks readers to reflect on their own childhood occupation of play and examine how it contributed to their skill development.

Natural Context of Preschool: Socialization, Emotional Growth, and Academic Readiness Opportunities

Within the context of preschool, the importance of play is generally accepted but undervalued. Many curricula have begun to separate play and learning activities in an attempt to achieve high-quality ratings for academic readiness (National Association for the Education of Young Children [NAEYC], 2009) under the belief that emphasizing academics at an earlier age ensures academic success. This trend to overachieve at such a young age pushes children to work beyond their level of neurodevelopmental readiness and can lead to patterns of inefficient and dysfunctional learning performance as well as elevated levels of anxiety. Less opportunity for play may also lead to apathetic learners and an increase in behavioral difficulties. Preschool should offer "play with a purpose": The environment and curriculum should include components that serve as the foundation for subsequent occupational engagement and participation across the developmental lifespan. Through interaction with others during play, children learn to express affection, develop trust, practice basic communication and reciprocation, and explore the world in the confines of a safe environment (Barnett, 1991; Bronfenbrenner, 1986; Slade & Wolf, 1994).

Social and Emotional Aspects of Preschool Play

Playing teaches you to be nice . . . no yelling, how to take turns, and share. Play helps you make friends.

—Maia B. Grove, age 6

Successful play experiences serve as the medium for achieving success and social competency (Reynolds & Jones, 1997). During the preschool years, children begin to show interest in developing friendships and in recognizing gender differences. Selective pairing and grouping of children during play is important for inclusive practices as well as for further development of social roles. Group activities, particularly with mixed-age groups, provide younger children with models and allow older children to serve as leaders. Both play initiation and play response are highly desirable elements of interactive play (Tanta, Deitz, White, & Billingsley, 2005); by pairing children with and without functional play skills, delays in play interactions can be naturally diminished.

The preschool stage of development is characterized by a challenging struggle for autonomy and an inability to delay gratification, which can make turn taking and sharing difficult (Douglas & Richman, 1985). Despite these challenges, an attitude of respect for the child must be established and maintained. Children need to develop a sense of independence, self-discipline, and responsibility (Perry & Perry, 2000). They need to feel secure and loved to support self-esteem. When children are stressed, the learning centers in the brain begin to shut down (University of California–Irvine, 2008). Incorporation of rules and daily routines is critical to help children develop a sense of time; order; and organization of activities, materials, and themselves. In addition, clear and consistent behavioral expectations are necessary, because children age 5 and younger tend to be long on feelings and short on reasoning (Perry, 2001). Fears are often present and should be taken seriously, because children may not be fully able to distinguish between reality and fantasy or dreams. Fluency with emotional expression is beginning to emerge alongside language, so patience is necessary as the child learns to cope with anxiety, frustration, and failure.

Academic Readiness

Three- to 5-year-olds like to wiggle and explore. Academic learning should be playful and exploratory, with academic goals and objectives woven into the context of play-based activities. Children cannot sit still long enough to follow a traditional style of passive learning. Learning processes in the brain share motor pathways, so the combination of learning paired with movement lends itself to more reliable acquisition of skills and is inherently less stressful and more fun.

To develop conceptual understanding and application of skills, children should be given the opportunity to explore materials; adults should be available to facilitate thinking and problem-solving skills (by asking open-ended questions) and support vocabulary and language development by commenting (NAEYC, 2009). Adults should use caution to avoid intervening too quickly, which may limit play interactions and foster dependence on adult support. Literacy (reading and writing) can be embedded through the use of stories, visual supports, and music within the classroom environment, whereas science and math can be addressed by means of cooking, block play, and sand and water play.

Remember this. . . .
Once external constraints are placed on play, it begins to be perceived as work (Mogford, 1977; Rast, 1986; Wade, 1985).

Play as a Therapeutic Context and Outcome

Play is often used within the context of therapy to work toward achievement of projected goals. Because a therapist controls aspects of the therapeutic environment, however, a paradox with the essence of play itself is created (Rast, 1986). Once external constraints are placed on play, it begins to be perceived as work (Mogford, 1977; Rast, 1986; Wade, 1985). Play is used as a treatment modality within occupational therapy practice, but it can also be identified as a desired treatment outcome of the therapeutic process.

Couch, Deitz, and Kanny (1998) surveyed pediatric occupational therapists and found that 92% of occupational therapists who responded used play as a modality to elicit motor, sensory, or psychosocial outcomes; 2% used play primarily as a free-choice activity or reward at the end of a therapy session; 4% used play equally as modality and reward; and 2% used play as an outcome in and of itself. Non–school-based occupational therapists reported that they used child-directed play along with a sensory integration treatment approach more often than did school-based occupational therapists. Results of this study represent practice patterns of the time at which the study was conducted and, for this reason, should be interpreted with caution.

This dichotomy of "play in therapy" versus "play as therapy" (Knox & Mailloux, 1997, p. 189) can be differentiated on the basis of frames of reference that may be selected and used by the occupational therapist. In the *developmental* frame of reference, play materials and activities are used to develop skills in cognitive, social, emotional, and physical areas, whereas a *functional* frame of reference emphasizes play as a way to engage a child to meet supportive component outcomes, such as increased range of motion in a child recovering from burns. Both approaches are applied as "play in therapy." In direct contrast, the *sensory integration* frame of reference is used to facilitate the development of play—in this scenario, the child chooses among activities following setup or manipulation of the environment by the occupational therapist. Likewise, an *occupational science* frame of reference emphasizes play as an outcome and an occupation determined by the child's interaction with the environment, thus supporting "play as therapy" (Knox & Mailloux, 1997).

Most educational approaches use play materials and activities to facilitate a child's development in specific skill domains (e.g., cognitive, motor, social, and emotional) or to address discrete skills (e.g., standing balance or tripod grasp). When embracing play as a measured outcome of intervention, however, the child is viewed as a dynamic system that interacts with the environment on the basis of his or her individual inner drive and desire for participation and mastery.

The differences in conceptual understanding of the construct of play within a therapeutic context are important for teams of professionals to consider, because they will guide evaluation and subsequent development of targeted goals and objectives for the child.

Learning Activity 7.2 asks readers to compare and contrast frames of reference with respect to their conceptual approach to play and apply them to a case study.

Learning Activity 7.2. Framing Play

The reader may wish to refer to the "Occupational Therapy Decision-Making Process" (Handley-More & Chandler, 2007).

1. Select one frame of reference using a play-in-therapy approach and one using a play-as-therapy approach.
2. Compare and contrast your purpose and approach to play using each frame of reference within the context of occupational therapy for the following case study:

   Shelley is a highly active soon-to-be 4-year-old who loves to move around and interact with others. She loves to run with her peers on the playground. She dislikes sedentary activities, and her teacher from the Head Start program reports that she demonstrates intense emotional reactions in the classroom when asked to follow rules and routines for completing less active school tasks.

Evaluation of Play in Preschool

If we cannot assess, implement, and promote play, we do not take it seriously.

—Anita C. Bundy (1993)

Formal evaluation of play in occupational therapy did not occur until the 1960s. Although occupational therapists often incorporate play into the evaluation process as a method for observing underlying developmental skills (Stone, 1991), it is also evaluated as an occupation in which a child engages. A more routine and systematic approach to assessment is necessary to measure play as an occupation, including playfulness, a child's abilities, and opportunities to play (Bundy, 1993).

Several formal and informal methods currently exist for assessing play. Most commonly used instruments rely on direct observation or parent interview. No matter which instrument is used, evaluation should be conducted in the most natural and effortless setting possible for the child and family using familiar play experiences with toys and objects to which the child is accustomed (Pellegrini, 2001). Functional observation of children at play without the use of formal instruments should not be discounted as providing valuable, if not the most valuable, insight into occupational engagement and participation.

The Play History (Takata, 1974) uses a semistructured interview of qualitative, open-ended questions to assess a child's interests, skills, and quality of play over time. It specifically examines the materials the child plays with, the actions a child uses to play, how the child plays with others, and when and where the child plays to establish a timeline of past and present play skills and patterns.

The Revised Knox Preschool Play Scale (Knox, 2008) is an observational assessment designed to give a description of typical developmental aspects of play behavior in children birth to age 6 by examining space management (how a child manages bodies and space around him or her through experimentation and exploration), material management (how a child handles and uses materials with purpose to control and use objects), pretense–symbolic factors (how a child gains understanding of the world through imitation and learns to separate reality from fantasy), and participation (how a child interacts with people in the environment, how frequently, and with what degree of independence and cooperation). Observations using this assessment must be completed across two 30-minute sessions in both indoor and outdoor settings that are natural and familiar where peers are also present.

By contrast, the Test of Playfulness (Bundy, Nelson, Metzger, & Bingaman, 2001), in combination with the Test of Environmental Supportiveness (Bronson & Bundy, 2001), allows for a person–environment–occupation–based approach to measuring play and playfulness for children ages 6 months to 18 years when observed during free play in both indoor and outdoor settings. The tests specifically examine the fit between the child's motivations, caregivers, playmates, objects, play spaces, and sensory environment. Validity studies of these measures have been conducted across cultural groups including African-Americans and Hispanics from the United States and Central America (Griffith, 2000; Phillips, 1998; Porter & Bundy, 2000).

In a survey of pediatric occupational therapists (Couch et al., 1998), 62% of respondents indicated that they evaluated play behaviors, whereas 38% did not evaluate play. In addition, 79% of non–school-based respondents evaluated play behaviors, compared with 54% of those working in schools. Most occupational therapists reported that they evaluated play using clinical observations, but 62% who did use assessments relied on norm-referenced measures; 59% used criterion-referenced measures; and 25% assessed using other means, such as parent report or site-specific play checklists (Couch et al., 1998). Readers are again cautioned to consider the date of this study.

A wide variability continues to exist in how play is evaluated; however, occupational therapists who use play as a method of intervention also document goals that include a play component (Couch et al., 1998). Knowledge of a child's skills, interests, and play style can assist with establishment of goals and subsequent implementation of intervention. Bundy (1993) suggested several considerations when observing children at play that support the process of goal development and intervention planning:

- In what activities does the child become completely absorbed?
- Does the child routinely engage in activities in which he or she feels free to vary the process, product, or outcome of in whatever manner he or she desires?
- Does the child have the ability, permission, and supports necessary to do what he or she chooses to do?
- Is the child capable of socially giving, receiving, and interpreting messages such as "This is play; this is how you should interact with me now"?

Case Study: Joshua

Joshua, age 2 years, 6 months, lives with his parents and his baby sister in a house in a rural area. He is a curious and active youngster who spends the balance of his day at his home with his mother and sibling. At his last regular visit to the family doctor, however, his mother identified some delays in his language and fine motor skills on his developmental screening. The pediatrician referred Joshua to the local early intervention program. His mother was concerned that Joshua had a fleeting attention span, so an observational play assessment was chosen as one method of evaluation. The Revised Knox Preschool Play Scale (RKPPS) was chosen, and two 30-minute observations were scheduled to take place in the family's play room as well as in the backyard on the play equipment.

Joshua was observed to enjoy gross motor activity, including running, jumping, climbing, and riding toys. He maneuvered the backyard play equipment and movement toys with ease and precision across uneven surfaces, including grass and mulch, as he guided them around trees and the family dog. On the space management dimension of the RKPPS, he demonstrated skills at the 36-month level.

In material management, Joshua had difficulty stringing beads, and he avoided toys that required fine motor precision, such as puzzles, preferring instead to push and roll cars and trains. He interacted with a variety of textures during play and quickly moved from one toy to another, playing for no more than 1 minute at a time independently. He stacked, took items apart, and placed them together when objects were medium to large in size. He demonstrated skills on the material management dimension at the 18-month level.

In the family play room, Joshua was noted to engage in some imitative behavior surrounding ADLs. He swept the floor with a toy broom and pretended to wash his cars with a washcloth. When his mother was writing at the table, he found paper and crayon and began to make marks on paper. Joshua demonstrated skills at the 24-month level on the pretense–symbolic dimension.

Finally, on the participation dimension, Joshua scored at the 18-month level, because he was beginning to interact with his baby sister by playing peek-a-boo but primarily demanded attention from his parents by means of crying and screaming; occasionally, he would point or gesture to indicate his wants and needs. After analyzing results from the RKPPS, it was determined that the intervention plan should emphasize material management and participation. More information on Joshua can be found later in this chapter.

Learning Activity 7.3 asks readers to complete a naturalistic play observation of children to examine the many factors that contribute to play as an occupation.

Development of Play-Based Goals, Objectives, and Outcomes

Some children play for the sake of play. However, some children need assistance and support to develop skills that support play as an outcome. When play is identified as an outcome of interest by parents and professionals, it is important to document play as a goal to be achieved within the child's preschool or early intervention experiences. Play has been described as a goal of intervention in the occupational science and sensory integration frames of reference as well as in the *Occupational Therapy Practice Framework: Domain and Process, 2nd Edition* (American Occupational Therapy Association, 2008; Knox, 2005).

Whether play is used as an intervention in and of itself or as an outcome of intervention, development of goals should be based on comprehensive and specific evaluation information. (*Note.* The term *outcome* is used in early intervention to denote both the goal and the end point of intervention, rather than only the end point, as it is used in most health and human service literature.) Individualized education programs under Part B of IDEA 2004 are required to outline special education supports and services; goals are derived from the Present Level of Academic and Functional Performance, which provides a baseline measure of a child's current performance. IFSP outcomes for infants and toddlers are derived from parental concerns and eligibility evaluation data. ISFPs should note areas of strength and areas of concern. Areas of concern should serve as the springboard to developing desired outcomes (targeted goals and objectives) and identifying areas of strength used as facilitators.

Learning Activity 7.3. Community-Based Play Observation

Travel to a local indoor or outdoor playground or play area.

- Observe children at play.
- Examine the interdependent variables of child and environment (human and nonhuman) and the impact of each on engagement and participation in play.
- Be sure to consider all elements or aspects of play.

Consider the following questions when developing goals as a team:

- Are the goals related to documented areas of need or difficulty?
- Are the goals realistic for the child to achieve in the given time frame?
- Are the goals measurable, observable, objective, and functional?
- Do the goals represent relevant and necessary priorities for the child as stated by the family and the early intervention or preschool team?

When working as a member of a team of professionals and parents, preplanning is important to establish a streamlined and comprehensive approach to goal or outcome development. Goals or outcomes should be written collaboratively, and all members of the team should support the individual goals. A team approach to goal or outcome writing is more likely to support replication of skills across team members and settings to ensure generalization of skills. Goals that are not shared by the team or connected in some way to the child's daily experiences are more likely to result in fragmented services (Hanft & Place, 1996).

Supportive Preschool Play Environments

A supportive play environment should offer imagination potential, physical and social possibilities and boundaries, physical and emotional safety, comfort, and fun (Chandler, 1997, p. 160). The environment may be planned, unplanned, or a combination thereof, but it should be stimulating to all the sensory systems and include child-sized furniture and a variety of materials for exploring. It should provide for continual adjustment to physical and cognitive needs with allowances made for responding to the actions of the child. Choices should be inherent to allow for freedom, creativity, challenges, and mastery while providing an adequate range of experience with some measure of control remaining in place (Dattner, 1969). The physical environment should invite movement and activity but be orderly. Defined areas of the room should support purposeful engagement in physical play (drawing, puzzles and manipulatives, gross motor); social play (drama); self-care; and ADLs such as sweeping, washing, and food and meal preparation (Perry & Perry, 2000). The environment should be language rich to include word games, songs, conversation, and books as a foundation for reading and writing.

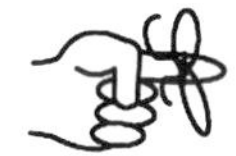

Remember this. . . .
A supportive play environment should offer imagination potential, physical and social possibilities and boundaries, physical and emotional safety, comfort, and fun (Chandler, 1997, p. 160).

Adults should be available to facilitate play experiences but should also stand back and give the child enough freedom to develop himself or herself within the environment. Activities should be child centered and include a range of interesting activities for the child to select as well as a balance of structured and unstructured activities. Creative pursuits that allow the child to evolve and transform the play environment should be included (Chandler, 1997; Perry, 2001). Electronics should be minimized as much as possible; instead, adults should include ample outdoor time for walks, climbing, and gardening.

Occupational therapists can be instrumental in supporting environmental design within the context of the preschool classroom to support engagement in play. Care must be given to consider whether the classroom will be housed in a public school setting to serve students with special needs or in a private, community-based preschool designed to meet the needs of larger numbers of students who are not disabled with inclusion of a smaller number of children with disabling conditions.

Rapport building with teaching staff is critical, because teachers often feel a sense of ownership over the classroom environment.

Selection and Adaptation of Toys, Learning Materials, and Activities

Perceptual–motor development is an essential component of development and reflects directly on a child's self-concept, cognitive, and social development (Perry, 2006). It is also used as a means to access and manipulate the classroom environment, whereby toy use serves as an environmental modification. The following are common activities and materials that support play-based development for preschool-age children:

- Open space for running and ball play
- Climbing, sliding, and riding equipment (tricycle)
- Tumbling mats
- Balance equipment (balance beams, balance boards, stilts)
- Ropes, parachutes, and a variety of balls (T ball, basketball, soccer ball, tennis balls)
- Trampoline, Hippity-Hop, therapy balls, Sit-n-Spin
- Sand and water play
- Boxes and packing cases for construction work and imaginative play
- Pretend play areas (housekeeping)
- Manipulative play (puzzles, beads, blocks)
- Music and rhythm instruments and materials
- Art supplies and creative materials (paper, paint, crayons, scissors)
- Books, song recordings, and finger plays for emergent literacy.

Children with atypical physical and sensory capabilities and resulting secondary social, emotional, or psychological limitations may experience several challenges to the learning opportunities afforded by play (Missiuna & Pollock, 1991). Physical limitations and environmental barriers may interfere with a child's ability to access, move, or grasp to manipulate toys and play materials. Limitations may be imposed by caregivers or professionals who are overprotective in allowing the child to explore, make decisions, and take risks. By contrast, *environmental deprivation* (total lack of toys or lack of age-appropriate toys) or *environmental indulgence* (too many toys or an overabundance of electronics) can lead to difficulties in the development of play skills. As a result of any of these factors, decreased skill practice, decreased sense of mastery, or a lack of intrinsic motivation based on perceived difficulty or past failure can promote a child's withdrawal from participation in play activities. Social challenges are more often present for children with disabilities (Clarke, Riach, & Cheyne, 1977/1982; Philip & Duckworth, 1982), because they are easily excluded from play and as a result may have poorly developed social skills. The tremendous value of play may be discounted by the belief that play that is not productive toward a developmental end is not of inherent value to the child.

Adaptations to overcome identified challenges or barriers to play are almost limitless but may involve considerations such as positioning for play; mobility aids (use of an adapted tricycle instead of a wheelchair); adaptations of size, shape, and weight of toys and materials; and technology- or computer-adapted options (e.g., modified power switches or keyboards, use of sound or visual aids). Additional adult facilitation may be necessary to assist with social barriers, but the support should not interfere with the natural spontaneity or interaction with peers (Missiuna & Pollock, 1991). Play materials and toys should have an air of familiarity with an added bonus of novelty to encourage exploration with gradual pacing of activities to the next appropriate developmental level (Ellis, 1973).

Individual Versus Group Play

Parten (1932) outlined the developmental stages of preschool social play that continue to offer consistent classification applicable to contemporary social play development (Table 7.1).

Group play can be accomplished in several ways; however, some children may need preparation and a slow transition into the group setting to be successful. The group may begin with two children and can expand accordingly. Cooperative play can be more challenging, because the potential for exclusion exists. Adults can use several strategies to promote social inclusion in play, such as assigning group membership for specific activities, assigning buddies for play activities each day, choosing two children (one with social difficulties and one who can model) to play with an adult in a special activity, and using adult-facilitated practice of group play entry skills with individual children (Widerstrom, 2005).

Many classrooms are organized around learning stations or centers; physical areas are designated as activity specific (e.g., housekeeping, art, books, manipulatives). Activities can be adult directed or child initiated as needed, allowing small groups of children to work together semi-independently. Learning activities are easily embedded within centers (Pretti-Frontczak & Bricker, 2001, 2004), although it is important to change the activities at each center on a regular basis to

Table 7.1. Developmental Stages of Preschool Social Play

Age (Years)	Class	Description
2–3	Parallel activity	Child plays independently but alongside another child without interacting, using toys that are similar.
2.5–3.5	Onlooker	Child watches others at play and engages with them verbally without physically entering into play.
4–5	Solitary independent play	Child pays alone with toys that are different from those of nearby children without making any effort to interact.
4–6	Associative play	Child plays with other children in a common activity but continues to act independently of others in the group with no division of labor present.
4–6	Cooperative play	Child plays in an organized group to engage in purposeful play with children taking on different roles (division of labor).

Note. Ages are approximate.
Source. Parten (1932).

maintain interest and motivation. Obstacle courses are another structured way to engage groups of children in play and can be adjusted to allow increasing physical challenge.

Self-initiated free play is spontaneous, intrinsically motivated, and self-regulated and requires expressive personal involvement of the child (Calder, 1980; Garvey, 1977; Gunn, 1975; Yawkey, Dank, & Glossenger, 1986). Free play may be viewed as a prerequisite to competence in occupational roles later in life and is vital for successful child growth and development (Reilly, 1974). Play serves as an antecedent for work and adult leisure pursuits, and the use of free play shapes later occupational success by fostering creativity, flexibility, and the development of social skills, all of which are valued in adult society. Free play is made easily accessible by providing materials that allow the child to choose, explore, create, and respond to change. Some options include boxes, blankets and pillows, dress-up clothes, sticks, pots and pans, and recycled containers.

Expanding Play Environments Into the Home and Community

Direct communication with families is important to bridge the child's development across home and preschool environments. Hanson and Beckman (2001) suggested using interest surveys in collaboration with parents to incorporate the child's favorite items and activities in play at home and school as well as inviting parents to volunteer and participate in play activities with the child at preschool. Professionals who serve as part of the early intervention or early childhood team (see Chapter 4) may wish to develop a toy lending library or toy exchange system, hold parent workshops to make toys or practice play skills, and design parent newsletters that describe what the child is learning at preschool along with suggested materials or activities to reinforce concepts at home.

Community-based instruction (CBI) and class field trips that occur within the context of the preschool program can be the first step to generalizing play skills to the community setting and can be an opportunity for parents to join in playful activities alongside their child. Who doesn't love an annual trip to the pumpkin patch, which offers myriad activities onsite as well as many follow-up activities? CBI should involve advanced planning to align the community experience with goals and objectives that need to be addressed. Preteaching may occur before the actual CBI trip to expose children to thematic aspects and vocabulary associated with the community environment. Follow-up and review of the excursion should also occur afterward to assist the children in reflection on their experience and assessment of the learning that will have occurred.

Sharing information on the success of CBI trips and other community resources with parents, such as public library story hours, play groups, recreation programs, or accessible playgrounds, provides opportunities for families to engage in play with children outside of the home (Widerstrom, 2005). Assisting parents in setting up play dates based on natural friendships that may have been established in the classroom can be as simple as sharing parental contact information. Some parents may need additional coaching on how to structure a play date (e.g., activities, length of time, number of children, location).

Supporting Play Through Collaborative and Transprofessional Models

Collaboration occurs when people come together as a team on a consistent basis to interact and share information and solve problems to directly benefit a child or children (Sandall & Schwartz, 2002). Interdisciplinary or transdisciplinary models of service delivery are often present in early childhood school-based settings. Because occupational therapy (and other therapies) and teaching are considered professions and not disciplines, however, the terms *interprofessional* or *transprofessional* are applied here to describe the collaborative process used when working with young children in a preschool setting (Mu & Royeen, 2004).

Several guiding principles lay the groundwork for successful transprofessional collaboration (Sandall & Schwartz, 2002):

- Participation by all team members
- Adequate time for the team to meet
- Sense of trust
- Positive, effective, and open communication
- Respect for everyone's contribution
- The ability to identify problems and develop goals and strategies to address them.

Early on, teams should develop an operational plan by having a conversation about the team model, shared goals of the team, and membership necessary for various tasks that need to accomplished (Sandall & Schwartz, 2002). Team members may include parents, child care and teaching staff, occupational therapists, physical therapists, speech therapists, nurses, service coordinators, and administrators.

Learning to apply professional knowledge in concert with interpersonal skills to blend traditional hands-on services for children with greater team, family, and school system supports is critical to effective collaboration (Hanft & Shepherd, 2008). It is essential for occupational therapists (who embrace play as a childhood occupation) to collaborate with parents, other professionals, and educational staff (whose primary purpose is to teach children) to establish a common vision for using play to support educational outcomes. The impact of having multiple practitioners with different professional approaches to intervention can result in significant confusion for parents as how to best promote their child's development.

Collaboration has been described as both an art and a science. The science focuses on team operations and management as well as its direct benefit to the child's performance in school, whereas the art of collaboration is a direct result of how seamlessly team members interact to balance direct service to children along with greater team and system supports (Idol, 1990). Through collaboration, occupational therapists can plan with, model for, and coach alongside educational staff to facilitate learning experiences that are supported through the modality of play.

The educational literature is filled with models for collaborative teaching. Common models that lend themselves to a partnership between teaching and related services professionals in the preschool setting are as follows (Friend & Cook, 2003):

- *Teacher monitor:* One professional teaches while another monitors the class to ensure that students are engaged, provides individual help as needed, or collects data on specific students. Using this model, an occupational therapist may run or lead a music and movement group with an entire preschool class of students while the teacher floats among the children providing help to those in need.
- *Interactive teaching:* One professional teaches while another demonstrates, provides clarifying information, asks questions, provides prompts, and elicits responses from children. Professionals may switch roles at any time during a lesson or activity. Using this model, a teacher may provide verbal instructions to the class on how to maneuver through an obstacle course while the occupational therapist simultaneously demonstrates the physical act of traveling through the obstacle course.
- *Parallel teaching:* Professionals work with small groups on the same task or activity at a similar pace, or each professional can teach a different part of the same lesson with students switching groups partway through. Using this model, a class may be broken into two smaller groups, with the teacher leading one group and the occupational therapist leading the other.
- *Alternative teaching:* One professional works with a large group while another works with a small group to preteach, reteach, or provide enrichment. Often, an occupational therapist using this model will serve the children on his or her caseload in a small-group setting using the same activity that the teacher is using with the remaining students in the class with extended time or additional modifications to the task provided.
- *Station teaching:* Professionals present different activities or tasks at various workstations, and students rotate among stations. This model can include small groups and opportunities for independent group work. In this model, the teacher and occupational therapist have usually planned various activities with an emphasis on specific skills at each station (e.g., the occupational therapy station may focus on fine motor skills or self-care).
- *Team teaching:* Professionals work in the same room using comprehensive cooperation and collaboration to co-plan and co-implement lessons and activities and provide support for accommodations and learning strategies to address the needs of all students in the classroom. Neither professional is viewed as an expert because roles are completely blurred. With this model, an occupational therapist may be committed to large amounts of time in a classroom to provide an ongoing presence and support for students who have more intensive needs (e.g., a specialized preschool classroom designed for students with autism in which an occupational therapist is available for 50% or more of the time each week).

Collaborative educational practices require shared responsibilities, joint planning time, and clear expectations and roles on behalf of team members. Unique systemic needs and models of service provision should be taken into account when considering a change in service provision models and may require administrative support and approval. The type of preschool setting may have a potential impact on how readily staff members are willing to collaborate. Some states and localities that do not offer preschool to all children have established public school–based early childhood special education preschool classrooms that reside within elementary or center-based sites to serve students who are identified with a disabling condition under IDEA 2004. Other states and localities serve preschool children with disabilities in the preschool classroom with students without disabilities in accordance with the least restrictive environment requirement of IDEA 2004. In other circumstances, students with a disabling condition may attend a private, community-based preschool, Head Start, or child care facility in which most children are typically developing. The skills of teachers in these settings for addressing the needs of a child with disabilities vary greatly. Some states offer preschool services in the home. The occupational therapist must adapt his or her role to the idiosyncrasies of the system in which he or she is providing educational support.

Learning Activity 7.4 asks readers to partner with an early childhood teacher to co-plan a lesson.

Case Study: Melina

Melina is a new occupational therapist working in a preschool classroom. She had previous experience during her Level II fieldwork in a pediatric outpatient center that specialized in offering monthly play clinics to families in need of training and support. The preschool teacher is very friendly and eagerly asks Melina to assist with establishing a baseline measure of play for all the students in her classroom. Melina feels a little nervous at first, because not all the students in the classroom receive special education services or occupational therapy as a related service. The school, however, is implementing Response to Intervention activities, and Melina's work in this classroom can be viewed as both Tier I and Tier II interventions, depending on individual child responses. She wants to do her best as an itinerant service provider to balance her school-based caseload, which is quite different from her experience in the outpatient center.

Melina agrees to help, but she asks the teacher for clarification as to what exactly she means by a "baseline measure of play." Melina had worked with teachers at the outpatient center during monthly play clinics, but she had never had the opportunity to establish a play program that would be carried out on site instead of in a family's home. The teacher invites Melina to have lunch with her staff to talk more about the project. At lunch, Melina meets the other professionals on the team, and they begin to chat about the children in the classroom. Melina begins to take note

Learning Activity 7.4. Teaming up for Play

- Recruit an early childhood teacher to be your partner.
- Select two collaborative teaching models, and design a lesson or treatment plan based on a preschool classroom learning theme of insects.
- Include a description of the objective(s) for the lessons and activities, materials needed, your role as an occupational therapist in relation to the role of the classroom teacher, and the desired outcome(s).
- Indicate your reasons for choosing these teaching models and your comfort level with implementation.

of children's specific interests and preferences as described by staff members, areas of strength and weakness, and desires of staff for how to expand the play repertoire of the various children. She is able to ask clarifying questions throughout the course of the conversation.

After lunch, she completes a file review of all the children before beginning her observational assessments. She wonders whether she should consider using any formal assessments, as she did in the clinic, but decides to wait until after her first clinical impressions have been established by observation. After 2 weeks of observation have been completed to account for all students in the class, she decides to schedule lunch again with the staff to share her thoughts. Melina summarizes areas of strength and weakness for each child and provides a spreadsheet highlighting the greatest areas of need alongside strengths and individual interests and preferences. She asks the team members how they feel goal planning and intervention should proceed by asking the following questions:

- What does the team want to accomplish related to play within the structure of the classroom?
- What types of individual play goals, if any, are needed for each of the children?

The team ponders Melina's questions and first establishes an overarching classroom goal: Each child will select and play independently or interdependently with peers for at least 10 minutes daily by school year's end. Then they establish individual play goals for the students in greatest need of specific play-based intervention. The team agrees, given the scope of the shared goal and vision, that collaborative planning should continue to occur weekly over lunch (everyone has to eat!). They discuss the various collaborative teaching service provision models that both Melina and the preschool teacher have used previously and agree to set up different stations for the children to rotate through as a place to begin.

Family-Centered Approach to Play: Sociocultural Awareness

Parents are a child's first teacher, and they serve a critical role in laying the groundwork for learning, education experiences, motivation, and behavioral adjustment (Esdaile, 1996). Parents with non-American cultural backgrounds may differ in their values and approaches to play. Beliefs about child development tend to be culturally bound and can affect the frequency of play, toys, space, and media available; number of children engaging in different types of play; and social play partners (Harkness & Super, 1986, 1996). Bazyk, Stalnaker, Llerena, Ekelman, and Bazyk (2003) noted that in rural, traditional Mayan families, children's ADLs are structured more around household work (e.g., chores, errands, and caring for younger siblings) and less around play.

In U.S. culture, parents are called on to strike an occupational balance between paid or unpaid work, household work, and play with their children. The occupation of caregiving involves two or more people (parent and child) as occupational participants, thus allowing parents to engage in co-occupations with their children (Zemke & Clark, 1996). Women are more likely than men to further enfold occupations by participating in multiple occupations and co-occupations at the same time (Bateson,

1996). This mosaic of occupations involves competing demands for both attention and time, because parents must orchestrate their children's occupations in addition to their own (Primeau, 1998; Primeau, Clark, & Pierce, 1989).

For these reasons, it is important for professionals to demystify the "expert" role and emphasize a family-centered, experiential approach to using play and toys to support child development within a culturally relevant context (Esdaile, 1996). Families should be viewed as a unit of intervention and be empowered by focusing on family-identified needs while building on their unique capabilities and strengthening their social network (Dunst, Trivette, & Deal, 1994). Through recognition that parents and siblings can play in a variety of ways, professionals can facilitate expanded opportunities for play within the natural context of daily, family routines (Dunst et al., 2001).

Occupational Therapist and Parent Partnerships

Just as roles need to be defined for the occupational therapist and family during the evaluation and goal-setting processes, roles need to be defined for the intervention process. The level of parent involvement will vary from early intervention (birth through age 2) to preschool (ages 3 to 5); early intervention has much more emphasis on direct involvement. Parents may continue to be involved in preschool through home and classroom visits as well as training opportunities offered by school staff, which may vary from one school district to another. Although the occupational therapist may provide direct intervention to the child in the absence of the parent in some situations, as noted previously, parents can take advantage of the many daily opportunities to promote their child's learning in the time between visits. On the basis of developmental models and supportive evidence-based data, infant–toddler home-based intervention programs such as Early Head Start, Parents as Teachers, Healthy Start, and Olds' Nurse Home Visiting Program have recognized the importance and effectiveness of incorporating the parent as an important participant in intervention (Olds et al., 2004; Peterson, Luze, Eshbaugh, Hyun-Joo, & Kantz, 2007; Sloper, 2004).

Supporting parent participation can occur through direct instruction, modeling (Chai et al., 2006), enhancing parent–child relationships (McCollum, Gooler, Appl, & Yates, 2001), or the active partnership between the occupational therapist and the parent (Campbell, 2004; Campbell & Sawyer, 2007; Rush & Shelden, 2005). Primeau (1998) identified two methods that parents use to fit play into the daily home routine: (1) strategies of segregation, in which play is interspersed with housework, and (2) strategies of inclusion, in which play is embedded in housework. Professionals may need to begin by modeling how to play with the child while encouraging parents or siblings to join in or pointing out the child's play strengths as a springboard for expanding play sequences and opportunities (Knox & Mailloux, 1997). Parents may need guidance on how to organize the play environment as well as recommendations for buying or adapting toys. Working with families as copartners, without being directive or judgmental, helps everyone to gain an understanding of the child within the context of the family's narrative story (Burke, Schaaf, & Hall, 2008) and will ultimately lead to successful and positive parent–child play interactions.

Dempsey and Dunst (2004) suggested that family-oriented models of service provision should emphasize capacity-building and participatory help-giving practices to enable parents and empower families. Modeling of parent participation in play activities is one example of how therapists can promote participatory help-giving practices. According to Bandura's (1992) model of self-efficacy, parents' participation with their child(ren) during play activities promotes their capabilities and confidence and, in turn, increases the time they spend promoting their child's development through play. Wilson, Holbert, and Sexton (2005) further defined three major elements that make up a capacity-building practice, as follows:

1. *Participatory learning opportunities* occur when the people providing intervention—in this case, occupational therapists—recognize and take advantage of parent participation in child play activities as a context for strengthening existing parent knowledge and skills, learning new knowledge and skills, and promoting parents' learning on their own behalf.
2 *Participatory help-giving* practices include the strategies and opportunities interventionists use during visits to promote parents' use of existing strengths and acquisition of new abilities that further their child's development. This element may include direct instruction, modeling, and observation of the parent and child together.
3. *Active learner participation* refers to practices that encourage the parent taking on the responsibility of planning (using his or her knowledge of the child's competencies and activities) and action (to generate solutions and strategies for determining goals and approaches) to accomplish desired outcomes.

Occupational therapists will recognize these three elements as the major parts of a therapeutic process, renamed. Intervention focused on promoting the parent's competency and participation as the primary provider of intervention supports requires professional competencies possessed by the occupational therapist (e.g., skill in interpersonal communication and relationship skills, self-reflection, clinical reasoning, role release, and facilitation of self-appraisal). A process of supporting parent capacity to promote the child's development has been termed *coaching* (Rush & Shelden, 2005). See Chapter 3 for a discussion of coaching as part of family-centered practices.

Case Study: Joshua

Background

Recall Joshua, the boy who lives with his parents and his baby sister in a rural area. Joshua is a curious and active youngster who spends the balance of his day at his home with his mother and sibling. At his last regular visit to the family doctor, his mother identified some delays in his language and fine motor skills on his developmental screening, and the family doctor referred him to the state Part C program.

The Story Continues

An early childhood intervention teacher, who is the service coordinator, and the occupational therapist conduct an eligibility evaluation and play evaluation with

Joshua in his home with both of his parents present. Before the assessment begins, Joshua's parents express concern with the limited number of words he uses and how little he is able to play independently and quietly in the house. They also note that he often cries and screams when it is time to pick up his toys for bedtime. The early intervention teacher explains what the team will ask Joshua to do during the assessment and invites the parents to be part of the play assessment.

Through interview questions and observations of Joshua during the play evaluation, the team, which includes the parents, identifies that Joshua loves to do the following activities:

- Run with the family dog
- Climb things
- Play peek-a-boo with his baby sister
- Sweep with a broom
- Dance to music with his father
- Play with toy cars
- Pretend to write with his mother's pen
- Go to the grocery store
- Stack cans of soup and vegetables
- Play in water with his cars and a washrag.

Play observations also indicate that although Joshua enjoys drawing and coloring, he resists directions his mother gives him when coloring pictures and does not stay engaged in a coloring activity or with a book for very long. After the assessment, the team discusses possible goals to focus on. Joshua's parents identify that they want Joshua to play by himself while they are busy preparing food for the family, caring for Joshua's baby sister, or completing other household work. They also want him to stop screaming and crying when he is upset and use words to convey his feelings.

The team reviews which activities are both interesting to and successful for Joshua and his family and which other daily routines offer opportunities for Joshua's parents to promote his play capabilities and language. Bath time and mealtime are identified as two of Joshua's favorite activities. They offer interesting play opportunities for Joshua and opportunities for his parents to support his learning. A plan is developed for the next week that incorporate these activities.

With only one working parent, the family has limited income to purchase toys, and few, if any, age-appropriate toys are available. The occupational therapist identifies common household objects and materials that can be used to encourage Joshua's capabilities during his bath time, such as cups, spoons, and different-sized sponges to allow Joshua to scoop and pour water while bathing. Because Joshua enjoys shopping and playing with cans of foods, the parents decide to move the canned goods to a lower shelf and engage Joshua's participation in putting the canned goods into the cupboard when the family returns home from shopping. The early childhood teacher demonstrates using simple phrases and verbal modeling strategies during the grocery shopping to promote Joshua's vocabulary. Strategies for elaborating and extending Joshua's water play with sponges and washrags to helping to clean up after meals in the kitchen are shared with the parents.

The following week, the early childhood teacher returns to Joshua's home and reviews with the family which activities and strategies were successful, which they wished to continue, and which new activities they would like to include. The mother states that she has figured out that doing the same thing as Joshua will keep his attention long enough for her to show him new things he can try with the spoons and cups. She also reported that Joshua had started to sing "Twinkle, Twinkle Little Star" after she showed him he could bang on a kitchen pot like a drum.

Strategies are modeled for Joshua's mother on how to cook with Joshua by allowing him to pour, mix, and transfer ingredients with her help and guidance while she is cooking as well as how to set his place at a child-sized table using shatterproof serving pieces and utensils.

Joshua's mother states that he has not really increased his vocabulary during grocery time but has become more interested in putting his favorite foods into the shopping cart. The early childhood teacher and Joshua's mother discuss focusing the parents' language modeling on his favorite foods. Joshua's mother decides to keep the same activities as the previous week, offer him some opportunities to help with cooking, and to focus only on favorite food words for the next week.

After 3 months of weekly plans, Joshua begins to name and ask for favorite foods and people consistently, has a consistent role in preparing meals, has extended cleaning up to include before bedtime, and is attempting to wash himself during bath time. He has begun to identify family foods in the weekly newspaper grocery store coupon insert as well.

Conclusion

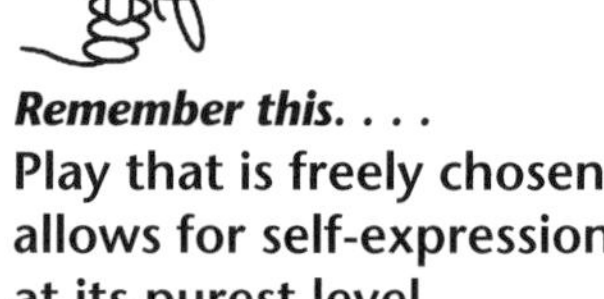

Remember this. . . .
Play that is freely chosen allows for self-expression at its purest level.

People of all ages engage in various occupations to support health and participation in life. The balance of occupational engagement and its distribution across areas of occupation changes across the lifespan; play is the primary occupation of childhood. Inherent at every stage of life is the need to engage in pleasurable activities in the form of play and leisure. Play that is freely chosen allows for self-expression at its purest level while building skills in decision making, problem solving, flexibility, creativity, self-esteem, social interactions, and conflict resolution. The benefits of play as a foundation for child and later adult development and performance clearly represent skills, traits, and values that support the many roles of adulthood, including those of parent and caregiver, spouse and partner, worker, and the like. It is through play that we as humans are able to suspend the consequences of everyday reality to provide holistic balance to our existence.

How Very Far We Have Come: Grace and Lydia and a Good IDEA (1979–1993)

Grace had started attending the neighborhood public school when she entered kindergarten. Annie thought of how, despite much work, it had been relatively easy to address Grace's needs compared with what her parents had had to do when she and Danny were born. She remembered her mother's endless work to get the schools to admit students with disabilities. She also remembered the long car rides to the hospitals and Danny being away from home as a little boy and then having to go away to school at 15 so he could graduate from an accredited school. She had never forgotten the look on his face when she got on the school bus the first time, and he had not.

Now, the schools were attentive to Grace's needs, developing individualized programs to address her specific needs and sending home weekly progress reports to inform Annie and Coleman. Grace also had therapy to help her achieve in school, and it was paid for by Annie's and Coleman's and all the other citizen's tax dollars, just as education for "regular" children always had been. The year of Grace's birth, Congress passed legislation that had its roots in the laws that had convinced Dan and their parents to have him attend the state school. The Education of All Handicapped Children Act (EHA) was passed in November 1975, just a month after Grace was born.

The advocacy of Lydia and countless others had finally come to fruition. Their children could attend school alongside their brothers, sisters, cousins, and neighbors. It had taken 19 years since Danny should have entered school to gain the right for children with disabilities to be there. He had finished both school and college by then. How many others had been working for far longer? How far back in time did the effort go?

Questions

1. At the time of its passage, it was said that the EHA was the most heavily lobbied bill that had ever been considered by Congress. What are several possible reasons for this?
2. Why was this time period right for the passage of this bill?
3. In what ways can the disabilities rights movement be seen as part of the civil rights movement?

References

Ainsworth, M. D. (1969). Object relations, dependency, and attachment: A theoretical review of the infant–mother relationship. *Child Development, 40,* 969–1025.

Alessandrini, N. A. (1949). Play—A child's world. *American Journal of Occupational Therapy, 3,* 9–12.

American Occupational Therapy Association. (2008). Occupational therapy practice framework: Domain and process (2nd ed.). *American Journal of Occupational Therapy, 62,* 625–683.

Bandura, A. (1992). Social cognitive theory. In R. Vasta (Ed.), *Six theories of child development: Revised formulations and current issues* (pp. 1–60). London: Jessica Kingsley.

Barnett, L. A. (1990). Developmental benefits of play. *Journal of Leisure Research, 22,* 138–153.

Barnett, L. A. (1991). Developmental benefits of play for children. In B. L. Driver, P. J. Brown, & G. E. Peterson (Eds.), *Benefits of leisure* (pp. 216–247). State College, PA: Venture.

Bateson, M. C. (1996). Enfolded activity and the concept of occupation. In R. Zemke & F. Clark (Eds.), *Occupational science: The evolving discipline* (pp. 5–12). Philadelphia: F. A. Davis.

Bazyk, S., Stalnaker, D., Llerena, M., Ekelman, B., & Bazyk, J. (2003). Play in Mayan children. *American Journal of Occupational Therapy, 57,* 273–283.

Berretta, S., & Privette, G. (1990). Influence of play on creative thinking. *Perceptual and Motor Skills, 71,* 659–666.

Brazelton, T. B., & Cramer, B. G. (1990). *The earliest relationship: Parents, infants, and the drama of early attachment*: Toronto, ON: Addison-Wesley.

Bronfenbrenner, U. (1986). Ecology of the family as a context for human development: Research perspectives. *Developmental Psychology, 22,* 723–742.

Bronson, M., & Bundy, A. C. (2001). A correlational study of the Test of Playfulness and the Test of Environmental Supportiveness. *OTJR: Occupation, Participation and Health, 21,* 223–240.

Bruner, J. S. (1972). Nature and uses of immaturity. *American Psychologist, 27,* 687–708.

Bryze, K. C. (2008). Narrative contributions to the play history. In L. D. Parham & L. S. Fazio (Eds.), *Play in occupational therapy for children* (pp. 2–21). St. Louis, MO: Mosby.

Bundy, A. (1993). Assessment of play and leisure: Delineation of the problem. *American Journal of Occupational Therapy, 47,* 217–222.

Bundy, A., Nelson, L., Metzger, M., & Bingaman, K. (2001). Validity and reliability of a test of playfulness. *OTJR: Occupation, Participation and Health, 21,* 276–292.

Burke, J. P. (1998). Play: The life role of the infant and young child. In J. Case-Smith (Ed.), *Pediatric occupational therapy and early intervention* (2nd ed., pp. 189–205). Woburn, MA: Butterworth-Heinemann.

Burke, J. P., Schaaf, R. C., & Hall, T. B. L. (2008). Family narratives and play assessment. In L. D. Parham & L. S. Fazio (Eds.), *Play in occupational therapy for children* (pp. 195–215). St. Louis, MO: Mosby.

Caillois, R. (1961). *Man, play, and games.* New York: Free Press.

Calder, J. E. (1980). Learn to play—Play to learn. In J. K. Atkinson (Ed.), *Too late at eight: Prevention and intervention, young children's learning difficulties* (pp. 163–188). Brisbane, Queensland, Australia: Fred and Eleanor Schonell Educational Research Centre.

Campbell, P. H. (2004). Participation-based services: Promoting children's participation in natural settings. *Young Exceptional Children, 8*(1), 20–29.

Campbell, P. H., & Sawyer, L. B. (2007). Supporting learning opportunities in natural settings through participation-based services. *Journal of Early Intervention, 29*(4), 287–305.

Chai, A. Y., Zhang, C., & Bisberg, M. (2006). Rethinking natural environment practice: Implications from examining various interpretations and approaches. *Early Childhood Education Journal, 34*(3), 203–208.

Chandler, B. E. (Ed.). (1997). Where do you want to play? Play environments: An occupational therapy perspective. In B. E. Chandler (Ed.), *The essence of play: A child's occupation* (pp. 159–172). Bethesda, MD: American Occupational Therapy Association.

Clarke, M. M., Riach, J., & Cheyne, W. M. (1982). Handicapped children and preschool education [Report to Warnock Committee on Special Education, University of Strathclyde]. In M. Philip & D. Duckworth (Eds.), *Children with disabilities and their families.* Windsor, England: NFER–Nelson. (Original report published 1977)

Coleman, P. K., & Karraker, K. H. (2003). Maternal self-efficacy beliefs, competence in parenting, and toddlers' behavior and developmental status. *Infant Mental Health Journal, 24*(2), 126–148.

Coleman, P. K., Trent, A., Bryan, S., King, B., Rogers, N., & Nazir, M. (2002). Parenting behavior, mothers' self-efficacy beliefs, and toddler performance on the Bayley Scales of Infant Development. *Early Child Development and Care, 172*(2), 123–140.

Cook, R., Tessier, A., & Klein, D. (2000). *Adapting early childhood curricula for children in inclusive settings* (5th ed.). New York: Charles E. Merrill.

Couch, K. J., Deitz, J. C., & Kanny, E. M. (1998). The role of play in occupational therapy. *American Journal of Occupational Therapy, 52,* 111–117.

Csikszentmihalyi, M. (1990). *Flow: The psychology of optimal experience.* New York: Harper Perennial.

Dattner, R. (1969). *Design for play.* New York: Van Nostrand Reinhold.

DeCasper, A., & Fifer, W. (1980). Of human bonding: Newborns prefer their mothers' voices. *Science, 208*(4448), 1174–1176.

Dempsey, I., & Dunst, C. J. (2004). Help-giving styles and parent empowerment in families with a young child with a disability. *Journal of Intellectual and Developmental Disability, 29,* 40–51.

D'Eugenio, D. (1997). Infant play. In B. E. Chandler (Ed.), *The essence of play: A child's occupation* (pp. 65–77). Bethesda, MD: American Occupational Therapy Association.

Dewey, J. (1902). *The child and the curriculum.* Chicago: University of Chicago Press.

Dewey, J. (1938). *Experience and education.* New York: Crowell–Collier–Macmillan.

Douglas, J., & Richman, N. (1985). *Coping with young children.* Harmondsworth, England: Penguin Books.

Dunst, C. J. (2006). Parent-mediated everyday child learning opportunities: I. Foundations and operationalization. *CASEinPoint, 2*(2), 1–10. Retrieved January 10, 2009, from www.fippcase.org/caseinpoint/caseinpoint_vol2_no2.pdf

Dunst, C. J., Bruder, M. B., Trivette, C. M., Hamby, D., Raab, M., & McLean, M. (2001). Characteristics and consequences of everyday natural learning opportunities. *Topics in Early Childhood Special Education, 21,* 68–92.

Dunst, C. J., Hamby, D., Trivette, C. M., Raab, M., & Bruder, M. B. (2000). Everyday family and community life and children's naturally occurring learning opportunities. *Journal of Early Intervention, 23*(3), 151–164.

Dunst, C. J., Trivette, C. M., & Deal, A. G. (Eds.). (1994). *Supporting and strengthening families: Volume 1: Methods, strategies, and practices.* Cambridge, MA: Brookline.

Education for All Handicapped Children Act of 1975, Pub. L. 94–142, 20 U.S.C. § 1400 *et seq.*

Ellis, M. J. (1973). *Why people play.* Englewood Cliffs, NJ: Prentice-Hall.

Erikson, J. (1996). The Infant–Toddler Developmental Assessment (IDA). In S. J. Meisels & E. S. Fenichel (Eds.), *New visions for the developmental assessment of infants and young children* (pp. 147–168). Washington, DC: Zero to Three

Esdaile, S. A. (1996). A play-focused intervention involving mothers of preschoolers. *American Journal of Occupational Therapy, 50,* 113–123.

Frank, L. K. (1955). Therapeutic play techniques symposium: Play in personality development. *American Journal of Orthopsychiatry, 25,* 576–590.

Friend, M., & Cook, L. (2003). *Interactions: Collaborative skills for school professionals* (4th ed.). Boston: Allyn & Bacon.

Garvey, C. (1977). *Play.* Cambridge, MA: Harvard University Press.

Greenspan, S. I., & Lewis, N. B. (1999). *Building healthy minds* (pp. 375–381). New York: Perseus.

Greenspan, S. I., & Meisels, S. J. (1996). Toward a new vision for the developmental assessment of infants and young children. In S. J. Meisels & E. S. Fenichel (Eds.), *New visions for the developmental assessment of infants and young children* (pp. 11–26). Washington, DC: Zero to Three.

Griffith, L. R. (2000). *Hispanic American children and the Test of Playfulness.* Unpublished master's thesis, Colorado State University, Ft. Collins.

Gunn, S. L. (1975). Play as occupation: Implications for the handicapped. *American Journal of Occupational Therapy, 29,* 222–225.

Handley-More, D., & Chandler, B. (2007). Occupational therapy decision-making process. In L. L. Jackson (Ed.), *Occupational therapy services for children and youth under IDEA* (3rd ed., pp. 59–87). Bethesda, MD: AOTA Press.

Hanft, B., & Place, P. (1996). *The consulting therapist.* Austin, TX: Pro-Ed.

Hanft, B., & Shepherd, J. (2008). 2 . . . 4 . . . 6 . . . 8 . . . How do you collaborate? In B. Hanft & J. Shepherd (Eds.), *Collaborating for student success: A guide for school-based occupational therapy* (pp. 1–33). Bethesda, MD: AOTA Press.

Hanson, M. J., & Beckman, P. J. (2001). *Me too! series: My new friends.* Baltimore: Brookes.

Harkness, S., & Super, C. (1986). The cultural structuring of children's play in a rural African community. In K. Blanchard (Ed.), *The many faces of play* (pp. 96–104). Champaign, IL: Human Kinetics.

Harkness, S., & Super, C. (1996). *Parents' cultural belief systems: Their origins, expressions, and consequences.* New York: Guilford Press.

Henry, A. (2008). Assessment of play and leisure in children and adolescents. In L. D. Parham & L. S. Fazio (Eds.), *Play in occupational therapy for children* (pp. 55–70). St. Louis, MO: Mosby.

Hirshberg, L. M. (1996). History-making, not history-taking: Clinical interviews with infants and their families. In S. J. Meisels & E. S. Fenichel (Eds.), *New visions for the developmental assessment of infants and young children* (pp. 85–124). Washington, DC: Zero to Three.

Idol, L. (1990). The scientific art of classroom consultation. *Journal of Educational and Psychological Consultation, 1,* 3–22.

Individuals With Disabilities Education Improvement Act of 2004, Pub. L. 108–446, 20 U.S.C. § 1400 *et seq.*

Knox, S. (2005). Play. In J. Case-Smith (Ed.), *Occupational therapy for children* (5th ed., pp. 571–586). St. Louis, MO: Mosby.

Knox, S. (2008). Development and current use of the Revised Knox Preschool Play Scale. In L. D. Parham & L. S. Fazio (Eds.), *Play in occupational therapy for children* (pp. 55–70). St. Louis, MO: Mosby.

Knox, S., & Mailloux, Z. (1997). Play as treatment and treatment through play. In B. E. Chandler (Ed.), *The essence of play: A child's occupation* (pp. 175–204). Bethesda, MD: American Occupational Therapy Association.

Lawlor, M., & Mattingly, C. (1998). The complexities embedded in family-centered care. *American Journal of Occupational Therapy, 52,* 259–267.

Lieberman, N. (1965). Playfulness and divergent thinking: An investigation of their relationship at the kindergarten level. *Journal of Genetic Psychology, 107*(2), 219–224.

Macy, M. G., & Bricker, D. D. (2006). Practical applications for using curriculum-based assessment to create embedded learning opportunities for young children. *Young Exceptional Children, 9*(4), 12–21.

Macy, M. G., & Bricker, D. D. (2007). Embedding individualized social goals into routine activities in inclusive early childhood classrooms. *Early Child Development and Care, 177*(2), 107–120.

Marakova, G., & Legerstee, M. (2008). How infants come to learn about the minds of others. *Zero to Three, 28*(5), 26–31.

McCollum, J., Gooler, F., Appl, D., & Yates, T. (2001). PIWI: Enhancing child interaction as a foundation for early intervention. *Infants and Young Children, 14*(1), 34–45.

Meisels, S. J. (1996). Charting the continuum of assessment and intervention. In S. J. Meisels & E. S. Fenichel (Eds.), *New visions for the developmental assessment of infants and young children* (pp. 27–52). Washington, DC: Zero to Three.

Meltzoff, A., & Moore, M. (1983). Newborn infants imitate adult facial gestures. *Child Development, 54*(3), 702–709.

Miller, E., & Kuhaneck, H. (2008). Children's perceptions of play experiences and play preferences: A qualitative study. *American Journal of Occupational Therapy, 62,* 407–415.

Missiuna, C., & Pollock, N. (1991). Play deprivation in children with physical disabilities: The role of the occupational therapist in preventing secondary disability. *American Journal of Occupational Therapy, 45,* 882–888.

Mogford, K. (1977). The play of handicapped children. In B. Tizard & D. Harvey (Eds.), *Biology of play* (pp. 170–184). Philadelphia: J. B. Lippincott.

Montessori, M. (1912). *The Montessori method: Scientific pedagogy as applied to early childhood education in Children's Houses.* New York: Frederick A. Stokes.

Mu, K., & Royeen, C. B. (2004). Interprofessional vs. interdisciplinary services in school-based occupational therapy practice. *Occupational Therapy International, 11*(4), 244–247.

National Association for the Education of Young Children. (2009). *Developmentally appropriate practice in early childhood programs serving children from birth through age 8* (Position statement). Washington, DC: Author. Retrieved December 9, 2009, from www.naeyc.org/files/naeyc/file/positions/PSDAP.pdf

Olds, D. L., Kitzman, H., Cole, R., Robinson, J., Sidora, K., Luckey, D. W., et al. (2004). Effects of nurse home-visiting on maternal life course and child development: Age 6 follow-up results of a randomized trial. *Pediatrics, 114*(6), 1550–1559.

Parham, L. D. (1996). Perspectives on play. In R. Zemke & F. Clark (Eds.), *Occupational science: The evolving discipline* (pp. 71–80). Philadelphia: F. A. Davis.

Parham, L. D. (2008). Play and occupational therapy. In L. D. Parham & L. S. Fazio (Eds.), *Play in occupational therapy for children* (pp. 2–21). St. Louis, MO: Mosby.

Parham, L. D., & Fazio, L. S. (1997). *Play in occupational therapy for children.* St. Louis, MO: Mosby–Year Book.

Parten, M. B. (1932). Social participation among preschool children. *Journal of Abnormal and Social Psychology, 27,* 243–269.

Pellegrini, A. D. (2001). Practitioner review: The role of direct observation in the assessment of young children. *Journal of Child Psychology and Psychiatry, 42*(7), 861–869.

Perry, D. (2001). *The child: What every caring parent needs to know.* Clarendon Hills, IL: MECA–Seton.

Perry, D. (2006). *Perceptual–motor development: At home and in the preschool.* Clarendon Hills, IL: MECA–Seton.

Perry, D., & Perry, C. P. (2000). *The child is a person: A parent's approach to educating the young child* (2nd ed.). Clarendon Hills, IL: MECA–Seton.

Pestalozzi, J. (1890). Letter to Heinrich Gessner about his orphanage at Stanz, Switzerland. In R. de Guimps (Ed.), *Pestalozzi, his life and work* (pp. 149–171). New York: Appleton. (Original work published 1799)

Peterson, C. A., Luze, G. L., Eshbaugh, E. M., Hyun-Joo, J., & Kantz, K. R. (2007). Enhancing parent-child interactions through home visiting: Promising practice or unfulfilled promise. *Journal of Early Intervention, 29*(2), 119–135.

Philip, M., & Duckworth, D. (1982). *Children with disabilities and their families.* Windsor, England: NFER–Nelson.

Phillips, H. A. (1998). *Guatemalan and Nicaraguan children and the Test of Playfulness.* Unpublished master's thesis, Colorado State University, Ft. Collins.

Piaget, J., & Inhelder, B. (1969). *The psychology of the child.* New York: Basic Books. (Original work published 1966)

Pollock, N., Stewart, D., Law, M., Sahagian-Whalen, H. S., & Toal, C. (1997). The meaning of play for young people with physical disabilities. *Canadian Journal of Occupational Therapy, 64,* 25–31.

Porter, C. A., & Bundy, A. C. (2000). Validity and reliability of three tests of playfulness with African American children and their parents. In S. Reifel (Ed.), *Play and culture studies. Vol. 3: Theory in context and out* (pp. 315–334). Westport, CT: Ablex.

Pretti-Frontczak, K., & Bricker, D. (2001). Use of the embedding strategy during daily activities by early childhood education and early childhood special education teachers. *Infant–Toddler Intervention: The Transdisciplinary Journal, 11*(2), 111–128.

Pretti-Frontczak, K., & Bricker, D. (2004). *An activity-based approach to early intervention* (3rd ed.). Baltimore: Brookes.

Primeau, L. A. (1998). Orchestration of work and play within families. *American Journal of Occupational Therapy, 52,* 188–195.

Primeau, L. A., Clark, F., & Pierce, D. (1989). Occupational therapy alone has looked upon occupation: Future applications of occupational science to pediatric occupational therapy. *Occupational Therapy in Health Care, 6*(4), 19–32.

Raab, M. (2005). Interest-based child participation in everyday learning activities. *CASEinPoint, 1*(2), 1–5. Retrieved January 10, 2009, from www.fippcase.org/caseinpoint/caseinpoint_vol1_no2.pdf

Rast, M. (1986). Play and therapy, play or therapy. In C. Pehoski (Ed.), *Play: A skill for life* (pp. 29–41). Bethesda, MD: American Occupational Therapy Association.

Reilly, M. (1974). *Play as exploratory learning.* Beverly Hills, CA: Sage.

Reynolds, G., & Jones, E. (1997). *Master players: Learning from children at play.* New York: Teachers College Press.

Rocco, S. (1996). Toward shared commitment and shared responsibility: A parent's view of developmental assessment. In S. J. Meisels & E. S. Fenichel (Eds.), *New visions for the developmental assessment of infants and young children* (pp. 27–52). Washington, DC: Zero to Three.

Rovee-Collier, C. (1987). Learning and memory in infancy. In J. D. Osofsky (Ed.), *Handbook of infant development* (pp. 98–148). New York: Wiley.

Rush, D. D., & Shelden, M. L. (2005). Evidence-based definition of coaching practices. *CASEinPoint, 1*(2), 1–5. Retrieved January 10, 2009, from www.fippcase.org/caseinpoint/caseinpoint_vol1_no6.pdf

Sameroff, A. J., & Fiese, B. H. (2000). Transactional regulation: The developmental ecology of early intervention. In J. P. Shonkoff & S. J. Meisels (Eds.), *Handbook of early childhood intervention* (2nd ed., pp. 135–159). Cambridge, England: Cambridge University Press.

Sandall, S., & Schwartz, I. S. (2002). *Building blocks for teaching preschoolers with special needs.* Baltimore: Brookes.

Schaaf, R., & Burke, J. (1997). What happens when we play? A neurodevelopmental explanation. In B. E. Chandler (Ed.), *The essence of play: A child's occupation* (pp. 79–105). Bethesda, MD: American Occupational Therapy Association.

Segal, M., & Webber, N. T. (1996). Nonstructured play observations: Guidelines, benefits, and caveats. In S. J. Meisels & E. Fenichel (Eds.), *New visions for the developmental assessment of infants and young children* (pp. 207–230). Washington, DC: Zero to Three.

Shonkoff, J. P., & Phillips, D. A. (Eds.). (2000). *From neurons to neighborhoods: The science of early childhood development.* Washington, DC: National Academies Press. Retrieved January 20, 2009, from http://books.nap.edu/openbook.php?record_id=9824&page=1

Slade, A., & Wolf, D. P. (Eds.). (1994). *Children at play: Clinical and developmental approaches to meaning and representation.* New York: Oxford University Press.
Sloper, P. (2004). Facilitators and barriers for coordinated multi-agency services. *Child, Health, and Development, 30,* 571–580.
Smith, M. B. (1974). *Humanizing social psychology.* San Francisco: Jossey-Bass.
Spariosu, M. (1991). *God of many names: Play, poetry, and power in Hellenic thought from Homer to Aristotle.* Durham, NC: Duke University Press.
Stern, D. N. (2002). *The first relationship: Infant and mother, with a new introduction.* Cambridge, MA: Harvard University Press.
Stone, F. (1991). *A descriptive study of the use of play in occupational therapy.* Unpublished master's thesis, University of Illinois at Chicago.
Takata, N. (1974). Play as prescription. In M. Reilly (Ed.), *Play as exploratory learning* (pp. 209–246). Beverly Hills, CA: Sage.
Tanta, K. J., Deitz, J., White, O., & Billingsley, F. (2005). The effects of peer–play level on initiations and responses of preschool children with delayed play skills. *American Journal of Occupational Therapy, 59,* 437–445.
Teti, D. M., & Gelfand, D. M. (1991). Behavioral competence among mothers of infants in the first year: The mediational role of maternal self-efficacy. *Child Development, 62*(5), 918–929.
University of California–Irvine. (2008, March 13). Short-term stress can affect learning and memory. *Science Daily.* Retrieved February 7, 2009, from www.sciencedaily.com/releases/2008/03/080311182434.htm
U.S. Department of Education. (2004). *Part C—Infants and Toddlers With Disabilities, Sec. 632 definitions.* Retrieved October 30, 2009, from http://idea.ed.gov/explore/view/p/,root,statute,I,C,
Vygotsky, L. (1978). *Mind in society: The development of higher psychological processes.* Cambridge, MA: Harvard University Press.
Wade, M. (1985). *Constraints on leisure.* Springfield, IL: Charles C Thomas.
Widerstrom, A. H. (2005). *Achieving learning goals through play: Teaching young children with special needs* (2nd ed.). Baltimore: Brookes.
Wilson, L. L., Holbert, K., & Sexton, S. (2005). A capacity-building approach to parenting education. *CASEinPoint, 2*(7), 1–9. Retrieved January 10, 2009, from www.fippcase.org/caseinpoint/caseinpoint_vol2_no7.pdf
Wilson, L. L., & Mott, D. W. (2006). Validity of the Asset-Based Context Matrix. *CASEinPoint, 1*(4), 1–4. Retrieved January 10, 2009, from www.fippcase.org/caseinpoint/caseinpoint_vol1_no4.pdf
Wilson, L. L., Mott, D. W., & Batman, D. (2004). The Asset-Based Context Matrix: A tool for assessing children's learning opportunities and participation in natural environments. *Topics in Early Childhood Special Education, 24*(2), 110–120.
Wolfberg, P. J. (1999). *Play and imagination in children with autism.* New York: Teachers College Press.
Yawkey, T. D., Dank, H. L., & Glossenger, F. L. (1986). *Playing: Inside and out.* Lancaster, PA: Technomic.
Zeanah, C. H., Larrieu, J. A., Heller, S. S., & Valliere, J. (2000). Infant–parent relationship assessment. In C. H. Zeanah, Jr. (Ed.), *Handbook of infant mental health* (2nd ed., pp. 222–235). New York: Guilford Press.
Zemke, R., & Clark, F. (1996). *Occupational science: An evolving discipline.* Philadelphia: F. A. Davis.

CHAPTER 8

Assistive Technology and Young Children: Laying a Foundation for the Future

Judith Schoonover, MEd, OTR/L, ATP

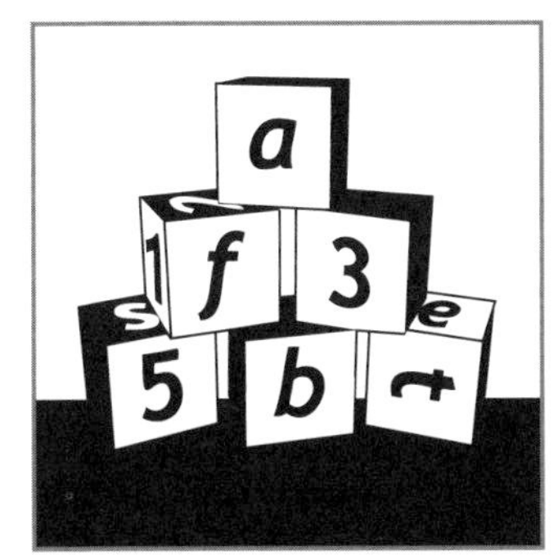

Learning Objectives

After reading this material and completing the examination, readers will be able to

- Identify four purposes of assistive technology (AT) in early childhood services for children with disabilities;
- Identify mandates, policies, and resources pertaining to AT in early intervention and in early childhood special education;
- Identify the guiding theories that influence decisions about AT;
- Delineate a child- and family-centered approach to evaluation, selection, and implementation of AT;
- Recognize cultural differences and their potential impact on the acceptance of AT;
- Delineate the importance of evidence-based practices throughout the AT service delivery process; and
- Identify optimal training and technical assistance practices for establishing and knowledge to support children's use of AT.

> *Much like the rock that sits poised on the top of a hill, assistive technology is potential energy in its purest form. While devices can be described as "assistive technology," "adaptive equipment," etc., it is the user who sets them free, and in reverse, it is the device that essentially returns the favor.*
>
> —J. Schoonover

During early childhood, children undergo continuous changes and expand on skills that will directly influence their independence, attitudes, and success in adulthood

(Mistrett, 2005). The learning that takes place in the early months and years through meaningful interaction with people and objects in and aspects of the environment is critical to later understanding and development. A key to the rapid, significant advancement in cognitive, perceptual, and motor abilities associated with early childhood is children's exploration of their surroundings through manipulation and mobility (Galloway, Ryu, & Agrawal, 2008). Children who are unable to participate in natural learning opportunities because of challenges involving motor, cognitive, sensory, social, or communication skills or environmental factors miss out on vital experiences that can have long-lasting effects developmentally and influence quality of life (Moore & Wilcox, 2006.)

For young children with disabilities and their families, assistive technology (AT) redefines possibilities and opportunities, saying, "Yes, you can!" and establishes a foundation for future successes. AT is a means rather than an end in itself (Pierce, n.d.). It is used to diminish the effects of disabilities and allow children improved alternatives to participate through movement, communication, and interaction with materials relevant to the activity (Mistrett, 2005). The possibilities are endless:

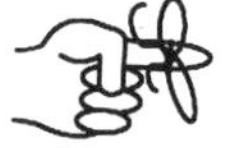

Remember this. . . .
AT can serve as a door opener and provide access for all who encounter barriers in their natural environments.

- An adaptive switch to activate a toy is a means to more independent play.
- A computer touch screen or interactive whiteboard is a means to create sounds and colors and can help children gain an understanding of the effect their actions can have on the world.
- Accessible and meaningful pictures to point to are a means for children with communication difficulties to interact with other children and family members.
- A weighted toy shopping cart to push is a means to independent mobility for a child unable to stand unaided.
- Spring-loaded scissors eliminating the need for hand-over-hand assistance are a means of facilitating independent participation in art activities.

AT can serve as a door opener and provide access for all who encounter barriers in their natural environments. The early introduction and judicious use of AT can provide young children with disabilities birth through age 5 and their caregivers with natural learning opportunities for child-centered movement, play, communication, and self-care experiences paralleling those of typically developing children. "Given the prominence technology holds in today's schools and society, it seems crucial to explore its use and function in home environments for [children] with disabilities, particularly when considering everyday technology such as 'smart' toys, computers, and communication devices" (Bouck, Okolo, & Courtad, 2007, p. 43).

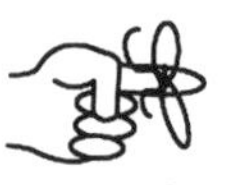

Remember this. . . .
AT can bridge the gap between potential and participation.

Occupational therapists working with children may be more familiar with the continuum of AT devices to support meaningful participation in many occupational roles, including daily living skills, learning, play and leisure, and work, than are other service providers (Post, Hartmann, Gitlow, & Rakowski, 2008). In a survey of state department of education leaders, district personnel, building administrators, special education teachers, parents, and students conducted by the National Assistive Technology Research Institute (NATRI; Ault, 2006) to learn more about AT implementation, occupational therapists were rated as having the highest level of

Learning Activity 8.1. Top 10 Things Everyone Should Know About Assistive Technology for Young Children

After reviewing the Top 10 list in Appendix 8.A (Zabala, 2009), make your own list of your top 10 beliefs about assistive technology (AT; or what you would like others to know about AT). In a second column, list the top 10 AT topics you wish you knew more about. Add to your list or cross-reference it with information gained as you read through this chapter. Many resources are included in the body of this chapter as well as in its conclusion.

It is impossible to list all the AT devices available for young children. New products and methodologies are being developed at an ever-increasing pace. By the time this book goes to press, there will be changes to the AT knowledge base. To learn more about AT products, resources, and rehabilitation equipment, visit the ABLEDATA Web site (www.abledata.com). This AT database provides information and resources on assistive devices and rehabilitation equipment products for people with disabilities as well as detailed information on products for use in all aspects of independent living, including personal care, transportation, communication, and recreation. Custom searches provide specific information on products, including generic and brand names, description, manufacturer, availability, and cost. In addition, the site provides resources and links, a library of AT-related articles, and a consumer forum. Appendix 8.B provides additional Internet resources.

---

expertise, secondary only to AT specialists, many of whom are occupational therapists. Yet a national survey of pediatric occupational therapists found that they rated their preparation in the arena of AT as less than adequate and themselves as having low confidence in terms of delivering AT and AT services (Long, Woolverton, Perry, & Thomas, 2007). Long et al. (2007) found that the therapists surveyed wanted training that is accessible and affordable in the areas of receiving funding for technology and services; collaborating with families and other service providers; and accessing reliable, knowledgeable vendors. The identified training needs are consistent with a survey of early intervention practitioners conducted by Moore and Wilcox (2006), who found that although occupational therapists expressed confidence in their ability to conduct or participate in AT assessments and their ability to use AT in interventions, they were less confident in their ability to obtain and use AT resources and support services.

This chapter is designed to provide basic information and resources relating to AT for occupational therapists working with children birth through age 5. Special educator and AT pioneer Joy Zabala issued "Ten Things Everyone Needs to Know About Assistive Technology in 2009" (Zabala, 2009); a modified version of the list is presented in Appendix 8.A.

"Top 10" lists are a recognizable, popular, and quick way to manage, relay, or digest data without information overload. In Learning Activity 8.1, readers are encouraged to develop a Top 10 list to guide their own self-study of assistive technology.

AT and the Law

Although the user is essential to all aspects of AT, an understanding of the mandates, policies, and resources pertaining to AT is important for service providers to access necessary devices and services. According to Zabala (2009), "Assistive technology is essentially a legal term" (p. 1). Several laws have been designed and authorized to support considering the need for, the procurement of, and the use of AT for people with disabilities (Table 8.1). The first AT law passed by Congress was the Technology-Related Assistance for Individuals With Disabilities Act of 1988. Also known as "the Tech Act," this law provided the first legal definitions of AT *devices* (item) and *services*

Table 8.1. Assistive Technology (AT) Laws

Law and Link for More Information	Description
Rehabilitation Act of 1973 (Amended) www.hhs.gov/ocr/504.html www.section508.gov/index.cfm?FuseAction=Content&ID=12	Section 504 of the Rehabilitation Act was the first civil rights law for people with disabilities. It requires federally funded activities and programs to offer reasonable accommodations to facilities and programs to ensure that people with disabilities have equal access and opportunity to derive benefits. Section 508 established requirements for electronic and information technology developed, maintained, procured, or used by the federal government. It requires electronic and information technology that is developed and used by federal agencies to be accessible to people with disabilities.
Technology-Related Assistance for Individuals With Disabilities Act of 1988 ("Tech Act")	This law first defined AT and established resource centers and information systems regarding obtaining and maintaining AT; some states supported training or establishment of central directories to facilitate access to AT; goals are to foster interagency cooperation, develop funding strategies, and promote access to AT throughout the lifespan.
Americans With Disabilities Act of 1990 (ADA) www.usdoj.gov/crt/ada/cguide.htm#anchor62335 www.ada.gov	The passage of the ADA raised public awareness of the civil rights of people with disabilities. This law has four sections (i.e., titles) and prohibits discrimination on the basis of disability in employment, state and local government, public accommodations, commercial facilities, transportation, and telecommunications.
Assistive Technology Act of 1998 ("AT Act") For a list of state projects funded under the act, visit www.ataporg.org/atap/	Grants funded through AT Act Title I support public awareness; promote interagency coordination; and provide technical assistance, training, and outreach support to statewide community-based organizations. Title II national activities provide increased coordination of federal efforts and authorizes funding to support AT grants. Title III awards grants to states to help establish alternative funding, including loans, for AT for people with disabilities.
Developmental Disabilities Assistance and Bill of Rights Act (2000) www.acf.hhs.gov/programs/add/ddact/DDACT2.html	Provides grants to states for developmental disabilities councils, university-affiliated programs, and protection and advocacy activities for people with developmental disabilities; provides training and technical assistance to improve access to AT services.
Individuals With Disabilities Education Improvement Act of 2004 (IDEA 2004) http://idea.ed.gov/	Originally passed as the Education for All Handicapped Children Act of 1975, IDEA has been amended several times. The act guarantees eligible children a free appropriate public education (FAPE). IDEA in 1990 outlined school district responsibility to provide AT equipment and services to children with disabilities by the public agency (e.g., public school, state-funded early intervention program) serving them. IDEA was most recently amended in 2004.
Medicaid (with Medicare, signed into law with the Social Security Amendments of 1965) www.disability.gov/digov-public/public/DisplayPage.do?parentFolderId=5106	Medicaid is an income-based program; eligibility and services differ from state to state. The federal government sets general program requirements and provides financial assistance to states by matching expenditures; largest funding source of AT benefits among all funding programs.

Sources. Cook and Polgar (2008); Family Center on Technology and Disability (2010).

(or series of actions to support the use of the device). Those definitions have been used in all subsequent laws that include the provision of AT. The main purpose of the Tech Act was to provide federal funds to assist states in the development of training and delivery systems for AT devices and services.

The Tech Act was replaced with the Assistive Technology Act ("AT Act") in 1998. The AT Act continued to provide discretionary grants, funding AT programs in all 50 states, the District of Columbia, and the U.S. territories to assist in developing and implementing programs of technology-related assistance for people of all ages who have disabilities, including AT in the early intervention services available to families and children (see the Association of Assistive Technology Act Programs Web site, www.ataporg.org/atap/index.php).

The Individuals With Disabilities Education Improvement Act of 2004 (IDEA 2004) defines *AT devices* as

> any item, piece of equipment, or product system, whether acquired commercially off the shelf, modified, or customized, that is used to increase, maintain, or improve the functional capabilities of a child with a disability. The term does not include a medical device that is surgically implanted, or the replacement of such device. (20 U.S.C. § 1401(1))

IDEA 2004 defines an *AT service* as "any service that directly assists a child with a disability in the selection, acquisition, or use of an assistive technology device" (20 U.S.C. § 1400(2)), including

- Evaluating needs and skills for AT;
- Acquiring ATs;
- Selecting, designing, repairing, and fabricating AT;
- Coordinating services with other therapies; and
- Training both people with disabilities and those working with them to use ATs effectively.

According to IDEA 2004, the need for AT must be considered for any child (from birth to age 21) who has a disability and is eligible for early intervention or special education, every 6 months during the development of an individualized family service plan (IFSP) and at least annually during the development of an individualized education program (IEP). If AT is determined to be necessary, it is included as part of the IFSP or IEP.

AT for Young Children Defined

AT refers to a broad range of devices, services, strategies, and practices used to address functional problems, such as communication, mobility, and self-help, encountered by people who have disabilities (Cook & Polgar, 2008). According to Blackhurst and Lahm (2000):

> Assistive technologies include mechanical, electronic, and microprocessor-based equipment, non-mechanical and non-electronic aids, specialized instructional materials, services, and strategies that people with disabilities can use either to (a) assist them in learning, (b) make the environment more

> accessible, (c) enable them to compete in the workplace, (d) enhance their independence, or (e) otherwise improve their quality of life. These may include commercially available or "homemade" devices that are specially designed to meet the idiosyncratic needs of a particular individual. (p. 7)

Appropriate AT devices and services can help improve, increase, or maintain performance for the users to complete or develop functional skills, access learning materials, become more efficient learners, or bypass lack of skills (Baush, Ault, & Hasselbring, 2006). Examples of AT devices are as varied as the people who use them, contexts in which they are used, and needs they support, but they may include positioning supports (a cushion to help a child sit upright in a shopping cart), mobility devices (a walker to navigate the home, community, or preschool classroom), specialized utensils such as "sporks" or utensils with built-up handles, communication devices (picture boards or voice output devices), toy adaptations, switches, pencil grips, and alternative clothing fasteners.

AT services include collaboration for evaluating the needs of the child and family, selecting and acquiring the appropriate device, training the family and other caregivers, and monitoring the use of the device. AT services begin with a discussion about family goals and outcomes, the child's developmental level, strengths and weaknesses, and how AT might help reduce impediments and increase active and meaningful involvement in valued roles and routines. For every child with a disability, the need for AT must be considered on an individual basis along with developmental, educational, therapeutic, and social service needs.

Integration of AT into naturally occurring roles and routines provides alternatives for young children with disabilities and their families; it can enhance capabilities and circumvent barriers in the natural contexts of home, child care, preschool, and the community. Independence and quality of life begin with enriching opportunities, strong emotional support, positive social interactions with peers and adults, and differentiated instruction.

AT Under Part C as Part of the Individualized Family Service Plan

Under Part C, AT devices and services are defined as part of supports and services necessary to meet the desired outcomes as stated on the IFSP (U.S. Department of Education, 2007). IDEA 2004 requires IFSP teams to consider AT for increasing function and for providing access to learning and functional opportunities within home community settings, including child care. Part C requires that "to the maximum extent appropriate to the needs of the child, early intervention services must be provided in natural environments, including the home and community settings in which children without disabilities participate" (34 C.F.R. § 303.12(b)).

Early intervention programs receive federal and state funds to pay for basic early intervention services, including service coordination. Part C of IDEA, however, does not guarantee funding to pay for AT, leaving it up to each state to determine how funds are allocated. Under Part C of IDEA, if AT is included as part of a child's IFSP, it must be provided at no cost, unless subject to 34 C.F.R. § 303.520(b)(3), yet Part C programs are "payers of last resort," so Part C monies can only be used if the family has exhausted all other possible sources of funding (34 C.F.R. § 303.527). If an IFSP team agrees that AT is needed, early intervention programs will seek reimbursement from Medicaid and private insurance for AT and other services. Early intervention service costs are not covered by Part C except for service coordination and initial assessment, so follow-up support and training for AT may be limited, depending on how the states choose to use their allocated monies.

AT recommended under Part C is intended for use in the natural environment and would reside with the child. Much of the AT used in early intervention is through lending libraries maintained by regional technology centers with the understanding that a child will use the device as needed and that the device will be returned to the lending center to be loaned to another child. This use of devices is realistic because children grow rapidly, and their needs change.

AT Under Part B as Part of the Individualized Education Program

Under Part B, the intent of AT is to facilitate the student's IEP goals and achievement in the least restrictive environment. Devices provided under Part B are directly related to the education program and typically belong to the school. They may or may not go home with the student, depending on the need for the equipment at home to meet educational goals. Considering the need for AT is not designed to be a fishing expedition to see what's out there; rather, it is a deliberate determination by the team members that all supports and accommodations necessary to provide access to learning opportunities are in place to achieve the goals developed. It is tempting for some members of the IEP team (families, educators, related service providers) to request the "latest and greatest" device on the basis of a description in a catalogue, yet matching a person to the right device is a process that requires an assessment of skills and needs in the natural context. The law requires that AT deemed necessary to implement the IEP and support academic achievement must be provided at no cost to the family, but it leaves the device selection to each IEP team. Specific devices are not named, leaving it to the discretion of the team to match the user to the appropriate intervention.

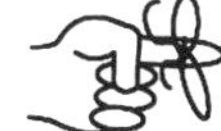

Remember this. . . .
AT is related to function rather than to specific disability categories (Zabala, 2009, p. 1).

AT and the User

AT is related to function in performance areas rather than to specific disability categories (Zabala, 2009, p. 1). Therefore, one might assume that many children eligible to receive AT services need equipment or product systems to maintain or improve their functional performance. The ultimate goal of AT is to provide the most appropriate tool for an individual, minimizing disruption to customary roles and routines and resulting in enhanced quality of life (Scherer, 1996). AT is potential energy in its purest form.

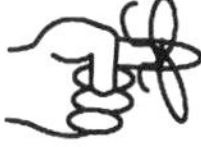

Remember this. . . .
AT is potential energy in its purest form.

Because a tool actually becomes AT through the successful and meaningful participation of its user, it is difficult to determine what AT supports exist in a given environment. For example, most homes and preschool classrooms have materials and tools, such as crayons and computers, that enrich literacy experiences but are not necessary to accomplish a specific task or goal. Yet, children with disabilities might *need* to use crayons or computers or use them with modifications to participate in literacy activities. This need redefines common environmental tools as AT. Therefore, it is important to consider what a tool does for a child and whether that child can participate without it. It would be unfortunate to eliminate the aspects of everyday items as AT just because they cannot be ordered from a specialty catalogue or labeled AT. The old adage "necessity is the mother of invention" could be referring to the process by which an everyday item found in the natural context becomes AT for a child who needs it to do something meaningful. For example, a child who uses a scooter board as a mobility device to navigate the household is using AT if it removes barriers and enhances access to roles and environments that are meaningful.

Although legislation defines AT, it by no means describes or encompasses the vast array of specialty, off-the-shelf, or adapted tools that can be used to positively change occupational performance. Some of the most basic tools that can be used to facilitate independence are the very tools that are found in the natural context of the home, preschool, or community settings of a young child. Those tools may be the result of improvisations based on available resources and immediate needs. Detection of "everyday AT" requires keen observation skills, an awareness of environmental resources, and a knowledge of the child's needs and desires. Learning Activity 8.2 provides an opportunity to reflect on your use of "detection skills" to discover or appreciate everyday AT.

The way in which tools are adapted and used defines them as AT. For example, it is an innate drive for children to move, explore, and communicate (Stoller, 1998). On the basis of their experience with movement or communication attempts or the response they receive, their next course of action is determined. Children need to be able to interact with their environment to explore it and learn from it. Positioning a child who is unable to lift his or her head so that he or she can view mother's face, a beloved toy, or a family pet may involve simple items easily overlooked as AT devices (e.g., rolled towels, foam wedge) and services (training caregivers in positioning the child or setting up the device). The following examples are all methods of increasing independence in an effort to allow for exploration of the environment.

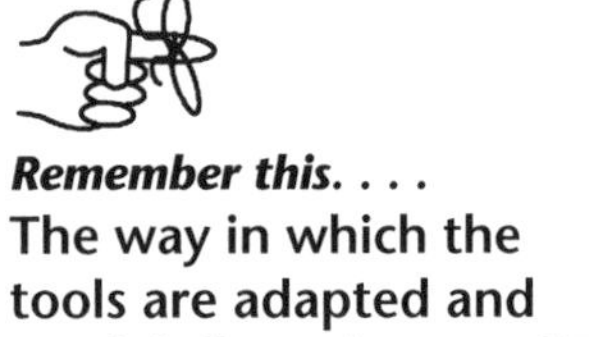

Remember this. . . .
The way in which the tools are adapted and used defines them as AT.

- A spoon with a built-up handle, a plate with nonskid material beneath it, and a cup with one end cut are all AT items that can be used to assist the caregiver or the child to have a more independent and satisfying mealtime experience.
- A tricycle with a backrest to decrease fatigue or improve positioning, a bolster to support the chest so that arms can be used for reaching rather than propping, a rolled towel to position an arm so that contact is made with a toy are all AT devices allowing for increased mobility.
- Pictures, objects, drawings, and clip art used to create simple communication tools are AT devices to facilitate or improve exchange of information.

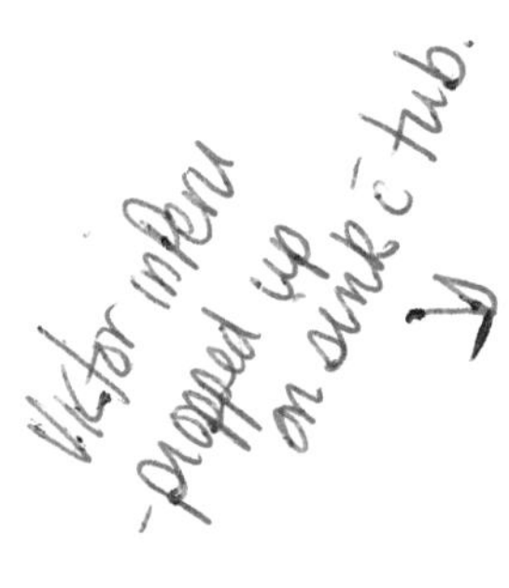

Learning Activity 8.2. Looking at the World Through "AT-Colored Glasses"

Have you or a client ever experienced an "assistive technology (AT) moment," in which the right device in the right environment for the right user made the difference between passivity and participation?

- How did you arrive at that moment?
- What actions did you take?
- What did you learn from the experience that shaped your next encounter?
- Was there anything you would have done differently?
- How will you use this information in the future? Try looking at the world through "AT-colored glasses" and discover the possibilities!

AT and the Individualized Family Service Plan

With the legal parameters in place to support widespread application of AT and the efficacy of its use, the field of early intervention is challenged to increase the necessary awareness of and skill development in considering AT as a means of paving the way to full access for young children in their daily routines and learning situations. Despite the benefits of AT and AT services for infants and young children, AT remains underdocumented, underused, and inconsistently integrated in service plans for young children. The U.S. Department of Education (1997–2001) reported that fewer than 4% of infants and toddlers had AT devices or services listed on their IFSP, yet service providers use a wide variety of tools and scaffolds to assist infants and children in interacting with their environment. A study by the Technical Assistance Project (2000) found a slightly higher percentage (approximately 7%) of children who received early intervention services throughout the country also received AT and AT services. Note that a national survey of parent and provider perspectives on AT use in early intervention found that only high-tech devices are listed on the IFSP; AT services and devices may have come to be viewed only as devices considered to be high tech or durable medical equipment (Wilcox, Bacon, & Campbell, 2004).

Clearly, parents and providers need more information regarding the broad range of AT in use. It is heartening to note that 2 years later, when a group of early childhood special educators completed surveys to assess what AT tools they found most useful for working with young children with disabilities, the results indicated that communication and low-tech devices, such as picture symbol display books for communication and calendars, adapted scissors, and pencil grips, were considered most useful (Judge, 2006).

Social Context of AT

Key people who provide assistance to a child using AT, including family members, teachers, paraprofessionals, and related service providers, have a direct effect on how and when it is used and accepted across environments (e.g., home, day care, school, and community). The service aspect of AT, such as training, can empower and provide them with a greater understanding of the user's strengths and weaknesses and how the AT provides support. People directly or indirectly interacting with an AT user (e.g., families, day care providers, teachers) are considered part of the social context of AT. The effect of the social context of AT use cannot be underestimated, because the social environment, including the attitudes of others, often creates more barriers than the physical context (Cook & Polgar, 2008) and may directly influence acceptance or rejection of the device. The social stigma of a disability and the additional attention a device might attract can be reduced when people within the social environment support use of the technology.

Benefits of AT for Young Children

AT tools, including switches, voice output devices, and computers, can help young children acquire important developmental skills or provide compensatory experiences. These tools help young children learn and practice cause and effect and early choice making, fine motor and visual–motor skills, and self-help. Assistive devices and services can influence the growth and development of infants and young children with disabilities, thereby providing opportunities to learn and interact with the environment in ways that might not otherwise be possible and allowing participation in family, school, and community activities (see Box 8.1 for a case example; Learning Activity 8.3 is based on the case). Appendix 8.C illustrates how AT can support infants and toddlers.

Continuum and Interrelationship Between No-Tech and High-Tech Solutions

AT has been categorized in several different ways, including by user, functional application, availability (commercial or custom), and setting (e.g., home, school, rehabilitation setting). AT devices range from simple to complex. Blackhurst (2001) made the following distinctions when describing the continuum of AT:

- *No-tech* solutions are those that make use of procedures, services, and existing conditions in the environment that do not involve the use of devices or equipment. These might include services such as physical therapy or occupational therapy or the services of other specialists.
- *Low-tech* items are less sophisticated and can include devices such as adapted spoon handles, non-tipping drinking cups, and Velcro fasteners.
- *Medium-tech* devices are relatively complicated mechanical devices, such as wheelchairs.
- *High-tech* devices incorporate sophisticated electronics or computers.

Devices and solutions from simple to complex should be considered when deciding on the appropriate technology for a child to use to accomplish different tasks and in a variety of settings. Often, practitioners who recommend AT tend to start at the upper end of the technology continuum when a simpler solution might be available. One reason might be that simple solutions are not identified and recognized as AT because of the common association of the word *technology* with complicated equipment requiring a complex skill set by the user and caregiver. With regard to infants and toddlers, for whom natural settings are especially important, devices from across the continuum should be considered and matched to the different environments in which the devices are needed. For example, although a low-tech device like a rolling stool or a weighted toy shopping cart might work well in the home environment as a mobility aid, a walker or wheelchair might be safer, more appropriate, or preferred in the day care or preschool setting, and a stroller or wheelchair might be used while out in the community. Similarly a gesture, sign, or a facial expression may serve as a no-tech form of communication in the home environment with familiar communication partners, whereas pictures or a voice output device might be used in the classroom, child care, or community to allow social interaction and expression of needs to and among a more varied number of communication partners, including peers.

Definitions of AT in the Occupational Therapy Literature

> *Occupational therapists . . . deliver assistive technology–related services in a variety of settings . . . in a variety of roles.*
>
> —American Occupational Therapy Association (AOTA; 2004a, p. 679)

Box 8.1. Case Example: Rafael

An assistive technology (AT) evaluation was requested for Rafael, age 4, who is homebound because of a medically unstable condition. The individualized education plan (IEP) team requested AT support to address a goal of choice making using a switch.[1] When the AT evaluators (in this instance, an occupational therapist and a special educator) entered the home, they found Rafael seated in a KidCart completely supported, unable to lift his arms or legs or turn his head. Rafael's eyes followed the evaluators, and he smiled responsively to the sound of their voices. During the course of the evaluation, his mother described Rafael's routine as follows:

- Wake up between 3:00 a.m. and 4:30 a.m.
- Medications and nebulizer
- Bathing
- G-tube feeding
- Story
- Nap
- Positioning and side lying
- Upright for 1 hr
- Positioning and side lying
- Tube feeding
- Cuddling
- Story and bed.

When asked about her goals for Rafael, his mother replied, "I want him to be able to swing on the swing in the backyard and ask for more swinging. I want him to be able to socialize with his sister and the children in the neighborhood and play games. I want him to be able to ask his big sister how her day at school went."

Although the education team had determined that choice making was the educational goal for which they were seeking AT support, Rafael's mother identified the essential aspects of childhood—play and interaction—as her own priorities. Therefore, when the AT report was completed, it included recommendations focusing on what occurred in Rafael's educational environment (his home), what was important to his family, and how those priorities related to educational goals. Because communication and social skills are educationally and functionally related, Rafael's IEP was revised to include additional communication goals, including responding to questions and making requests. AT for play and leisure and increasing social interaction was recommended, including an adapted swing that could be attached to the family's backyard swing set to allow Rafael to swing with his sister and other children in the neighborhood. In addition, the evaluators recommended the following strategies:

1. Explore the use of voice output augmentative communication devices to engage in functional communication exchanges for choice making, requesting, rejecting, and greeting. To enhance communication opportunities during various school activities (which took place by means of a teacher providing services in the home), consider the following:
   a. A single-cell voice output device (a switch or button that, when activated, plays back recorded sounds or words) could be used during story or song time. A symbol or photo from the story, when pressed, could start playback of one of the repetitive lines in a story such as *Brown Bear, Brown Bear, What Do You See?* or a repetitive phrase in a song, such as "E-I-E-I-O" in "Old MacDonald." A single-cell voice output device could have pictures or photos with associated voice recordings for arrival and departure greetings as well as choice making, requesting, and rejecting.
   b. A single-cell voice output device could have a message recorded on it for Rafael to activate, such as "I'm here" or "Guess what I did last night?" so that others can engage him further in conversation and he can respond using yes–no responses.
   c. A one-button sequential messaging device could be used to deliver news, tell jokes, or make comments.
2. Consider using a yes–no board to provide a visual cue for responding to yes–no questions with eye gaze or vocalization.

---

[1]Some educators believe that the AT should not be named according to the goal of what the child is going to do and that it should instead be included in the supports the child needs to accomplish the goal. The goal should state what the child is going to do, and the supports that are required should be listed under the supports or accommodations section of the IEP. Typically, AT should not drive the goal; rather, the targeted behavior (making a choice) should drive the choice of AT.

(*Continued*)

Box 8.1. Case Example: Rafael (*cont.*)

3. Consider use of an eye-gaze board for choice making, requesting, or rejecting. The portability of an eye-gaze board would allow for quick communication exchanges during walks in the community or other outdoor play opportunities when reprogramming or setting up a voice output device is not time efficient.
4. Consider the use of a switch for Rafael to access the computer and expand his opportunities for engaging in cause-and-effect and choice-making activities. To support development of these skills, further explore computer-based activities:
   a. Multimedia presentation software, such as PowerPoint, can be used to create talking or musical interactive activities. This multimedia tool allows the author to incorporate text, graphics, picture symbols, digital photos, videos, narration, sound effects, music, and animation. PowerPoint presentations can also be read aloud by using PowerTalk, a free download available for computers with Windows operating systems (http://fullmeasure.co.uk/powertalk).
   b. A variety of highly interactive Web sites and online storybooks provide visual and auditory input and can engage Rafael's interest.
5. Further explore the use of adaptive switches to operate battery-operated devices. Using switches can reinforce cause-and-effect relationships, choice making, eye–hand coordination, and peer socialization and provide more opportunities for learning through play. Also, consider using a switch-activated PowerLink (AbleNet, Inc., Roseville, MN 55113) for a variety of activities. In addition to turning on the television or tape player, it can be used to turn on other appliances, such as a blender to make smoothies or shakes (Figure 8.1), a popcorn popper, holiday lights, a lamp, a fan (to operate a pinwheel, wind chimes, or a bubble wand), battery-operated light-up toys, or an overhead projector. Two switches and two appliances can be used with the PowerLink for choice making. Although Rafael is tube fed, helping his mother in the kitchen is a typical childhood occupation and one that his mother valued as a routine associated with her occupation as mother.
6. Consider using a talking photo album with story inserts to allow Rafael's kindergarten-age sister to "read" to him by pressing the buttons on each page and activating a recorded passage (more information on talking photo albums can be found at www.augcominc.com/index.cfm/talking_photo_album.htm).

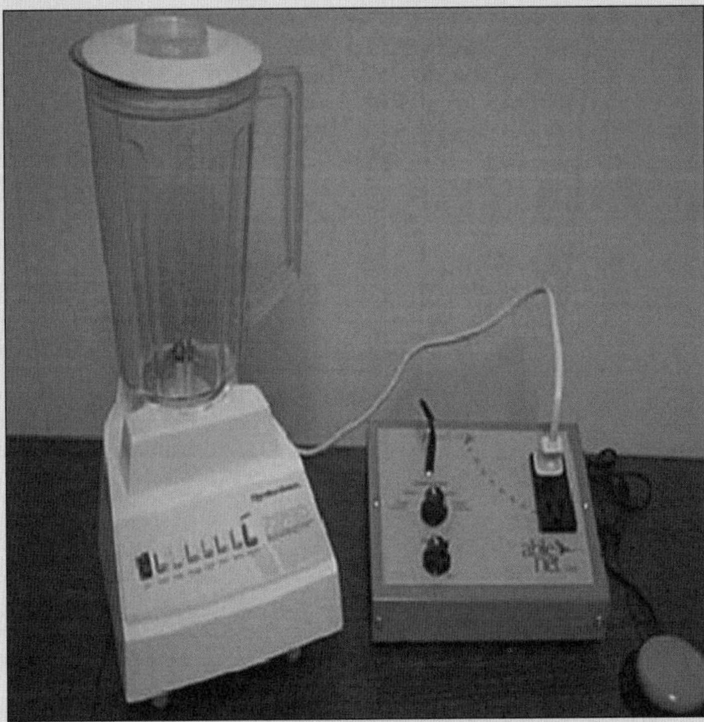

Figure 8.1. Blender; PowerLink (environmental control unit) from AbleNet, Inc., Roseville, MN; and switch to activate blender.

Source. Personal collection of J. Schoonover.

Learning Activity 8.3. Talking It Over

With a special education colleague, review the recommendations made for Rafael in the case study in Box 8.1.

- Identify the (clinical) reasoning process used by the therapist and teacher (the assistive technology team). What frames of reference seem most apparent in the recommendations? What educational perspective is most evident?
- Discuss the reasoning process presented with your colleague. How do these recommendations fit with the education and functional needs of Rafael and the setting in which his special education occurs?

Occupational therapists who typically work with infants and toddlers use AT every day, whether they realize it or not. The word *assistive* suggests providing help, and the word *technology* implies a deliberate action based on skill. AT "enables or enhances a person's ability to be independent" (Trefler & Hobson, 1997, p. 486). Interestingly, the root of the word *technology* is Greek and translates as "art," "skill," or "craftsmanship" and "the totality of the means employed to provide objects necessary for human sustenance and comfort" (Techno-, 1990). The tools used to improve mobility, facilitate caregiving, increase independence, and enhance learning are all considered AT. Before the words *assistive technology* became commonplace, words such as *adaptive equipment* were used to describe performance-enhancing tools. Stoller (1998) proposed that the following definition be used by the profession of occupational therapy, with the emphasis on how devices are used to enhance the essence of occupation:

> Assistive/adaptive equipment refers to the provision of special devices or structural changes that promote a sense of self-competence, the further acquisition of developmental skills into occupational behaviors or an improved balance of time spent between the occupational roles in an individual's life as determined by the individual's goals and interests and the external demands of the environment. (p. 6)

Creating, modifying, or adapting devices or tools to meet the individual needs of a client is intrinsic to the practice of occupational therapy, yet it is a proficiency or service for which occupational therapists often fail to give themselves credit or distinguish as AT (Schoonover & Smith, 2007).

"The occupational therapist provides a broad range of services in the application of technology, including evaluation, recommendation, justification of need, advocacy, awareness of funding resources, fabrication, customization, training, integration, and follow-up" (AOTA, 2004a, p. 679). AT may be considered a specialty area, yet occupational therapists infuse their practice with both basic, or low-tech, AT devices (e.g., toys and utensils with built-up handles, slant boards) and complex, or high-tech, AT devices (e.g., custom seating and mobility systems, adapted computer access, environmental control units; Schoonover & Smith, 2007). To reiterate, although various tools are described as AT or adaptive equipment, it is the action of the user that sets him or her free, and in reverse, it is the tools that essentially return the favor. "Occupational therapy practitioners' understanding of their clients' daily occupational needs, abilities, and contexts make them ideal collaborators in the

Learning Activity 8.4. Which Model Is Right for You?

With a study group, explore the following Web sites and the decision-making models presented. Compare and contrast the models. What are the advantages of each? Are there disadvantages?

- **Educational Tech Points (Bowser & Reed, 1995)**
  www.educationtechpoints.org/manuals-materials/education-tech-points-manual
  Questions relate to assistive technology (AT) used by professionals at various points in the assessment process to help teams effectively select AT and implement AT services.
- **Human, Activity, Assistive Technology (HAAT; Cook & Polgar, 2008)**
  This model considers the skills of the AT user, the task that the person is expected to perform, and the context or constraints on the activity.
- **Matching Person and Technology (MPT model; Scherer, 1991, 2004)**
  www.matchingpersonandtechnology.com
  The MPT model is a user-driven, person-centered process for matching people with technologies. The model consists of a series of questionnaires that consider the environment, the user's preferences, and the functions and features of the AT.
- **Student, Environment, Task, and Tools (SETT; Zabala, 1995)**
  www.otap-oregon.org/Documents/Forms/AllItems.aspx
  This collaborative process assists teams in building consensus on a child's need for AT, the type of AT needed, and the interventions needed to support the AT.

To view 52 models and taxonomies, see www.r2d2.uwm.edu/atoms/archive/technicalreports/fieldscans/fs7/tr-fs-taxonomiesmodels-resource.html.

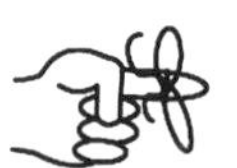

Remember this. . . .
"Occupational therapy practitioners' understanding of their clients' daily occupational needs, abilities, and contexts make them ideal collaborators in the design, development, and clinical application of new or customized technological devices" (AOTA, 2004a, p. 678).

design, development, and clinical application of new or customized technological devices" (AOTA, 2004a, p. 678).

Frameworks and Models Influencing AT

Before beginning this section, readers are challenged to type the words *assistive technology frameworks* or *assistive technology models* into an Internet search engine and skim the results. It is clear that an ever-expanding number of frameworks and models are influencing AT. Edyburn (2002) reviewed 12 AT models relating to technology use in special education. In analyzing the function or purpose of each model, he found three patterns: (1) AT consideration, (2) technology-enhanced performance, and (3) developmental models that describe specific aspects of technology use in special education. Because of the individualized circumstances of each AT user (what he or she wants to do, where the user wants or needs to use AT, why it is important to do so, and how it can most easily be accomplished with the least amount of disruption and the most benefits), models will likely continue to proliferate. When all is said and done, at the heart of each model is the user.

Frameworks and models serve an important purpose: They provide structure and a frame of reference to guide an intervention approach or decision making. Incorporating various perspectives when making decisions about AT is not always easy, yet a collaborative decision results in richer, more comprehensive solutions that exemplify best practice. Learning Activity 8.4 provides information for you to compare and contrast models of AT decision making. Understanding the use of decision-making models in AT is a fundamental skill that all occupational therapists should have.

Successful Play Experiences With Toys and Other Children

Play as an occupation has long been recognized as the foundation for the development of fine motor, gross motor, perceptual, social, communication, and cognitive

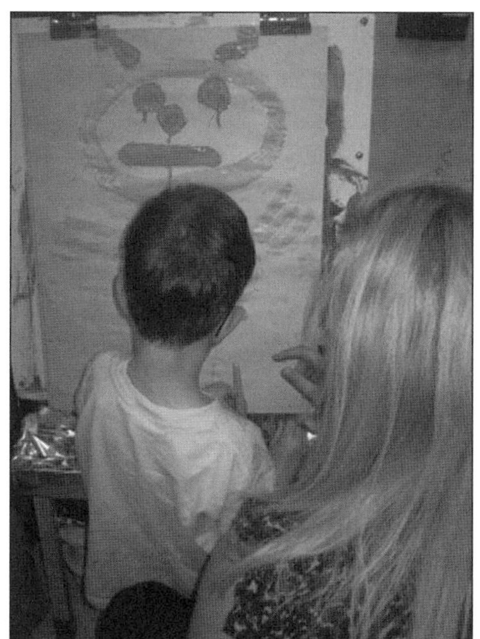

Figure 8.2. Child painting using an adapted paintbrush with paper placed at or above eye level to encourage reach and visual regard.

Source. Personal collection of J. Schoonover.

skills. Creativity on the part of the occupational therapist in adapting both tools and the environment can result in successful play experiences (Figure 8.2). The reader is referred to Chapter 7 for a more detailed perspective on play in early childhood. Play experiences, and the learning that results, contribute to the development of each child. An "inborn drive to discover and learn" (Burkhart, 2002, p. 1) motivates children to understand the word around them, strive for independence and sense of self, and connect socially with others. The goal of facilitating play requires occupational therapists not only to consider the potential for skill development but also to consider and engineer the environment to support playful interactions and reduce barriers (Hamm, 2006) by creating motivating activities, developing opportunities for active participation, presenting information and materials using multiple modalities, and using authentic learning scenarios in natural contexts (Burkhart, 2002). AT can facilitate engagement in developmentally appropriate experiences that might otherwise be impossible and can create exciting opportunities for children to explore, interact, and function in their environments. AT for young children, however, is likely underused because of a lack of awareness by parents and providers and limited opportunities for service providers to increase their knowledge of and skills in incorporating AT strategies into clients' daily routines (Sawyer, Milbourne, Dugan, & Campbell, 2005). Cost of items may be another barrier.

Remember this. . . .
Children who lack the opportunity to actively explore their environment and learn the consequences of their actions run the risk of becoming passive.

When a child has special needs, a more deliberate approach is necessary in using typical, adapted, or specialized toys and self-care and mobility equipment to facilitate meaningful participation in family and community life. Children who lack the opportunity to actively explore their environment and learn the consequences of their actions run the risk of becoming passive. Interventions should include direct interaction with the child and with the child's caregivers as well as the opportunities provided by the environment. Training of parents, caregivers, and service providers in effective ways to promote play in children and making changes in the physical environment can encourage participation in the occupation of play (Hamm, 2006).

This is such an important message to convey to parents

Hamm (2006) found that parents prioritized the following outcomes of play:

- Increased variety of play options
- Improved specific play skills
- Sensory exploration

- Independent play
- Play with others.

Because of any number of factors, including sensory and mobility issues, children with disabilities may have difficulty accessing, exploring, manipulating, and using play materials. How the toys are presented and the manner in which the child is positioned have a direct impact on the child's interactions (Mistrett, 2000). Hamm (2006) found that parents chose functional (off-the-shelf) toys over specialty toys. Simple adaptations to off-the-shelf toys can make them easier for a child to use:

- *Attachers,* such as hook-and-loop fabric, curtain rings, and elastic are materials that are used to bring items closer to the child, making reaching, grasping, and playing less work.
- *Extenders,* such as knobs on puzzle pieces and foam roller handles, are materials that can be used to build up certain access features. They help children press too-small buttons or keys or make markers easier to hold.
- *Stabilizers,* such as suction cups and nonskid shelf liners, support play by preventing a toy from moving out of reach.
- *Confiners,* such as box lids and raised-edge trays, keep toys from moving too far away from a child. Items such as hula hoops, box tops, or planter bases help a child control his or her immediate play environment (Mistrett, Lane, & Goetz, 2000).

See Web resources pertaining to play and tips for buying toys for children with disabilities in Appendixes 8.B and 8.D.

Mobility and Positioning for Participation and Exploration

Typically developing children experience life around them by physically interacting with their environment through movement. Their motor, cognitive, and social development, as well as their sense of autonomy, is influenced through opportunities to experience and see things from different perspectives and to discover the effects of their actions. An infant or child who cannot move independently can experience needed positioning for function or mobility through AT devices and services. In addition, AT can play an important role in caregiving by providing support in the daily management of the child at home, school, or the community. When a child has special needs, a more deliberate approach is necessary using typical, adapted, or specialized toys and self-care and mobility equipment to facilitate meaningful participation in family and community life. Comfortable positioning and mobility for the child may also provide relief for the caregiver, reducing physical demands to allow for more meaningful interaction.

Appropriately selected and individualized positioning and seating equipment provides increased stability and may facilitate improved control of head, arms, and hands while minimizing the effects of abnormal muscle tone and preventing injury or skeletal deformity (Cook & Polgar, 2008). AT devices for positioning, seating, and mobility can include car seats, bath chairs, high chairs, scooters, tricycles, strollers, and wheelchairs. Positioning and mobility devices can contribute to improved

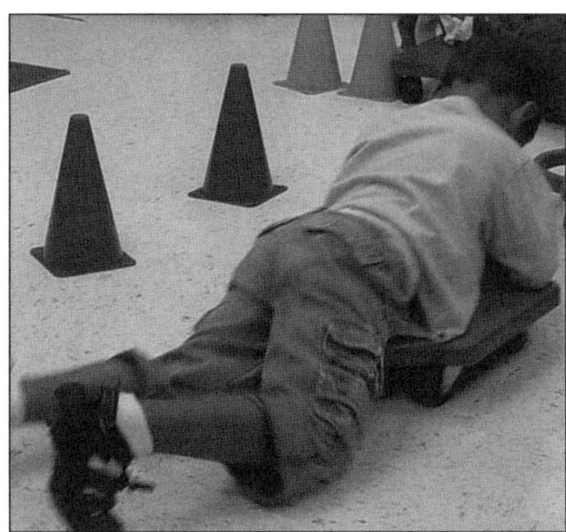

Figure 8.3. A scooterboard allows this child, who is nonambulatory, the opportunity to engage in play with peers, develop motor planning strategies, explore his environment, and see things from different perspectives.

Source. Personal collection of J. Schoonover.

function, comfort, safety, and quality of life by allowing children to be placed in positions allowing for greater participation in occupational roles of childhood. Figure 8.3 demonstrates how a typical scooterboard can act as a mobility device, allowing a child who is unable to walk an opportunity to move and play independently.

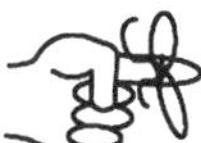

Remember this. . . .
Positioning and mobility devices can contribute to improved function, comfort, safety, and quality of life by allowing children to be placed in positions allowing for greater participation in occupational roles of childhood.

Many options are available, ranging from off-the-shelf to customized equipment and systems, to support infants and young children with disabilities with positioning and mobility. The consideration of positioning and mobility begins with an awareness of physical (e.g., narrow doorways, steps) and cultural (e.g., family belief system that prohibits placing child on the floor) barriers to performance and potential assets (e.g., existence of baby equipment that can be modified). A child's position may be modified with or without additional equipment using rolled towels, wedges, and bolsters to stimulate developmental milestones, such as head–neck–trunk extension, prone propping, and supported sitting. Effective positioning can assist with improved respiratory function, oral–motor control, and fine motor skills. Short-term versus long-term benefits should be reviewed, keeping in mind that some families or educational teams may be unwilling or unable to adjust to the needs of one person. Generally, typical baby equipment is preferred over specialized equipment. For example, a child's potty chair may be modified with a tray, abduction posts, armrests, backrests, or footrests, emphasizing proximal stability for comfort and to normalize tone while approximating what typically developing children are using. Familiar materials, as opposed to specialized equipment, may translate to increased use.

A poor match of user to equipment can result in discomfort, disuse, and potential for injury. For example, ignoring a child's head, neck, and trunk position when a placing a child with low tone in a walker can elicit inappropriate compensatory skills or poor quality of performance. Occupational therapists' understanding of the biomechanical forces and physiologic factors that influence posture and movement plays an essential role in determining the "just-right" challenge when selecting and modifying equipment. They also have a responsibility to educate clients using the equipment to prevent misuse, which is the service aspect of AT.

It is important to have a back-up plan for any intervention in the event that the equipment breaks or is unavailable. More than one device may be needed, depending on the environments in which the device is used. For example, if a child's home has any steps to the entrance, a manual or power chair may have to stay at school or in the car, requiring a separate activity chair or stroller for the home. The Delaware

Assistive Technology Initiative Center for Applied Science and Engineering (n.d.) suggested considering the following points when deciding on positioning, seating, and mobility aids:

- Can customary environments be navigated using this equipment?
- Is more than one kind of mobility device required on the basis of daily routines and contexts?
- In what environment will the equipment be used?
- Does the child's condition vary in severity from day to day?
- What funding resources are available for the purchase?
- What are the child's strengths, limitations, and preferences?
- What are the family's (or educational team's) preferences?
- Is the mobility device comfortable?
- Can the child or caregivers operate the selected equipment safely and well?

Communication

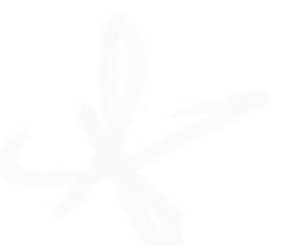

All persons, regardless of the extent or severity of their disabilities, have a basic right to affect, through communication, the conditions of their own existence.

—National Joint Committee for the Communication Needs of Persons With Severe Disabilities (1992, p. 4)

The preceeding statement represents a basic tenet of human existence. It was written by a joint committee of people representing several national organizations, including AOTA, involved with services for people with disabilities. (See the full text in Appendix 8.E.) Communication is a life skill necessary for interaction with others; it is based on a set of complex behaviors. Three major components of language—*form* (sound, order, and parts of words), *content* (vocabulary), and *function* (pragmatics, how and why language is used)—contribute to the ability to read and write (Cooper, Chard, & Kiger, 2006). Communication requires one or more partners because its purpose is to exchange and share information with others.

Skau and Cascella (2006) estimated that 4% to 7% of young children have a specific language impairment. A range of performance levels related to receptive and expressive language may be observed in children with disabilities. Many tools, strategies, and techniques provide alternatives to speaking, writing, and motor performance and address communication needs including sign language, picture or symbol communication board, adapted books, and low- and high-tech voice output devices. Augmentative and alternative communication (AAC) can support people by overcoming barriers to speak or understand spoken or written language (Cook & Polgar, 2008). The American Speech–Language–Hearing Association (2002) defined *AAC* as follows:

> AAC is, foremost, a set of procedures and processes by which an individual's communication skills (i.e., production as well as comprehension) can be maximized for functional and effective communication. It involves supplementing or replacing natural speech and/or writing with aided (e.g., picture communication symbols, line drawings, Blissymbols, and tangible objects)

> and/or unaided symbols (e.g., manual signs, gestures, and finger spelling). Whereas aided symbols require some type of transmission device, unaided symbols require only the body to produce. Many individuals with severe communication and cognitive impairments can benefit from nonsymbolic forms of AAC such as gestures (reaching for a desired object) and vocalizations that convey different emotions. (p. 2)

Children with a wide range of communication disorders can benefit from AAC (Beukelman & Mirenda, 1992). As with all AT interventions, AAC should be dynamic and include not only the individual child but also his or her primary communication partners (Cook & Polgar, 2008). To support the development of language and emergent literacy, enhance participation in educational settings, facilitate social relationships, and support interactions with family members and people in the greater community, a collaborative approach is essential. Each contributor to the process of evaluating and implementing AAC brings a unique perspective based on knowledge of the child and area of expertise. For example, the child, family, and other caregivers will have the best understanding of daily communication needs, priorities, and routines; early interventionists and preschool teachers will have knowledge related to literacy, instruction, and classroom activities; speech–language pathologists provide expertise in language acquisition; and occupational and physical therapists are experts in positioning and physically accessing the AAC system (Cook & Polgar, 2008).

One must consider the continuum of AT options available to support communication at any level. For example, visual representation can be used to increase comprehension, communication opportunities, and social connectedness. Visual representation can take many forms, including objects, photographs, realistic drawings, line drawings, and written words, and may vary depending on the environment and the circumstances under which they are being used. From the low-tech standpoint, *tangible symbols* (Rowland & Schweigert, 2000) provide simple symbolic representation of language, thereby allowing communicators to relate to objects and experiences beyond their immediate context. Two- and three-dimensional manipulatives (objects, parts of an object, associated objects, textures or shapes, or line drawings that are based on the user's own experience and represent progressively more abstract concepts) are used to convey meaningful information to the user or represent his or her communicative intent. For example, a small belt might indicate "going for a ride," or a circle formed from a pipe cleaner might indicate "morning circle." Figure 8.4 shows a variety of low-tech visual representations, including an actual object (pretzel), photos, and line drawings.

Bloomfield (2000) recommended the use of true object–based icons (TOBIs) for people experiencing difficulty understanding one-dimensional visual representation systems such as photos, drawings, and graphics (see Figure 8.4 for examples of TOBIs). TOBIs provide visual and tactile cues to the communicator and can be made from line drawings, pictures, photos, or product labels cut out in the shape or outline of the item they represent. Hodgdon (1995) advocated the use of *visual bridges* to help children connect two environments and communicate information about themselves to other people in other environments through the use of printed words, objects, photos, picture symbols, clip art, or other visual cues.

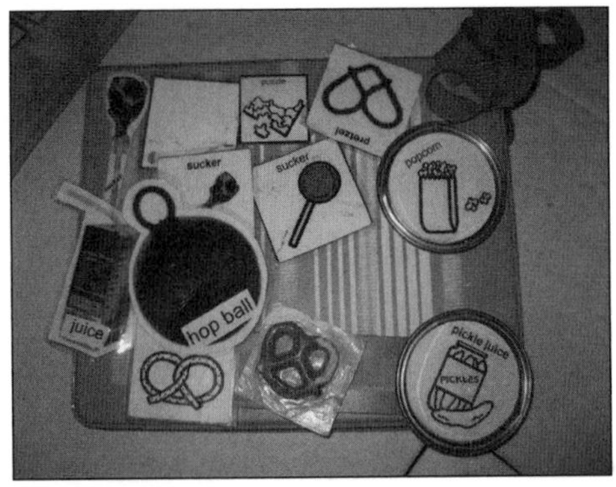

Figure 8.4. Communication supports, including real objects, photos, picture symbols, and symbols paired with words.

Source. Personal collection of J. Schoonover.

Visual supports can be used during the development of schedules, augmentative communication systems, games, sequencing, and academics. The use of a simple "first–then" board can assist a child in understanding the sequence of activities and begin developing temporal awareness. Occupational therapists' understanding of motor control, sensory sensitivities, and visual perception can assist teams in developing devices the child can access, choosing access sites and methods, and designing the size and appearance of visuals. Activities to support oral language development include reading aloud, dramatic play, puppetry, songs and poems, word play, and elaboration of sentences (Cooper et al., 2006).

Remember this. . . .
True object–based icons provide visual and tactile cues to the communicator and can be made from line drawings, pictures, photos, or product labels cut out in the shape or outline of the item they represent.

Attitude and acceptance of AAC and training of communication partners play a role in the quality and function of interactions. Interventionists should take a family-centered approach, in which AAC is integrated into the child's daily experiences and interactions to ensure caregiver support of its use (Light & Drager, 2002). AAC systems, such as communication boards and voice output devices, must be designed with layout and messages that match the child's desires, preferences, abilities, skills, and environmental contexts. For example, placing a choice board with preferred snacks within reach on the refrigerator can allow a child to communicate food preferences to a caregiver. Although some parents and professionals believe that AAC will interfere with speech development, it has actually been found to enhance it (Blackstone, 2006).

Literacy

> *Literacy is about more than reading and writing—it is about how we communicate in society. It is about social practices and relationships, about knowledge, language and culture.*
>
> —*UNESCO Statement* (2003, p. 1)

The recognition that words correspond to speech and that words are made up of sound is the foundation for literacy. Literacy is acquired through experience and exposure, from bedtime stories to signs in the grocery store. The term *emergent literacy* represents a belief that in a literate society, children as young as ages 1 and 2 are in the process of becoming literate (DeCoste & Glennen, 1997). *Functional literacy* is "the application of literacy skills and the use of a variety of literacy tools (such as listening and technology) to accomplish daily tasks in the home, school, community, and work settings" (Koenig & Holbrook, 2000, p. 265). According to Koppenhaver, Evans, and Yoder (1991), literacy skills affect the likelihood of successful competitive or supported employment. Nonreaders are at risk for failure at societal integration, difficulty managing information, difficulty in academic skill acquisition, and poor quality of life in today's text-based society.

Children with significant disabilities experience limited emergent reading and writing opportunities, putting them at considerable risk for lifelong literacy learning problems (Hanser, 2006). Therefore, children who may face barriers to literacy experience because of motor, behavioral, cognitive, or sensory differences require early and accurate assessment of their strengths and weaknesses and appropriate tools and experiences to circumvent the barriers. Emergent literacy activities for children involve offering opportunities to experience conceptual information. They include helping children understand that pictures and words have meaning and can be used to communicate and helping children create stories using pictures and words (Wershing & Symington, 1998). Daily exposure to literacy in natural environments, such as looking at and listening to books, seeing signs and labels, and using writing tools, demonstrates the importance of words. Assistive and instructional technology—including adapted books, switches, computer software and hardware, and alternative input devices—provides a set of powerful tools to provide access to learning opportunities across developmental domains and curriculum (Hutinger, Bell, Daytner, & Johanson, 2006).

According to Hanser (2006), children with multiple disabilities may have limited experience with print, including writing, for a variety of reasons. Demanding schedules of care and therapy, limited information regarding substitutions or tool adaptations for writing, a child's inability to communicate verbally, and the erroneous assumption that prerequisite writing readiness skills may contribute to fewer opportunities to actively engage in the writing process. Adapting books, a methodology that should be familiar to occupational therapists, provides print access to support emergent literacy that follows using the universal design for learning (UDL) framework. Books can be stabilized using book holders, rubberized shelf liner, nonslip mats, hook-and-loop strips, and magnets. Pages can be made easier to turn by "fluffing" them with weather stripping, clothespins, craft sticks, cotton balls, or beads. Definition can be added to pictures by outlining, removing background, adding texture, or changing colors. Content or concepts can be emphasized with tangible items and sounds (Figure 8.5). Page appearance and text can be simplified by reducing words on pages or supplementing words with rebus pictures; these are all forms of AT. Books can also be adapted and viewed electronically by scanning the pages or finding comparable clip art

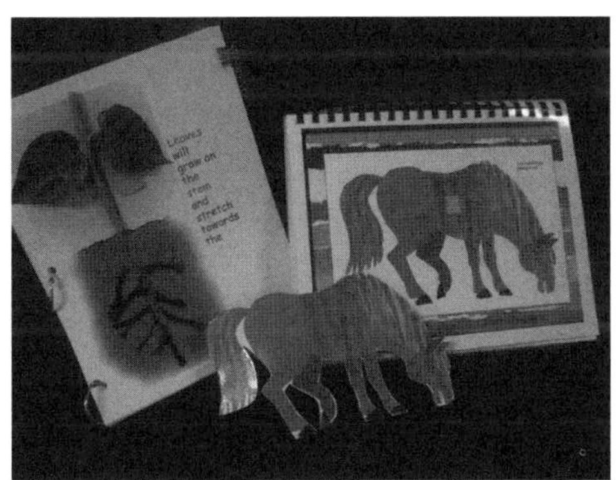

Figure 8.5. Books can be adapted with yarn, fabric, and objects to engage the reader and provide additional tactile cues. Duplicate pages can be cut apart to create matching activities. Placing pages on rings allows the amount of pages explored to be modified to ensure successful literacy experiences.

Source. Personal collection of J. Schoonover.

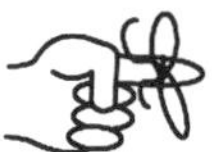

Remember this. . . .
Adapting books, a methodology that should be familiar to occupational therapists, provides print access to support emergent literacy that follows using the universal design for learning framework.

and assembling it in a multimedia slide show. Standard computer features can be used to add sound, read a story, add animation, change the visual contrast, slow down, speed up, or alter the story to improve comprehension.

All children have something to say, and it is up to service providers to provide them with opportunities for self-expression. (Readers may wish to review "A Literacy Bill of Rights"; Yoder, Erickson, & Koppenhaver, 1997.) Hanser (2006) described AT that can promote active manipulation of and experimenting with letters while accommodating for individual physical and sensory abilities through a range of "alternative pencils":

- Attaching a marker to a toy car activated with a switch so that when the car moves, a mark is made on paper
- Using an alphabet flip chart and a communication partner so that a child unable to write can select letters to be transcribed by the partner
- Using alternative keyboards and software programs to provide prewriting "scribbles"
- Using an eye-gaze frame with letters or pictures placed on it so that the child can tell or retell a story.

Hanser (2006) pointed out that alternative access tools are effective only when the writing activity is perceived as meaningful.

Sowing the Seeds of Self-Determination With AT

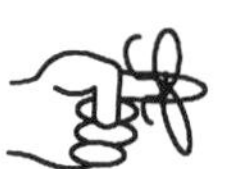

Remember this. . . .
Learned helplessness at a young age is difficult to overcome.

The term *self-determination* "refers to the right of individuals to have full power over their lives regardless of illness or disability" and "encompasses concepts such as free will, civil and human rights, freedom of choice, independence, personal agency, self-direction, and individual responsibility" (University of Illinois at Chicago National Research and Training Center [UICNRTC] on Psychiatric Disability & the UICNRTC Self-Determination Knowledge Development Workgroup, 2002, p. 1). To achieve greater control over their lives, children with disabilities should be provided with opportunities to exert control and make choices, the supports and accommodations needed for greater independence, and opportunities to develop new skills to increase participation (Wehmeyer, 2002). Learned helplessness at a young age is difficult to overcome. Often, parents and people who work with children with disabilities see their role as a protector or enabler and contribute to learned helplessness. It should be the goal of every AT intervention to build opportunities for self-determination to begin the first time it is used, even before a child is physically, cognitively, or communicatively capable. Self-determination can begin with the explanation of the device: how it works, how to charge it, what kind of batteries it uses, and what it is compatible with.

In a society where the idea of "person first" competes with the convention of "wheelchair bound," it is important to recognize that independence takes many forms. "Individuals are independent when they perform tasks themselves, when they perform tasks in an adapted environment, and when they appropriately oversee task completion by others on their own behalf" (AOTA, 1995, p. 1014). The revised AOTA position paper *Broadening the Construct of Independence* supported the expanded definition of independence as follows: "Independence is a self-directed state of being characterized by an individual's ability to participate in necessary and preferred occupations in a satisfying manner, irrespective of the amount or kind of external assistance desired or required" (AOTA, 2002, p. 660). Although the paper has been rescinded, the concept of independence and autonomy even when eternal assistance is provided is an essential aspect of occupation. Even a child who does not have the motor skills to care for a device can direct another child to complete the task. Equally, teaching a child how to direct someone else in adjusting his or her positioning or assisting with access will help that child learn to speak up in other circumstances.

Skills should be developed in the area for which the AT was chosen (e.g., positioning, mobility) as well as in use and care of the device, appropriate times for using it, and the social implications and responsibilities of using the device (Castellani & Bowser, 2006). Successful transitions from home to school and from school to the community will be enhanced through the development of self-determination skills to ensure that AT becomes an integrated part of typical routines (Castellani & Bowser, 2006).

Bremer, Kachgal, and Schoeller (2003) offered the following tips for families and professionals for promoting self-determination in children with disabilities, which are in alignment with the philosophy of occupational therapy service provision:

- Promote choice making.
- Encourage exploration of possibilities.
- Promote reasonable risk taking.
- Encourage problem solving.
- Promote self-advocacy.
- Facilitate development of self-esteem.
- Develop goal setting and planning.
- Help youth understand their disabilities. (p. 3)

Relationship Between Universal Design, Universal Design for Learning, and AT

Universal design is the design of products and environments to be usable by all people, to the greatest extent possible, without the need for adaptation or specialized design.

Ron Mace, 1941–1998 (Center for Universal Design, 2008b)

The late architect and visionary Ronald Mace, founder and program director of the Center for Universal Design (www.design.ncsu.edu/cud), used the term *universal design* to describe the philosophy of making all products and the built environment physically pleasing and usable to the greatest extent possible by everyone, regardless of their age, ability, or status in life (see Appendix 8.F). Everyday examples of universal design in the built environment include ramps, curb cuts, levered door handles, sensor-based flush toilets, and automated doors. Everyday examples of universally designed products include closed captioning, accessibility features in software products, remote controls, rubberized handles on kitchen tools, and hook-and-loop fasteners. Mace contracted polio as a child and used AT in the form of a wheelchair for mobility purposes. His work relating to accessible design influenced the passage of national legislation prohibiting discrimination against people with disabilities. One could view universal design as providing greater access to *all* people, whereas AT focuses on the needs of each person individually in the context of his or her unique circumstances. A common ground is found in the reduction of barriers through deliberate design. According to the Center for Universal Design (2008c),

> Though coming from quite different histories and directions, the purpose of universal design and assistive technology is the same: to reduce the physical and attitudinal barriers between people with and without disabilities.
>
> Universal design strives to integrate people with disabilities into the mainstream and assistive technology attempts to meet the specific needs of individuals, but the two fields meet in the middle. In fact, the point at which they intersect is a gray zone in which products and environments are not clearly "universal" or "assistive," but have characteristics of each type of design.

Or, as Mace stated,

> So, if you could separate barrier-free, universal, and assistive technology distinctly, they would look like this: *assistive technology* is devices and equipment we need to be functional in the environment; *barrier-free, ADA,* and *building codes* are disability mandates; and *universal design* is design for the built environment and consumer products for a very broad definition of user that encourages attractive, marketable products that are more usable by everyone. The reality, however, is that the three blend and move into each other. (Center for Universal Design, 2008a, italics added)

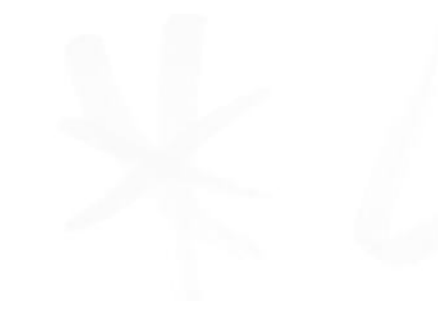

If a child can't learn the way we teach, maybe we should teach the way they learn.

—Ignacio Estrada, cited in Valdez (2003, p. 6)

Designing educational experiences that promote learning by all children regardless, of their abilities is the foundation of UDL. The term *universal design for learning* was inspired by the work and philosophy of Ron Mace. UDL is an approach to education that focuses on providing maximum flexibility in all aspects of teaching and learning to cater to the wide range of student needs and interests. It embraces three basic principles, rooted in the work of Vygotsky (1978) and Bloom (1956), who recognized individual learning differences and the teaching methodologies, including scaffolds, required to address them (CAST, 2008):

- Multiple means of representation to give learners various ways of acquiring information and knowledge
- Multiple means of expression to provide learners alternatives for demonstrating what they know
- Multiple means of engagement to tap into learners' interests, offer appropriate challenges, and increase motivation.

> A universally designed curriculum is a curriculum that has been specifically designed, developed, and validated to meet the needs of the full range of students who are actually in our schools, students with a wide range of sensory, motor, cognitive, linguistic, and affective abilities and disabilities rather than a narrow range of students in the "middle" of the population. (Hitchcock & Stahl, 2003, p. 45)

Universal design, UDL, and AT share a common goal of reducing barriers and facilitating participation. However, universal design and UDL do not replace AT. Children with disabilities will continue to need specific AT devices, such as communication aids, visual aids, wheelchairs, orthoses, and adapted toys, depending on their individualized strengths and challenges, to interact more fully with their environment. Building accessibility into new technologies and curricular materials as they are developed will help ensure the maximal inclusion of children with disabilities into the full array of learning opportunities available to all children (CAST, 2008). CAST (founded as the Center for Applied Specialized Technology) is a nonprofit research and development organization that provides an extensive collection of educational resources (see www.cast.org/research/index.html).

Creating Positive Learning Environments

Building Accessibility

Evaluating accessibility of homes and schools and recommending necessary changes are also considered AT and may include devices and services. Modifications may be required to allow children with physical or sensory impairments to navigate inside and outside using curb cuts, ramps, and door openers to enter. Labeling key areas with pictures, text, and Braille and providing accommodations for children of various sizes or who use wheelchairs to access restrooms, water fountains, playgrounds, and elevators can increase opportunities for participation. Identifying ways to improve performance and safety in the natural context of participation, to arrange resources, and to modify the environment to decrease or eliminate barriers is part of what occupational therapists do (Schoonover, Argabrite Grove, & Swinth, 2009).

In the educational setting, free, appropriate public education (FAPE) means that all students are able to get to school, enter the school, and use the building and facilities. AT might be needed to provide access to the school bus, classroom, playground, gymnasium, auditorium, or lunchroom or to the materials, furnishings, or equipment they contain. Local education agencies must meet the Americans With Disabilities Act of 1990 requirements for making information and events accessible to the community and to their staff and considering accessibility in the provision of services to students with disabilities. Safety and access to information must be provided to all who enter the school building. All safety information and diagrams depicting emergency exits must be made available to students in accessible format. Within the building, doors, walkways, handles, light switches, and stairs can be modified to provide equal access to all students. Outside the building, seating and playground modifications can allow or enhance participation in recreational activities (George, Schaff, & Jeffs, 2005).

According to Furey, Tedder, Welsh, and Wilson (2009),

> Occupational therapy practitioners' involvement in playgrounds can be as simple as helping parents find out if an accessible playground exists in or near their community, or as involved as creating or becoming an advocate for one. Practitioners can also recommend universal design equipment that can be added to an existing playground, and to educate parents and others on others on how the equipment can benefit all children. (p. 12)

Adapting and modifying a playground can create increased opportunities for mobility, socializing, and meeting sensory needs in typical environments. Learning Activity 8.5 encourages you to become active in the design and use of playgrounds in your neighborhood or area.

Social and Environmental Modifications

In addition to the obvious physical access, examining the climate of the environment while considering the individual skills and needs of the child can help determine what other supports might be required. For example, noise or clutter, fluorescent lighting, and standardized furniture may be problematic for some children whose sensory sensitivities or physical status might require alternatives for them to feel comfortable or be able to fully participate. The following are suggestions for providing environmental and low-tech supports at home and in the classroom:

- Offer choices at every opportunity. "Sabotaging" the environment to promote the need for communication works wonders. For example, hold a swing still and give the child a choice to "go" or "stop." Provide visuals in the form of pictures, items, symbols, or words to strengthen the expressive choices. Visuals can be used to provide a variety of communication opportunities. For example, during snack time or lunchtime, placemats with visuals for requesting and commenting can be created (Figure 8.6). In addition to the picture symbols that are included on the placemat, picture cards to request napkins, utensils, food, drink, need help, open, and the like should be available to use with an "I want" board.

Learning Activity 8.5. Designing Areas That Promote Play for All Children

As agents of change, occupational therapists are challenged to take a proactive role in recommending building design or modifications.

- Using what you have learned about universal design (UD), list the needs for or draw up plans for an accessible playground.
- Think about children who have mobility, behavioral, cognitive, or sensory challenges. What would a playground that these children and everyone could use look like?
- Look at the playgrounds in your local area. Are there elements of UD? How might these playgrounds be adapted for UD?
- Find out more! Go to Playgrounds for Everyone: www.danvilleambucs.com/projects/playgroundForEveryone.html

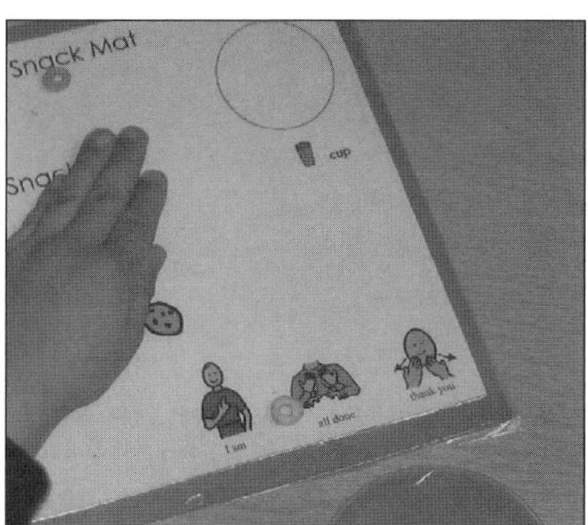

Figure 8.6. Shapes and picture symbols on a placemat provide matching and communication opportunities (cup goes on circle, "I am all done").

Source. Personal collection of J. Schoonover.

- Explore the use of voice output communication devices for labeling, requesting objects, and expanding commentary about the activity. These devices and accompanying visuals can be used to gain focus and provide auditory narration ("Pass it to me . . . pass it along").
- Provide positioning alternatives. Without proximal stability, it is more difficult to stabilize, converge eyes, and maintain a level of arousal. Think about having the children sit on the floor, and vary sitting positions according to their sensory needs.
- Use social situation stories to ease transition and aid in understanding of expectations (see examples at www.vanderbilt.edu/csefel/practicalstrategies.html). Social situation stories can be created using multimedia software, such as PowerPoint. They can be played repeatedly on the computer, with narration, sound effects, and animation, to encourage sustained attention and engagement. Hard copies can be printed and laminated for use in school and at home.
- Implement a behavioral management program. This technique involves introducing strategies that support children in understanding rules, recognizing and anticipating daily routines, completing the tasks, and learning to determine appropriate behaviors.

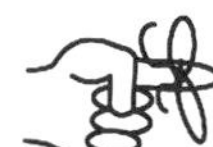

Remember this. . . .
Placemats with visuals for requesting and commenting can be created. In addition to the picture symbols that are included on the placemat, picture cards to request napkins, utensils, food, drink, need help, open, and the like should be available.

To support task completion, explore the use of a visual sequence card that depicts the steps involved in the task. The symbols can be attached to the card with hook-and-loop fasteners, then removed and placed into a "finished" envelope upon completion of each step, or each step can be checked off as it is completed. In addition to supporting task completion, this board can be used to provide communication opportunities when discussing the task.

Empowerment of Service Providers

A survey of early intervention providers (Wilcox, Guimond, Campbell, & Moore, 2006) solicited information about the respondents' views of AT for infants and toddlers with disabilities. The findings indicated that providers have a broad view of the continuum of AT and that training makes a positive difference in terms of consideration and use (Wilcox et al., 2006). Therefore, it is imperative to provide for and advocate for training opportunities in the area of AT. Moreover, occupational therapists should take every opportunity to identify the AT devices they are embedding in their service delivery in conversation, documentation, and training to create a common understanding of the continuum of devices and service that are considered AT.

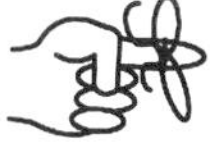

Remember this. . . .
Occupational Therapy + AT = Participation: Increasing Quality of Life.

> Six-month-old Jamal lies prone over a rolled towel. A bright red button switch is placed in front of him, which is connected by a cord to a battery-operated toy dog. Unable to support himself on his forearms independently because of decreased muscle tone, Jamal needs help to hold his head up to explore his environment and explore toys. Jamal reaches for the bright red button. When he contacts it, the toy dog in front of him begins to bark and walk. Jamal's eyes widen. For several seconds, the dog advances, then stops. Jamal looks expectantly. Finally, Jamal reaches for the bright red button. As the dog begins to moves again, Jamal chortles in delight.

The cause-and-effect event in which Jamal has just participated is the result of several AT interventions. The rolled towel provides him the support he needs to reach the switch. The switch provides access to a toy. Teaching people who provide services to Jamal how to position him and set up toys is a form of empowerment for everyone involved.

The National Institute on Disability and Rehabilitation Research (n.d.) suggested a "new paradigm" of disability:

> [D]isability is the result of an interaction between characteristics of the individual and those of the natural, built, communications (IT [information technology]), cultural, and social environments. Personal characteristics, as well as environmental ones, may be either enabling or disabling. The relative degree of this situation fluctuates, depending on condition, time, and setting. This view of disability suggests that one of the most effective ways to address particular disabilities may be through the removal of barriers and the provision of accommodation or assistive technology.

Occupational therapists "work in early intervention and school-based settings with children, parents, caregivers, educators, and other team members to facilitate the child's ability to engage in meaningful occupations" (AOTA, 2004b, p. 681). Play enhances social and cognitive performance, self-confidence, self-determination, and collaboration as well as motor skills (Ariel, 2002). In many instances, the foundation for all other ATs begins with equipment and strategies used for positioning, seating, and functional mobility. The need for (other) ATs can be assessed and tried once a stable position for optimal participation has been established (Post et al., 2008).

Transportation and AT

IDEA requires that for preschool, children with disabilities have access to related services, including transportation. Car and bus modifications for entry and exit and safe and appropriate seating can help with transportation to and from day care, school, and school-related activities, including field trips, sports, and recreation. Occupational therapists and other AT providers need to be knowledgeable about equipment options and assist transportation providers with the skills and resources necessary to provide adequately for the safety of young children while being transported. Infants and toddlers may be transported to Early Head Start programs or other child care facilities by a variety of transportation providers, including the public schools in some states. Infants, toddlers, and preschool-age children with special physical, cognitive, or behavioral needs present challenges and responsibilities for transportation providers, including physical handling, communication with young children, behavioral management, child safety seats, restraint systems, safety vests, wheelchairs and occupant securement systems, special equipment management, medical fragility and complex conditions, and more.

Determining what is required to safely transport young children with disabilities requires knowledge of available resources and collaboration with teams of families and professionals. The National Center for the Safe Transportation of Children with Special Healthcare Needs (www.preventinjury.org) serves as a resource for families, health care professionals, transportation providers, and child passenger safety advocates. One of the resources it provides is an occupational therapist trained to identify the appropriate child safety restraint required for a broad range of health conditions. The Rehabilitation Engineering Research Center on Wheelchair Transportation Safety at the University of Michigan (www.travelsafer.org) provides information pertaining to safe travel in motor vehicles for people seated in wheelchairs.

Critical Aspects of AT Assessment

Keep in mind that the AT literature uses the terms *assessment* and *evaluation* differently from IDEA, AOTA, or most early childhood literature. *Assessment* reflects ongoing intervention with continual changes made on the basis of client performance. *Evaluation* implies a static set of tests or a singular event at the beginning of service delivery.

In addition to the tangible aspect of AT in the form of devices or tools, AT can be an action or service requiring initial and ongoing assessment and intervention. Because of the dynamic interplay between the child, the activities, the tools, and the contexts that make up the essence of participation, evaluating a child's performance and AT needs is an ongoing process rather than a one-time event. Successful implementation of AT begins with individualized and contextual evaluations that lead to identification of appropriate solutions. Despite the fact that specialists have knowledge and experience about people with disabilities and tools to address barriers, it is the families of young children who have unique expertise regarding their child, their routines, and the environment in which they live. No standardized AT assessments have been created because of the highly individualized nature of AT use, although several inventories, checklists, and processes have been developed.

Evaluation begins with the identification of need. Because young children with disabilities frequently have needs involving several disciplines and environments, people contributing to the evaluation process might include family members; educators; therapeutic and related service providers; medical professionals; rehabilitation engineers (specialists in customizing a device); and social workers, service coordinators, and case managers. Ideally, the AT evaluation is completed by the team that will also provide the intervention or by a team that has been formed specifically for the purpose of conducting AT evaluations in the natural context. Because of the complexity of many AT systems, some hospitals, clinics, community agencies, and schools may have a designated AT team. In the event that separate teams are responsible for evaluation and intervention, they should collaborate to make decisions and recommendations.

Providing opportunities to try different types of AT is considered best practice for determining a good match between the child and family (or school personnel) and the AT device or system. Trials as a part of the assessment process can help prevent the costly procurement of an incorrect device and alert the family and school staff to any potential difficulties or need for further modifications. It is important to think beyond the purchase or loan of the device and to consider the ongoing costs for maintenance (e.g., batteries, parts, and additional devices required to operate or interact with the device), upgrades to the system, and repairs. Swinth (2001) recommended that teams ask themselves the following questions:

1. What financial resources are available to the family?
2. When the AT device is in need of repair, does the family have access to services?
3. Does the AT device significantly increase the child's level of independence and function?
4. Can the AT device be adapted to enable higher levels of function as the child grows and matures?
5. Can a less complex device meet the same needs just as well? (p. 583)

Appendix 8.G provides additional guiding questions for trialing and selecting an AT device.

The cost of AT and who pays for it will vary depending on the focus of the program, what the child needs, and where the needs occur. Costs have been identified as a barrier for families. The team discusses these issues and other issues that are unique to each family in deciding whether a system is a reasonable and appropriate investment that will increase the child's functional independence. The team should present the child and family with objective and realistic information regarding investment in and use of AT. After considering the options and alternatives described, the family and the team should make the final decision together as to what AT is implemented and how it is incorporated into the child's program (Schoonover et al., 2009).

AT Decision Making

Once the initial assessment process has been completed and a potential need for AT has been determined, it is important for team members to come to a consensus regarding the kind of intervention that will best meet the child's individual needs. Several approaches to AT decision making have been identified. Parette and Brotherson (2004) described interrelated considerations, including child characteristics, family issues, technology features, and service system concerns), that lead to an individualized and child-centered decision. Decision making should first include

- Consideration of whether AT is related to the child's goals;
- Whether the intervention would be practical for that particular child; and
- Whether devices are viewed from the perspective of the child's strengths and needs.

A focus on the family's needs, preferences, abilities, and experiences will help ensure the device's acceptance and use in the home and community. The team must also take into account the device's potential to increase performance as well as practical considerations such as cost, ease of use, comfort, dependability, transportability, adaptability, and durability. Finally, the service system's ability to provide needed AT devices and services must be reviewed. These services include financing options, protection from theft and damage, personnel training needs, transportation, and transition needs (Parette & Brotherson, 2004).

Understanding cultural and linguistic diversity can prevent alienation of family members whose participation could influence acceptance of AT devices and services (Parette & Brotherson, 2004). According to Kalyanpur and Harry (1999),

> the issue is not that we must have had the same experiences in terms of culture, ethnic background, race, socioeconomic status, or gender as the families we serve—because we cannot—but that we have the willingness to learn about and understand their experiences, that we are willing to understand how our own experiences have shaped us, and that we respect and accept these differences in our various experiences. (p. 131)

Parette and Brotherson (2004) found that when intervention focused on the client, the environment, and what the client wanted to do, the client was more likely to use the AT than when intervention focused on the tool or on what the tool could do. They cited Kalyanpur and Harry's (1999) four-step process involving collaboration with families from culturally and linguistically diverse backgrounds during AT decision making to determine the best match of AT with user:

> 1. Identify the values affecting the client's interpretation of his or her AT needs or the recommendation for services.
> 2. Determine whether the client values the AT provider's AT assumptions; if not, determine how his or her perceptions differ.
> 3. Acknowledge and respect any cultural differences identified, and fully explain the foundation of the AT provider's assumptions.
> 4. Determine the most effective way to adapt AT interpretations or recommendations to the client's value system. (Parette & Brotherson, 2004, p. 361)

Some of the fundamental skills an occupational therapist needs to participate in AT decisions, whether as the primary evaluator or as a member of a team, include an awareness of AT resources, an understanding of developmental milestones, a clear vision of the family's and child's desires, and an ability to work collaboratively with other professionals to determine child- and family-centered options, even when in direct conflict with personally held opinions of best practice.

AT Team

Clearly, working in teams is the best way to provide comprehensive AT services. Bodine and Melonis (2005) drew the following distinctions between the types of teams:

> 1. *Multidisciplinary* teams, often associated with the medical model of intervention, are made up of professionals of different disciplines who work independently of one another. Each assessment and recommendation is performed individually, and findings are reported to the group.

2. *Interdisciplinary* teams are made up of parents and professionals; each individual is responsible for his or her own area of expertise. Sharing ideas in interdisciplinary groups is common; however, communication can be affected by professional jargon and lack of awareness of the expertise of each member.
3. *Transdisciplinary or collaborative* teams exchange knowledge and information and may cross boundaries of expertise for the purpose of providing family- or client-centered services.

Copley and Ziviani (2007) used a pilot study to develop and trial a team AT assessment and planning process using questionnaires as assessment tools. Their findings indicated several benefits for teams, including development of more specific and achievable technology goals; increased knowledge, skills, and confidence of team members; more effective teamwork to assist in decision making; and better coordination of technology use between home and school (Copley & Ziviani, 2007). The role of the occupational therapist as part of the team is as follows:

1. Share information about the student's positioning and posture needs.
2. Assess the student and inform the team about the student's motor abilities and requirements (e.g., hand function, reach, keyboarding skills, computer access, material storage).
3. Provide information about the student's present mobility equipment (e.g., seating inserts, splints, standing frames, walkers, wheelchairs).
4. Provide information regarding any pending medical procedures for the student (e.g., medical reevaluations, orthopedic surgery).
5. Share technical expertise regarding alternative access (e.g., recommended devices, ergonomic considerations, adaptations, or modifications. (Special Education Technology–British Columbia, 2005, p. 8)

Although these recommendations are sound practices, the occupational therapist is encouraged to address all aspects of a person or the environment that support or impede occupational engagement by identifying and taking ownership of their role as agents of change, providing additional perspective on sensory, psychosocial, environmental, and behavioral aspects of performance.

Considering Family Roles, Routines, and Values

Occupational therapists use various interventions that enable people to engage in occupations and participate in daily life. Some of the interventions may require changing, eliminating, adding, or incorporating new and therapeutic activities into the daily routines (Segal, 2004). Everyone closely involved in the caregiving and lives of children using AT, as well as the child, if possible, should be involved in choosing the devices that will best meet the child's needs with a minimum of disruption to daily occupations and routines. To prevent possible abandonment of a device or practice in favor of more familiar routines and habits, the people involved in making decisions about AT devices and services must be sensitive to the effects of adapting apparently simple routines (Phillips & Zhao, 1993). Change may be more difficult to implement when families must shift and adapt elements of expressing and sharing their sense of identity (Segal, 2004). Therefore, the team must be aware of and sensitive to established roles.

Given a range of low- to high-tech options, it is not uncommon for families to select and use low-tech interventions, possibly because their appearance approximates typically found toys and materials and calls less attention to the child or reason it is needed (Mistrett, 2000). What is acceptable in the household in terms of appearance of equipment and alternative methods to accomplish a task (e.g., eating with feet) may not be considered acceptable during an excursion to a local restaurant. For children, the mixed message of what is acceptable in the public and private arena can be confusing.

The author of this chapter worked with a family whose child was unable to sit up or walk independently. Her first response was to suggest that the family get a wheelchair for the child. This suggestion was met with resistance from the family, who pointed out that not only did the neighborhood lack sidewalks on which to push the child, but that the main family goal was to have the child join them at the dinner table. In this situation, the lack of consideration of the physical environment of the home and outlying areas, the emotional culture of the family, and what was important to the family and their needs versus the therapist's need to do something could have resulted in abandonment of the device ordered and, of greater import, distrust in the service system offering support. The occupational therapist realized that she was imposing what she felt was the most important intervention (the provision of a mobility device) so that the child could be transported more easily around the house and in the community. As she continued to talk with the family, it became clear that their priorities were different. She instead suggested an adjustable seating insert, which allowed the child to join the family at the dinner table. Together, the occupational therapist and the family discovered that a side benefit of the insert was that it could be placed in a lightweight stroller, thereby providing a mobility option for trips outside the immediate neighborhood.

Role of Cultural Background in the Acceptance of AT

Carrying a child who is unable to walk is preferred by some cultures not only for the physical contact and interaction but also to mask the child's inability to move independently. In some cultures, it is perfectly acceptable for a child to be waited on and cared for, especially when disabled, such that supports for activities of daily living (ADLs) are not be highly valued. In other cultures, anything that would draw attention to the child, making him or her look "different," would be undesirable. Part C of IDEA mandates that services occur in the natural environment, which encompasses not only the physical environment of the home (e.g., furniture, crib, car seat) but also the cultural environment (e.g., parents' wants and needs for their children, their belief system). One role of the occupational therapist is to empower children and their families to be strong advocates for their needs to give them their best chance for success, keeping in mind that families do not always share the same concerns as those of the professionals. Families should know their rights, including consideration of the need for AT and the benefits of such devices and services, to place their child on the road to a successful, independent, and meaningful life. Continued research should be conducted so that providers of AT can understand the influence of cultural mores and acceptance or refusal of AT.

According to Suarez-Balcazar et al. (2009),

> *[c]ultural competence* is demonstrated when the practitioner understands and appreciates differences in health beliefs and behaviors, recognizes and respects variations that occur within cultural groups, and is able to adjust his or her practice to provide effective interventions for people from various cultures." (p. 499)

Being culturally competent can help AT teams develop client- and family-centered intervention approaches that recognize and include the effects of culture on the perspective on and decision making about AT. The emphasis placed on participation and engagement in various activities and life roles is influenced by each person's unique culture as well as by his or her interaction with others (Cook & Polgar, 2008). Although the reader is cautioned against cultural stereotypes, historically, some cultures do not place the same value on the independence that AT provides, or an AT device may not be chosen or used if it substitutes for a valued life role of another. Cultural factors must therefore be considered when providing AT devices and services.

The development of cultural reciprocity can assist people with the AT decision-making process to establish relationships of mutual respect. Cultural reciprocity (Harry, Kalyanpur, & Day, 1999) promotes a foundation of self-reflection and self-awareness. It begins when service providers develop insight into the values that are the basis of their understanding of a child's difficulties or in the kind of AT recommendations they make. Leake and Black (2005) described Harry et al.'s (1999) five key features of the posture of cultural reciprocity as follows:

1. Goes beyond awareness of differences to self-awareness
2. Aims for subtle levels of awareness of difference
3. Has universal applicability
4. Avoids stereotypical solutions
5. Ensures that both families and personnel are empowered. (pp. 25–26)

Potential for Abandonment

Failure to consider consumer preference and choice has been cited as the number one reason for device abandonment (Galvin & Scherer, 1996; Phillips & Zhao, 1993). There is a paucity of studies on this particular topic, and nearly all of them refer back to one of the oldest, Phillips and Zhao (1993). One might infer that the AT experts focus more on their knowledge of the tool and less on the hopes, dreams, and needs of the client and the reality of where and how the device is intended to be used. According to Scherer (1991), three aspects of AT use must be considered in preventing AT abandonment: (1) the milieu or situation in which the person uses the AT, (2) the personality and preferences of the user, and (3) the characteristics of the AT.

When participating in decision making about AT, it is essential that occupational therapists not only consider the attributes of the task, environment, and tool and the effect of the disability but also reflect on the user, the family, and their attitudes and feelings regarding assistive devices (Hocking, 1999), separating their personal from their professional values. Being alert to the social and cultural implications of assistive devices and of disability and emphasizing activities that hold purpose and meaning will promote the kind of AT service delivery for which occupational therapists are uniquely trained (AOTA, 2004a).

Hocking (1999) stated that occupational therapists need to

> broaden their focus from procedural reasoning about the characteristics of the task, environment, assistive device, and the effect of the disability, to conditional and interactive reasoning about the person and their attitudes and emotional responses and context to using assistive devices. This will require therapists to be alert to the social and cultural meanings of assistive devices and of disability, because these are the meanings that people with disability must negotiate in the processes of accepting both their disability and the need to use assistive technology, and establishing an identity in their social setting. (p. 8)

Learning Activity 8.6 encourages you to develop AT advocacy skills by creating an AT Bill of Rights.

Importance of Training and Support

Copley and Ziviani (2004) conducted a literature review of research on AT use by children to determine barriers to its implementation and integration in the educational setting. Barriers identified included lack of appropriate staff training and support, negative staff attitudes, inadequate assessment and planning processes, insufficient funding, difficulties procuring and managing equipment, and time constraints. Lack of training and knowledge about AT may limit its use with infants and young children (Dugan, Campbell, & Wilcox, 2006). Because of the lack of training that many early intervention providers and occupational therapists report, young children may not be acquiring the full benefit of interventions to enhance their performance of functional skills and participation in everyday activities and routines. Ideally, preservice training should include information about intervention methodologies and various forms of AT. Information is available to providers through federally funded programs supported by state and local agencies.

When providers are knowledgeable about and view AT as an effective way of intervening with infants and toddlers, children's participation will be enhanced. In the school setting, AT specialists are more likely to recommend AT devices for children, whereas those representing several disciplines, including early intervention

Learning Activity 8.6. Assistive Technology Bill of Rights

A bill of rights is a list of the human rights or privileges that are considered important and essential by the group of people it represents. After reviewing the top 10 list you created in Learning Activity 8.1, the Communication Bill of Rights (Appendix 8.E), and the sections discussing assistive technology abandonment, develop an "Assistive Technology Bill of Rights."

teachers, occupational therapists, physical therapists, and speech–language pathologists, are more likely to recommend AT devices and services for infants and toddlers (Dugan et al., 2006). It is postulated that evidence-based, individualized training may assist professionals in understanding the factors that influence their use of AT with young children and provide them with sufficient knowledge and resources to apply recommended practices (Dugan et al., 2006). A survey of early intervention providers suggested that training makes a positive difference in terms of AT consideration and use (Wilcox et al., 2006). People who use AT and their significant others must all be educated in the use and maintenance of the equipment and have continued support.

Overcoming the Obstacles of Funding

> Anita listens to the discussion about Maria's need for a communication device. A device that will help her daughter communicate sounds wonderful, but who is going to pay for such a thing when she can barely scrape enough together to put food on the table?

Funding for AT comes in many forms. Although federal mandates determine that a child receives the AT devices necessary to support the IEP, these devices almost always belong to the facility purchasing them. Therefore, when a child moves or changes environments, the device remains with the funding source. Other funding sources for equipment that should be accessible to the child at all times should be explored. Funding sources can be organized according to purpose, nature of equipment, age of user, location, and financial status. Medicaid, private insurance, service organizations, state loan programs, special interest groups such as Easter Seals, church groups, thrift shops, and charitable organizations such as the Make a Wish Foundation are all potential funding resources. The Regional (Technology Resource) Centers in each state are a primary source for locating equipment and identifying and working with funding sources.

Research has indicated that funding for AT devices is one of the biggest obstacles to the procurement of AT devices and service provision (Judge, 2000). Funding for AT comes from several sources, including Part B of IDEA; Medicaid; the Early and Periodic Screening, Diagnosis, and Treatment program; state AT loan programs; private insurance; community service organizations; and other agencies. Parents might be asked to share the cost of AT but are not required to do so if loss of benefits, increase in copay, or discontinuation of services may result. A survey of 48 Tech Act directors who oversee their state's programs funded under the AT Act indicated that most of their states had cash loan programs to finance AT, yet only 28% of them reported that the programs were used by infants and toddlers. Some of the reasons identified for the statistics were (1) use of cash loans more often for home or vehicle modifications, (2) no applicants for newer programs, or (3) low demand for the program (Campbell, Wilcox, Milbourne, & Bacon, 2004). Occupational therapists should familiarize themselves with the funding sources and mechanisms in their state for AT, particularly for infants and toddlers.

When a school or agency funds a device, it owns it, and the device might have to be returned when the child leaves the area or ages out of the program. In the case of Medicaid or private insurance funding, the device belongs to the family of the child. Depending on the state, before the child turns 3 years old, a transition plan that should include discussion of the child's AT needs and moving or acquiring equipment to the next placement must be developed. Care must be taken that the child has whatever equipment or services are necessary to meet IEP goals.

Implementation

> *Assistive technology implementation proceeds according to a collaboratively developed plan. . . . all those involved in implementation work together to develop a written action plan that provides detailed information about what will be done and who will do it.*
>
> —Quality Indicators of Assistive Technology Consortium (2004, p. 9)

NATRI surveyed state department of education leaders, district personnel, building administrators, special education teachers, parents, and students to learn more about AT implementation, resulting in a top 10 list of findings and a toolkit for schools: *Assistive Technology Planner: From IEP Consideration to Classroom Implementation.* (A reproducible AT implementation plan form is available to download from the NATRI Web site at http://natri.uky.edu/resources/ImpPlanform060807.pdf.) A "Tech Works" brief from the National Center for Technology Innovation and the Center for Implementing Technology in Education (2006) lists the top 10 findings from the NATRI data, which include the fact that although a variety of service delivery models were found across the country in schools, ranging from trained AT teams to building or district representatives to regional AT centers, no single service delivery model was found to be most prevalent.

Responsible (and Responsive) Data Collection

Data collection is an essential aspect of the AT service delivery system. It can give an indication of what's going right (and wrong) with a selected intervention. If monitored properly, it can stave off potential equipment abandonment and disillusionment by the user or caregivers and document, confirm, or justify a continuing need. The effectiveness of a chosen AT device or intervention can be measured using quantitative and qualitative information. Data collection begins with deciding what information is needed and what it looks like. For example, when developing a data sheet for switch activation, the team needs to consider what constitutes a deliberate versus an accidental contact, which part of the body will be used to activate the switch, whether and how much wait time will be allowed before a prompt is given, the type of prompt to be given (e.g., visual, verbal, hand over hand), and the definition of success for the given task (e.g., single-switch activation, activation or deactivation of an electronic device, holding a switch for a specified amount of time; Schoonover et al., 2009). During implementation planning, there should be consensus regarding who takes data, what kind of data are taken, how the data are collected, and how often they are reviewed. Data collection can take many forms, from hatch marks on sticky notes to a digital portfolio. Data collection methods should be intuitive enough that all team members, including family members, are able to record accurate information. A "go-to" person or people should be identified so that in the event of a question or equipment failure, the matter can be dealt with in a timely manner. The advent of new, versatile, and readily available tools for data collection, including handheld computers and cell phone features, makes it possible to embed data collection into familiar routines and activities.

One form of data collection, the use of a portfolio, is familiar to most educators. Work samples exemplifying the criterion measured are analyzed over time and baseline to document the effects interventions have on performance. Portfolios can be paper or electronic. One obvious advantage of electronic portfolios is their ability to add dimension to the snapshot of a child's performance using photos, scanned work samples, audio clips, video clips, and more. A digital portfolio can be stored and made available to others electronically and can serve as a historian over time to document introduced AT and subsequent effects on a child's performance. A digital portfolio can serve double duty as a means to share positioning and setup information for people who are unfamiliar with the child. Anyone with a passing familiarity with creating a digital slideshow using a multimedia software program such as PowerPoint can create a digital portfolio. Any number of Web sites can assist with this process.

Other technologies that can be used for data collection include digital cameras, cell phones (as picture takers and as memory joggers) that allow the caller to leave a voicemail that is turned into text and sent to a designated destination using e-mail, text message, or Web update), tape recorders, spreadsheets, and data collection forms available on the Internet. Some voice output devices contain a built-in language acquisition monitor (LAM) that records characters being selected and adds a time stamp. LAMs can be used to identify the number of times the device has been activated and the communication patterns used.

A collection of AT outcome measurement tools can be found at http://utoronto.ca/atrc/reference/atoutcomes. General outcome tools include the Canadian Occupational Performance Measure (Law et al., 2005) and the Occupational Therapy Functional Assessment Compilation Tool (Smith, 1995), which was created to standardize the collection and reporting of occupational therapy functional assessment data and outcomes.

Evidence-Based Practice

Evidence-based practice in early childhood education is characterized as "conscientious, explicit, and judicious use of current best practice in making decisions . . . integrating individual clinical expertise with the best available evidence from systematic research" while considering the needs of the child and family (Lowman, 2008, p. 3). More than a decade ago, AT research was characterized as "scattershot" (Okolo & Bouck, 2007). Because of the individualized needs of children and families, it is difficult to find large-scale studies. To evaluate the effectiveness of the intervention, focus should be placed on interplay among the user, the technology, the activities, and the context, rather than singularly looking at the device or service (Cook & Polgar, 2008). Outcomes studied should be related to the success experienced by the user on the basis of the AT system. Applying evidence-based practice can increase accountability and use information gathered from families and professionals to provide children and their families with interventions that are vetted with an anticipated outcome of greater user satisfaction and investment.

AT in Transition Planning

Susan and Rob came to their son Bobby's transition meeting with some trepidation. With Bobby entering an early childhood special education program at their neighborhood school at age 3, he will no longer receive services in their home. What will happen to the switches provided by the program that give him such pleasure operating the computer, and who will provide him with the special feeding equipment he uses at home?

Transitions can be described as "actions coordinated to prepare for or facilitate change, such as from one functional level to another, from one life stage to another, from one program to another, or from one environment to another" (AOTA, 1998, p. 866). Although transitions are an inevitable part of the growth and development of young children, the passages from early intervention services to preschool and from preschool to elementary school can result in a loss of continuity of services and interpersonal connections and may leave families feeling adrift. For a child with a disability and for family members, transitions can be stressful if the supports that the child needs to participate are not in place or do not fit the context of the new environment (Myers, Stephens, & Tabor, 2009). 34 C.F.R. § 300.124 describes the transition of children from the Part C program to preschool programs. (See Chapters 1 and 4 for specific requirements of the transition process from early intervention to preschool.)

Successful transitions begin with careful and coordinated planning involving representatives from different classrooms, child care settings, programs, buildings, or agencies involved with the child and family. When a child transitions from one environment to another, critical information as well as skill sets, strategies for interaction, and information regarding specialized technology may not be passed along from one setting to another. According to Myers (2008), occupational therapists practicing in early childhood programs may have a restricted view of their potential role in supporting families and children with special needs during the transition process; perceived barriers to support include lack of time, lack of employer support for participation, and inadequate training, yet the problem-solving and psychosocial perspective of an occupational therapist could prove invaluable to the success of the process.

IDEA mandates the provision of both AT services and transition services for people with disabilities. When a child requires AT to accomplish one or more functional skills, the use of that AT must be included in effective transition planning. Information on the kind of equipment needed, the way the child uses it, and the support services required is essential to ensure continuity and prevent abandonment. Occupational therapists' understanding of activity analysis and environmental adaptation and modification makes them uniquely qualified to make recommendations regarding potential equipment needs and regarding modifications to the context or task in the new environment; enhanced participation within the classroom setting is the ultimate goal (Myers, 2008). Self-advocacy, advocacy on behalf of the client, and implementation are critical issues for transition planning. Clearly, a strong argument can be made for the involvement of occupational therapy at such crucial life stages.

Explicit documentation is essential during all transitions to ensure that the transitioning child has the support he or she needs. Documentation can take the forms of text, photos, and videos. For children who require AT devices or services to receive FAPE, the transition plans should contain a statement of needed AT devices and services and indicate agency responsibilities and linkages, if appropriate. AT can accompany the child home or to other environments if it is considered necessary for FAPE.

Remember this. . . .
AT, including devices, switches, computer hardware and interactive software, and alternative input devices, provides a set of powerful tools to equalize learning opportunities for young children across developmental domains and content areas.

Susan and Rob are glad that Julia, the occupational therapist who has been working with Bobby in their home, has created a transition portfolio to share with his school-based occupational therapist and the IEP team. The intent is to use this portfolio to provide continuity in terms of how Bobby is positioned and what tools he is accustomed to using. With Susan and Rob's permission, Julia has taken pictures of Bobby's positioning in his high chair, his cut-out cup, and his built-up spoon. She has described how she slides the handle of his spoon over his index finger, under his middle finger, and over his ring finger, so the spoon stays in place even though he cannot grip it in a typical manner. Julia has used the portfolio to document Bobby's current level of performance as well as to inform those who will work with him in the future.

Keeping Current With AT Can Be a Daunting Task

Twenty-first century occupational therapists living in the digital age must develop their own strategies for keeping abreast of current practices and ensuring that implementation is consistent with national, state, and local policies. In their survey, Long et al. (2007) found that occupational therapists have identified a need for accessible and affordable training specifically in areas of funding AT devices and services and collaborating with families and other service providers. Exploring professional literature, the Internet, conferences, workshops, and AT e-mail lists is a good way to start. AOTA offers opportunities for therapists to connect with others through AOTA's members-only online forums (OT Connections, http://otconnections.aota.org/), blogs, galleries, public forums, and communities of interest. The Technology Special Interest Section provides a venue for occupational therapists to explore technology-related topics with their peers through online forums, conference offerings, and quarterly publications. AOTA (in press) has developed a Technology Knowledge and Skills Paper that outlines technology competencies. In addition, AOTA offers books and online courses on the topic of AT.

The Quality Indicators of Assistive Technology Listserv is a free tool that enables discussions with people of a wide variety of backgrounds (e.g., therapists, educators, parents, policymakers) who share an interest in AT. As previously mentioned, each state has a federally funded AT project that provides information and resources to its constituents. The projects are coordinated by RESNA through a National Institute for Disability and Rehabilitation Research grant (for more information, go to www.resna.org/projects/).

The decision to specialize in AT is typically made on the basis of personal interest and self-study or assigned as part of a job description. Current legislation does not list qualifications required to be regarded as an AT provider or specialist. No national-level organization oversees AT providers, and few publications focus specifically on AT service delivery for children. Certificate programs and advanced degrees in AT are offered by a growing number of universities. A mechanism for verifying a minimum level of competence for people acting as AT providers has been established by RESNA through an examination process that provides credentialing for people working as AT practitioners.

Conclusion

The contribution of occupational therapy practice to the health and well-being of children cannot be underestimated. As services to children with disabilities become more closely tied to the natural context, the need to understand the attributes, tasks, and tools necessary for successful participation increases. For young children with disabilities and their families, AT redefines possibilities and opportunities, says "Yes, you can!" and establishes a foundation for future successes. The early introduction and judicious use of AT can provide children with disabilities from birth through age 5 and their caregivers with natural learning opportunities for child-centered movement, play, communication, and self-care experiences paralleling those of typically developing children. Occupational therapists plan and implement strategies that promote participation in meaningful occupations by developing opportunities to establish, restore, or maintain skills. Occupational therapists need to stay abreast of trends in AT as well as recognize and document the adaptations and strategies they implement every day as AT.

Examples of AT devices are as varied as the people who use them, the contexts in which they are used, and the needs they support. AT services include collaboration for evaluating the needs of the child and family, selecting and acquiring the appropriate device, training the family and other caregivers, and monitoring the use of the device. AT is one of many tools occupational therapists use to promote or substitute for the acquisition of developmental skills and engagement in meaningful activities. It can serve as a door opener and provide access for all who encounter barriers in their natural environments, paving over the gap between potential and participation with possibilities.

Occupational therapists can and should

> advocate for universal design and environmental modifications that remove barriers in homes, schools, and communities to ensure access to supportive community services, including transportation, personal care, health care, education, employment, and other services, and to facilitate engagement in social and civic activities. (AOTA, 2008, p. 1)

By holistically considering the hopes and dreams of a child, the family, and caregivers, as well as attending to the natural context of early childhood, occupational therapists can guide the selection of appropriate AT devices and services (Schoonover et al., 2009).

How Very Far We Have Come: Luke (1993–2010)

Grace graduated from high school in 1993. Attending her graduation was a 2-year-old little brother, a surprise for Annie and Coleman in what they had thought would be their "relaxing years." Luke was born a month early, but he gained weight quickly and did not have any medical problems. What he did have were his days and nights reversed and a tendency to overreact to everything, crying inconsolably.

Annie had returned to teaching when Grace was in fifth grade, and she knew just where to turn. She called up the state's early intervention program. What she and Coleman needed (and Grace, as well, because she needed rest for all her high school activities) was definitely early intervention to help get Luke on the right track. Annie liked that the services were provided in the home, again remembering the day-long trips for Dan to be seen for 10 minutes. An occupational therapist worked with Annie to help her "read" Luke's cues as well as arrange his environment to be less stimulating until he could handle it. Within a few months, Luke was on track and growing well. Annie and Coleman decided with the early intervention providers that they would keep Luke in the program with monthly monitoring. This decision was a good one, because Luke was slow to talk in a manner that anyone could understand. He was frustrated, but he was not interested in signing (although he eventually did it, stomping his foot each time for emphasis). Luke made progress with speech therapy, but at age 3, he was still behind in his expressive language. He transitioned from the early intervention program to the preschool program provided by the public school. Again, Annie marveled at all the services that were available and how well they fit together.

Fifteen years later, Uncle Dan, now running his own accounting business, driving a car with adapted controls, using a lightweight one-arm-drive wheelchair, and serving on the city council of their hometown, was in attendance at Luke's high school graduation, sitting beside his own parents, Lydia and Sam, now 80. Lydia could not keep from crying and smiling as their grandson Luke gave the valedictory speech with perfect enunciation and expression. "How far, how very far, we all have come," she said.

Questions

1. The early intervention program is a discretionary state grant program in which states choose to participate. What are some of the reasons that all states currently participate? What are the reasons and needs stated for the program?
2. Look again at the titles of the laws. What do the changes in the words suggest? Why were these words chosen for each law, specifically for the Individuals With Disabilities Education Act?
3. This case study spans 60 years in the 20th and 21st centuries. Review the changes in perceptions of and services to people with disabilities.

References

American Occupational Therapy Association. (1995). Position Paper: Broadening the construct of independence. *American Journal of Occupational Therapy, 49,* 1014.

American Occupational Therapy Association. (1998). Standards of practice for occupational therapy. *American Journal of Occupational Therapy, 52,* 866–869.

American Occupational Therapy Association. (2002). Position Paper—Broadening the construct of independence. *American Journal of Occupational Therapy, 56,* 660.

American Occupational Therapy Association. (2004a). Assistive technology within occupational therapy practice. *American Journal of Occupational Therapy, 58,* 678–680.

American Occupational Therapy Association. (2004b). Occupational therapy services in early intervention and school-based programs. *American Journal of Occupational Therapy, 58,* 681–685.

American Occupational Therapy Association. (2008). *AOTA's societal statement on livable communities (attachment B.1.a).* Retrieved December 24, 2008, from www.aota.org/Practitioners/Official/SocietalStmts/Livable.aspx

American Occupational Therapy Association. (in press). Specialized knowledge and skills in technology and environmental intervention for occupational therapy practice. *American Journal of Occupational Therapy.*

American Speech–Language–Hearing Association. (2002). *Augmentative and alternative communication: Knowledge and skills for service delivery.* Retrieved July 12, 2009, from www.asha.org/docs/html/KS2002-00067.html

Americans With Disabilities Act of 1990, Pub. L. 101–336, 42 U.S.C. § 12101.

Ariel, S. (2002). *Children's imaginative play.* Westport, CT: Praeger.

Assistive Technology Act of 1998, Pub. L. 105–394, 29 U.S.C. § 2201.

Ault, M. J. (2006, March). *The National Assistive Technology Research Institute's "top ten" list of findings.* Paper presented at the annual meeting of the California State University, Northridge, Los Angeles.

Baush, M. E., Ault, M. J., & Hasselbring, T. S. (2006). *Assistive technology planner: From IEP consideration to classroom implementation.* Lexington, KY: National Assistive Technology Research Institute.

Beukelman, D. R., & Mirenda, P. (1992). *Augmentative and alternative communication: Management of severe communication disorders in children and adults.* Baltimore: Brookes.

Blackhurst, A. E. (2001). *What is assistive technology?* Lexington, KY: National Assistive Technology Research Institute. Retrieved January 2, 2009, from http://natri.uky.edu/resources/fundamentals/defined.html

Blackhurst, A. E., & Lahm, E. A. (2000). Foundations of technology and exceptionality. In J. Lindsey (Ed.), *Technology and exceptional individuals* (3rd ed., pp. 3–45). Austin, TX: Pro-Ed.

Blackstone, S. (2006). Young children: False beliefs, widely held. *Augmentative Communication News, 18*(2), 1–4.

Bloom, B. S. (1956). *Taxonomy of educational objectives.* Boston: Allyn & Bacon.

Bloomfield, B. C. (2000, May). *Icon to I can: A visual bridge to independence.* Paper presented at the TEACCH International Conference, Chapel Hill, NC.

Bodine, C., & Melonis, M. (2005). Teaming and assistive technology in educational settings. In D. Edyburn, K. Higgins, & R. Boone (Eds.), *The handbook of special education technology* (pp. 209–227). Whitefish Bay, WI: Knowledge by Design.

Bouck, E. C., Okolo, C. M., & Courtad, C. A. (2007). Technology at home: Implications for children with disabilities. *Journal of Special Education Technology, 22*(3), 43–56.

Bowser, G., & Reed, P. (1995). Education TECH points for assistive technology planning. *Journal of Special Education Technology, 12*(4), 325–338.

Bremer, C., Kachgal, M., & Schoeller, K. (2003). *Self-determination: Supporting successful transition.* Minneapolis, MN: National Center on Secondary Education and Transition. Retrieved January 20, 2009, from www.ncset.org/publications/viewdesc.asp?id=962

Burkhart, L. J. (2002). *Getting past learned helplessness for children who face severe challenges: Four secrets for success.* Retrieved October 10, 2005, from www.lindaburkhart.com/learned_helplessness.pdf

Campbell, P., Wilcox, M., Milbourne, S., & Bacon, C. (2004). Report of Technology Act Project Director's Survey. *Research Brief, 1*(1). Retrieved December 8, 2008, from http://tnt.asu.edu

CAST. (2008). *Universal design for learning guidelines* (Version 1.0). Wakefield, MA: Author.

Castellani, J., & Bowser, G. (2006, November). Transition planning: Assistive technology supports and services. *Technology in Action, 2*(3), 1–8.

Center for Universal Design. (2008a). *About the center—Ronald L. Mace: Last speech.* Retrieved December 6, 2008, from www.design.ncsu.edu/cud/about_us/usronmacespeech.htm

Center for Universal Design. (2008b). *About UD.* Retrieved February 4, 2010, from www.design.ncsu.edu/cud/about_ud/about_ud.htm

Center for Universal Design. (2008c). *About UD: Universal design history.* Retrieved December 6, 2008, from www.design.ncsu.edu/cud/about_ud/udhistory.htm

Cook, A., & Polgar, J. (2008). *Cook and Hussey's assistive technologies: Principles and practice* (3rd ed.). St. Louis, MO: Elsevier.

Cooper, J. D., Chard, D. J., & Kiger, N. D. (2006). *The struggling reader: Interventions that work.* New York: Scholastic.

Copley, J., & Ziviani, J. (2004). Barriers to the use of assistive technology for children with multiple disabilities. *Occupational Therapy International, 11*(4), 229–243.

Copley, J., & Ziviani, J. (2007). Use of a team-based approach to assistive technology assessment and planning for children with multiple disabilities: A pilot study. *Assistive Technology, 19*(3), 109–125.

DeCoste, D. C., & Glennen, S. L. (1997). *Handbook of augmentative and alternative communication.* San Diego, CA: Singular.

Delaware Assistive Technology Initiative, Center for Applied Science and Engineering. (n.d.). *Assistive technology facts: Seating, positioning, and mobility.* Retrieved January 1, 2009, from www.dati.org/info/seatposmob.html

Developmental Disabilities Assistance and Bill of Rights Act of 2000, Pub. L. 106–402.

Dugan, L., Campbell, P. H., & Wilcox, M. J. (2006). Making decisions about assistive technology with infants and toddlers. *Topics in Early Childhood Special Education, 26*(1), 25–32.

Education for All Handicapped Children Act of 1975, Pub. L. 94–142, 20 U.S.C. § 1400 *et seq.*

Edyburn, D. L. (2002). Models, theories, and frameworks: Contributions to understanding special education technology. *Special Education Technology Practice, 4*(2), 16–24.

Family Center on Technology and Disability. (2010). *Assistive technology laws* [Fact sheet]. Retrieved March 17, 2010, from www.fctd.info/factsheets

Furey, M., Tedder, C., Welsh, J., & Wilson, E. (2009). Promoting accessible playgrounds. *OT Practice, 14*(15), 8–12.

Galloway, J. C., Ryu, J. C., & Agrawal, S. K. (2008), Babies driving robots: Self-generated mobility in very young infants. *Journal of Intelligent Service Robotics, 1*(2), 123–134.

Galvin, J. C., & Sherer, M. J. (Eds.). (1996). *Evaluating, selecting and using appropriate assistive technology.* Gaithersburg, MD: Aspen.

George, C. L., Schaff, J. I., & Jeffs, T. L. (2005). Physical access in today's schools: Empowerment through assistive technology. In D. Edyburn, K. Higgins, & R. Boone (Eds.), *The handbook of special education technology* (pp. 355–377). Whitefish Bay, WI: Knowledge by Design.

Hamm, E. (2006). Playfulness and the environmental support of play in children with and without developmental disabilities. *OTJR: Occupation, Participation and Health, 26*(3), 88–96.

Hanser, G. (2006). Fostering emergent writing for children with significant disabilities: Writing with alternative pencils. *Technology Special Interest Section Quarterly, 16*(1), 1–4.

Harry, B., Kalyanpur, M., & Day, M. (1999). *Building cultural reciprocity with families.* Baltimore: Brookes.

Hitchcock, C., & Stahl, S. (2003). Assistive technology, universal design, universal design for learning: Improved opportunities. *Journal of Special Education Technology, 18*(4), 45–52.

Hocking, C. (1999). Function or feelings: Factors in abandonment of assistive devices. *Technology and Disability, 11,* 3–11.

Hodgdon, L. (1995). *Visual strategies for improving communication. Volume 1: Practical supports for school and home.* Troy, MI: Quirk Roberts.

Hutinger, P., Bell, C., Daytner, G., & Johanson, J. (2006). Establishing and maintaining an early childhood emergent literacy technology curriculum. *Journal of Special Education Technology, 21*(4), 39–54.

Individuals With Disabilities Education Improvement Act of 2004, Pub. L. 108–446, 20 U.S.C. § 1400 *et seq.*

Judge, S. L. (2000). Accessing and funding assistive technology for young children with disabilities. *Early Childhood Education Journal, 28*(2), 125–131.

Judge, S. L. (2006). Constructing an assistive technology toolkit for young children: Views from the field. *Journal of Special Education Technology, 21*(4), 17–24.

Kalyanpur, M., & Harry, B. (1999). *Culture in special education: Building reciprocal family–professional relationships.* Baltimore: Brookes.

Koenig, A. J., & Holbrook, M. C. (Eds.). (2000). *Foundations of education. Volume II: History and theory of teaching children and youths with visual impairments* (2nd ed.). New York: American Foundation for the Blind.

Koppenhaver, D. A., Evans, D. A., & Yoder, D. E. (1991). Childhood reading and writing experiences of literate adults with severe speech and physical impairments. *Augmentative and Alternative Communcation, 7,* 20–33.

Law, M., Baptiste, S., Carswell, A., McColl, M. A., Polatajko, H., & Pollock, N. (2005). *Canadian Occupational Performance Measure* (4th ed.). Toronto, ON: CAOT Publications.

Leake, D., & Black, R. (2005). *Essential tools: Cultural and linguistic diversity: Implications for transition personnel.* Minneapolis: University of Minnesota, Institute on Community Integration, National Center on Secondary Education and Transition.

Light, J., & Drager, K. (2002). Improving the design of augmentative and alternative communication technologies for young children. *Assistive Technology, 14,* 17–32.

Long, T. M., Woolverton, M., Perry, D. F., & Thomas, J. (2007). Training needs of pediatric occupational therapists in assistive technology. *American Journal of Occupational Therapy, 61,* 345–354.

Lowman, D. K. (2008) Applying EBP to the education setting. *The T/TAC Telegram, XIII*(1), 3. Retrieved October 2, 2009, from http://ttac.gmu.edu/assets/docs/TTAC/Newsletters/Sept_Oct_08.pdf

Mistrett, S. G. (2000). *Let's play! Project final report* (Final Report to OERS, No. H024B50051). Buffalo: State University of New York, Center for Assistive Technology.

Mistrett, S. G. (2005). Assistive technology helps young children with disabilities participate in daily activities. In C. Wilbarger (Ed.), *Technology and media for accessing the curriculum: Instructional support for students with disabilities* (pp. 29–38). Arlington, VA: Technology and Media Division.

Mistrett, S. G., Lane, S., & Goetz, A. (2000). *A professional's guide to assisting families in creating play environments for children with disabilities.* Buffalo: State University of New York at Buffalo, Center for Assistive Technology.

Moore, H., & Wilcox, J. (2006). Characteristics of early intervention practitioners and their confidence in the use of assistive technology. *Topics in Early Childhood Special Education, 26*(1), 15–23.

Myers, C. T. (2008). Descriptive study of occupational therapists' participation in early childhood transitions. *American Journal of Occupational Therapy, 62,* 212–220.

Myers, C. T., Stephens, L., & Tabor, S. (2009). Early intervention. In J. Case-Smith & J. C. O'Brien (Eds.), *Occupational therapy for children* (6th ed., pp. 681–711). Maryland Heights, MO: Elsevier.

National Center for Technology Innovation, & Center for Implementing Technology in Education. (2006). *The assistive technology planner: From research to implementation* ("Tech Works" Brief). Retrieved October 5, 2009, from http://ldonline.org/article/12375

National Institute on Disability and Rehabilitation Research. (n.d.). *Frequently asked questions about NIDRR.* Retrieved December 26, 2008, from www.ed.gov/about/offices/list/osers/nidrr/faq.html

National Joint Committee for the Communication Needs of Persons With Severe Disabilities. (1992). *Guidelines for meeting the communication needs of persons with severe disabilities.* Retrieved October 5, 2009, from www.asha.org/docs/html/GL1992-00201.html

Okolo, C. M., & Bouck, E. C. (2007). Research about assistive technology: 2000–2006. What have we learned? *Journal of Special Education Technology, 22*(3), 19–33.

Parette, H. P., & Brotherson, M. J. (2004). Family-centered and culturally responsive assistive technology decision making. *Infants and Young Children, 17,* 355–367.

Phillips, B., & Zhao, H. (1993). Predictors of assistive technology abandonment. *Assistive Technology, 5,* 36–45.

Pierce, P. (n.d.). Assistive technology and infants and toddlers. In P. Pierce (Ed.), *Baby power: A guide for families for using assistive technology with their infants and toddlers* (pp. 1–4). Chapel Hill: University of North Carolina, Center for Literacy and Disabilities Studies. Retrieved October 5, 2009, from www2.edc.org/ncip/LIBRARY/ec/Power_1.htm

Post, K. M., Hartmann, K., Gitlow, L., & Rakowski, D. (2008). AOTA's *Centennial Vision* for the future: How can technology help? *Technology Special Interest Section Quarterly, 18*(1), 1–4.

Quality Indicators of Assistive Technology Consortium. (2004). *Quality indicators for assistive technology service: Research-based revision, 2004.* Retrieved October 5, 2009, from www.matcoop.org/attransition06/7_QIAT_Revised_2005.pdf

Rehabilitation Act of 1973 Amendments, Pub. L. 95–602.

Rowland, C., & Schweigert, P. (2000). *Tangible symbol systems* (rev. ed.). Portland: Oregon Health Sciences University, Center on Self-Determination, Design to Learn Products.

Sawyer, B., Milbourne, S., Dugan, L., & Campbell, P. (2005). Assistive technology training for providers and families of children in early intervention. *Research Brief, 2*(1). Retrieved October 5, 2009, from www.asu.edu/clas/tnt/appendix/ATtrainingbrief2-8-05.pdf

Scherer, M. (1991). *Matching people with technologies.* Webster, NY: Scherer Associates.

Scherer, M. (1996). Outcomes of assistive technology use on quality of life. *Disability and Rehabilitation, 18*(9), 439–448.

Scherer, M. J. (2004). *Matching person and technology process and accompanying assessment instruments* (rev. ed.) Webster, NY: Institute for Matching Person and Technology.

Schoonover, J., Argabrite Grove, R., & Swinth, Y. (2009). Influencing participation through assistive technology. In J. Case-Smith & J. C. O'Brien (Eds.), *Occupational therapy for children* (6th ed., pp. 583–619). Maryland Heights, MO: Elsevier.

Schoonover, J., & Smith, M. (2007). ParticipATion: Finding the OT in AT. *OT Practice, 12*(16), 12–16.

Segal, R. (2004). Family routines and rituals: A context for occupational therapy interventions. *American Journal of Occupational Therapy, 58,* 499–508.

Skau, L., & Cascella, P. (2006). Using assistive technology to foster speech and language skills at home and in preschool. *TEACHING Exceptional Children, 38*(6), 12–17.

Smith, R. O. (1995). *OT FACT software system for integrating and reporting occupational therapy assessment* (Version 2.03) [Computer software and manual]. Bethesda, MD: American Occupational Therapy Association.

Social Security Amendments of 1965, Pub. L. 89–97.

Special Education Technology–British Columbia. (2005). *Alternate access technologies: A guide for school-based teams.* Retrieved October 5, 2009, from www.setbc.org/setbc/access/alternate_access_technologies_a_guide_for_school_based_teams.html

Stoller, L. C. (1998). *Low-tech assistive devices: A handbook for the school setting.* Framington, MA: Therapro.

Suarez-Balcazar, Y., Rodawoski, J., Balcazar, F., Taylor-Ritzler, T., Portillo, N., Barwacz, D., et al. (2009). Perceived levels of cultural competence among occupational therapists. *American Journal of Occupational Therapy, 63,* 498–505.

Swinth, Y. L. (2001). Assistive technology: Computers and augmentative communication. In J. Case-Smith (Ed.), *Occupational therapy for children* (4th ed., pp. 571–608). St. Louis, MO: Mosby.

Technical Assistance Project. (2000). Update on the use of assistive technology among infants and toddlers. *TAP Bulletin.* Retrieved October 5, 2009, from www.resnaprojects.org/nattap/library/bulletins/jul00.html

Techno-. (1990). In *Webster's ninth new collegiate dictionary.* Springfield, MA: Merriam-Webster.

Technology-Related Assistance for Individuals With Disabilities Act of 1988, Pub. L. 100–407.

Trefler, E., & Hobson, D. (1997). Assistive technology. In C. H. Christiansen & C. M. Baum (Eds.), *Occupational therapy: Enabling function and well-being* (2nd ed., pp. 483–506). Thorofare, NJ: Slack.

UNESCO Statement for the United Nations Literacy Decade, 2003–2012. (2003). Retrieved December 19, 2008, from http://portal.unesco.org/education/en/ev.php-url_id=22420&url_do=do_printpage&url_section=201.html

University of Illinois at Chicago National Research and Training Center (UICNRTC), & the UICNRTC Self-Determination Knowledge Development Workgroup. (2002). *Self-determination framework for people with psychiatric disabilities.* Chicago: Author. Retrieved from www.psych.uic.edu/uicnrtc/sdframework.pdf

U.S. Department of Education. (1997–2001). National Early Intervention Longitudinal Study (NEILS): Services received by families and children in early intervention. In *23rd Annual Report to Congress on Implementation of IDEA* (pp. 1–69). Washington, DC: Author.

U.S. Department of Education. (2007). Title 34: Education. Part 303—Early Intervention Program for Infants and Toddlers With Disabilities; Proposed Rules (72 FR 26456).

Valdez, C. (2003, January 6). Hidden messages: Ventriloquist uses power of laughter to teach children respect. *LBT Business Journal.* Retrieved October 19, 2009, from http://airwolf.lmtonline.com/lmtbusiness/archive/010603/jrnl6.pdf

Vygotsky, L. S. (1978). *Mind and society: The development of higher psychological processes.* Cambridge, MA: Harvard University Press.

Wehmeyer, M. L. (2002). Promoting the self-determination of students with severe disabilities. *ERIC Digest.* Retrieved June 8, 2008, from http://eric.ed.gov/ERICDocs/data/ericdocs2sql/content_storage_01/0000019b/80/29/d2/46.pdf

Wershing, A., & Symington, L. (1998). Learning and growing with assistive technology. In S. L. Judge & H. P. Parette (Ed.), *Assistive technology for young children with disabilities* (pp. 45–75). Cambridge, MA: Brookline Books.

Wilcox, M., Bacon, C., & Campbell, P. (2004). National Survey of Parents and Providers Using AT in Early Intervention. *Research Brief, 1*(3). Tots 'n Tech Research Institute. Retrieved March 3, 2010, from www.asu.edu/clas/tnt/presentations/ResBriefParProviSurv 9-16-04.pdf

Wilcox, M., Guimond, A., Campbell, P., & Moore, H. (2006). Provider perspectives on the use of assistive technology for infants and toddlers with disabilities. *Topics in Early Childhood Special Education, 26*(1), 33–49.

Yoder, D. E., Erickson, K. A., & Koppenhaver, D. A. (1997). *A literacy bill of rights*. Durham, NC: Center for Literacy and Disability. Retrieved March 3, 2010, from http://nationaldb.org/documents/products/conference/2008_topical_workshop/LiteracyBill.doc

Zabala, J. S. (1995). *The SETT framework: Critical areas to consider when making informed assistive technology decisions*. Houston, TX: Region IV Education Service Center. (ERIC Document Reproduction Service No. ED381962)

Zabala, J. (2009). *10 things everyone should know about assistive technology in 2009*. Retrieved December 13, 2009, from www.sst4.org/_upload//10Things_to_knowaboutAT_in_2009 (1).pdf

Appendix 8.A.
Top 10 Things Occupational Therapists Need to Know About Assistive Technology and Children

<table>
<tr><td>1. Assistive technology (AT) is a legal term.</td><td>AT Device
a. any item, piece of equipment or product system . . . that is used to increase, maintain, or improve functional capabilities of individuals with disabilities.
b. EXCEPTION: The term does not include a medical device that is surgically implanted or the replacement of such a device.
Pub. L. 108–446 § 602(1)

AT Service
Any service that directly assists a child with a disability in the selection, acquisition, or use of an assistive technology device.
Pub. L. 108–446 § 602(1)

Universal Design
Universal design has the meaning given the term in section 3 of the Assistive Technology Act of 1998, as amended, 29 U.S.C. § 3002.
A concept or philosophy for designing and delivering products and services that are usable by people with the widest possible range of functional capabilities which include products and services that are directly usable (without requiring assistive technologies) and products and services that are made usable with assistive technologies.</td></tr>
<tr><td>2. The primary purpose of AT is to enhance capabilities, remove barriers to participation, and improve quality of life and learning.</td><td>Individuals With Disabilities Education Act Amendments of 1997, Pub. L. 105–117, 20 U.S.C. § 1400 et seq.
• IDEA ensures a free, appropriate public education (FAPE).
• FAPE is defined by the individualized education program (IEP).
• AT required to implement the IEP and support achievement must be provided at no cost to the family.</td></tr>
<tr><td>3. AT is related to performance areas rather than disabilities.</td><td>Performance in areas of occupation include activities of daily living, instrumental activities of daily living, education, work, play, leisure, and social participation.</td></tr>
<tr><td>4. AT may be applicable to all ages and stages of growth and development</td><td>Although there may be prerequisite skills for the use of specific AT devices, there are no prerequisites for AT devices and services.</td></tr>
<tr><td>5. AT follows a child-centered process and requires a team approach.</td><td>• Texas Assistive Technology Network Training Modules: www.texasat.net
• Technology and Media Division of the Council for Exceptional Children Monographs: www.tamcec.org
• The Student Environment(s), Tasks, and Tools Framework: www2.edc.org/NCIP/workshops/sett/SETT_Framework.html
• Wisconson Assistive Technology Initiative: www.wati.org
• Institute for Matching Person and Technology: www.matchingpersonandtechnology.com</td></tr>
<tr><td>6. The foundations of assessment and intervention are a continuous process that ebbs and flows yet consists of systematic problem analysis and problem solving in context.</td><td>Assessment involves an analysis of performance skills and performance patterns. It is critical that intervention plans include documentation regarding AT use and ongoing assessments to ensure that AT solutions are appropriate for changes in the person, environment, occupational role, and physical growth and development.</td></tr>
</table>

7. When team members can describe the child, the context, and the activity demands, they can likely describe the tools and solutions to support participation.	After sharing information about the child, the context, and the activity demands, ask, "If there were something that would help this child participate, what would it be?" Remember to ask the child or his or her immediate caregivers and teachers.
8. The least complex solution (or restrictive environment) should be the first solution.	Technology should be viewed as a system of tools. High-tech solutions are often overemphasized when there are less complex and less expensive low-tech alternatives.
9. AT does not eliminate the need for instruction in skills pertinent to the activity.	Having a means to do something is not the same thing as knowing how to do it. AT enables children to participate.
10. There are many ways to do it right!	Effective decision making and good stewardship • Avoid device abandonment and underuse by being involved • Try before you buy • Plan for implementation • Identify expected change • Evaluate effectiveness. Quality indicators for AT services in schools (www.qiat.org) • Consideration • Assessment • IEP development • Implementation • Evaluation of effectiveness • Transition • Professional development • Administrative support.

Source. From "10 Things Everyone Should Know About Assistive Technology in 2009," by J. Zabala, 2009. Copyright © 2009 by Joy Zabala. Adapted with permission.

Appendix 8.B.
Internet Resources for Assistive Technology

Ablenet (www.ablenetinc.com) is a commercial Web site that primarily features devices sold by Ablenet. However, it includes good ideas on incorporating switches and switch-activated devices into fun activities for preschool and younger children.

AblePlay™ (www.ableplay.org/) provides information on toys for children with special needs. The site applies a rating system representing the depth of accessibility and application for children with disabilities for each product reviewed on the basis of the following disability categories: physical, sensory, communicative, and cognitive.

The Alliance for Technology Access (ATA; www.ataccess.org/resources/wcp/endefault.html) is a growing national and international network of technology resource centers, community-based organizations, agencies, individuals, and companies. "We Can Play," part of the Alliance for Technology Access Web site, presents 20 different activity ideas to use with children of all abilities.

Augmentative and Alternative Communication (AAC) Connecting Young Kids (YAACK; http://aac.unl.edu/yaack/) deals with issues related to AAC and young children. YAACK's purpose is to provide information and guidance to families, teachers, speech–language pathologists, and anyone else who is involved with a child with special communication needs.

Closing the Gap (www.closingthegap.com) provides AT resources for children and adults with special needs.

Every Kid Can: Technology Supports for Young Children (http://letsplay.buffalo.edu/AT/EKC-wheel.pdf) can be used by families, service providers, and other caregivers when considering technology supports for young children.

The Family Center on Technology and Disability (www.fctd.info/) is a resource designed to support organizations and programs that work with families of children and youth with disabilities.

LekoTek (www.lekotek.org/default.asp) is a nonprofit authority on toys and play for children with disabilities.

Let's Play (http://cosmos.buffalo.edu/letsplay/) is an informative Web site that includes pdf booklets and one-page idea sheets emphasizing play with infants and toddlers with special needs.

Let's Play! Projects (http://letsplay.buffalo.edu/) provide families with ideas and strategies to promote play through better access to play materials and use of AT, primarily involving low-tech AT. Find information on toy selection, toys for children with disabilities, adapting, locating specially designed toys, and other resources to promote play.

National Early Childhood Technical Assistance Center (NECTAC; www.nectac.org/) has extensive resources for states and systems about AT with young children.

Simplified Technology (www.lburkhart.com/handouts.htm) is special educator and AT expert Linda Burkhart's Web site. The link page goes directly to an index for "Make it Yourself" directions and workshop handouts, including "Make Your Own Talking Switch"; "Make a Mouse House"; "Computer Play: Using Computers With Young Children" and "What We Are Learning About Early Learners and Augmentative Communication and Assistive Technology." Other pages related to "Simplified Technology for Children With Disabilities" can be found on the site.

Technical Assistance Alliance for Parent Centers (www.taalliance.org) provides training and information to meet the needs of parents of children with disabilities living in the area served by the center.

Tots 'n Tech (http://tnt.asu.edu) is a national research program about AT and includes information about adaptations and devices for infants and toddlers, resource information, and links to many useful sites.

Note. This list is not exhaustive, and inclusion does not imply endorsement by the American Occupational Therapy Association/AOTA Press.

Appendix 8.C. How Assistive Technology Can Support Infants and Toddlers

Life Skill	Possible Solutions
Mealtime and snacking	Adaptive utensils (shortened, curved, or built-up handles; cutout, weighted, or handled cup), nonskid mat or suction cups, scoop dish or plate guard, sandwich holder, universal cuff, positioning aids, communication supports for making choices
Bathing and grooming	Bath mitts, bath chairs, vibrating toothbrushes, adapted bath toys, potty chair with positioning aids (head and back support, footrest, abduction post, armrests)
Play time	Nonskid mats, toys adapted with hook-and-loop fabric, cause-and-effect toys, built-up handles, switches, communication supports including social situation stories and visuals, simulation software
Bed time and dressing	Soothing music, lotion and massage, calming scents, predictable routines, and visual schedules Clothing adaptations (zipper pulls, hook-and-loop closures, slip-on shoes, elastic shoelaces)
Early reading	High-interest interactive picture books with predictable or repetitive text, sound, objects, or manipulatives (props, page fluffers); electronic storybooks; switch-activated recordings and software
Early writing	Adapted pencils and grips; eye-gaze boards; rubber stamps; universal cuff; multiple forms of representation; multimodal software offering words, sound, and animation; bendable waxed yarn
Early math	Manipulatives, abacuses, counting tubs, simulated math exploration software
Expressive arts • Drawing • Music • Dramatic play	Adaptive art materials such as large-handled drawing tools, spring-loaded scissors, visual "cue cards" for requesting materials, switch-activated art and music activities such as Spin Art and music software, musical instruments with alternative handles, puppetry, dress-up
Positioning	Rolled towels, bolsters, U-shaped infant support pillows, bean bag chairs, chair inserts, footrests, standers, straps, trays, weighted vests, T-stools, inflated sit disks, applied ergonomics
Mobility	Scooters, trike and bike modifications, walkers, specialized strollers, manual wheelchairs, wheelchairs, motorized chairs
Communication	Gestures and signing, objects, pictures and digital photos, clip art and visual symbol software, "talking" photo frames and albums, single- and multiple-cell voice output devices, dynamic screen devices
Computer use	Input devices—keyboard guards, alternative keyboards, mouse modifications, switches, touch screens, interactive whiteboards, head pointers Output devices (monitors, printers, multimedia) Software—cause and effect, early learning, digital storybooks, and Web sites for children
Hearing	Reducing ambient noise, preferential seating, earphones, sound amplification
Vision	Preferential seating, increased contrast, clutter elimination, flashlights or light boxes, enlarged materials, tactile and auditory cues
Adaptive materials	Attachers, confiners, extenders, highlighters, simplifiers, and stabilizers (see Let's Play Project: http://letsplay.buffalo.edu)

Source. From *Every Kid Can: Technology Supports for Young Children,* by S. Mistrett, A. Ruffino, S. Lane, L. Robinson, P. Reed, & S. Milbourne, 2004. Retrieved November 29, 2009, from http://letsplay.buffalo.edu/AT/EKC-wheel.pdf. Copyright © Let's Play Project (U.S. Department of Education Grant No. H327A030059). Adapted with permission.

Appendix 8.D.
10 Tips for Buying Toys for Children With Disabilities

1. **Multisensory appeal**
   - Does the toy respond with lights, sounds, or movement to engage the child?
   - Are there contrasting colors?
   - Does it have a scent?
   - Is there texture?
2. **Method of activation**
   - Will the toy provide a challenge without frustration?
   - What is the force required to activate the toy?
   - What are the number and complexity of steps required to activate it?
3. **Places the toy will be used**
   - Will the toy be easy to store?
   - Is there space in the home?
   - Can the toy be used in a variety of positions such as side-lying or on a wheelchair tray?
4. **Opportunities for success**
   - Can play be open ended with no definite right or wrong way?
   - Is it adaptable to the child's individual style, ability, and pace?
5. **Current popularity**
   - Is it a toy that will help the child with disabilities feel like "any other kid"?
   - Does it tie in with other activities like books and art sets that promote other forms of play?
6. **Self-expression**
   - Does the toy allow for creativity, uniqueness, and making choices?
   - Will it give the child experience with a variety of media?
7. **Adjustability**
   - Does it have adjustable height, sound volume, speed, and level of difficulty?
8. **Child's individual abilities**
   - Does the toy provide activities that reflect both developmental and chronological ages?
   - Does it reflect the child's interests and age?
9. **Safety and durability**
   - Does the toy fit with the child's size and strength? Does it have moisture resistance?
   - Are the toy and its parts sized appropriately? Can it be washed and cleaned?
10. **Potential for interaction**
    - Will the child be an active participant during use?
    - Will the toy encourage social engagement with others?

Source. From *Resources . . .Top 10 Tips for Choosing Toys,* by the National Lekotek Center, n.d. Retrieved July 18, 2009, from www.lekotek.org/resources/informationontoys/tentips.html. The National Lekotek Center, a division of Anixter Center, is a nonprofit organization with a national network of affiliates dedicated to making play and learning accessible for children with disabilities and provides supportive services for their families. For additional information on toys, play, and technology for children with disabilities, visit www.lekotek.org.

Appendix 8.E.
Communication Bill of Rights

All persons, regardless of the extent or severity of their disabilities, have a basic right to affect, through communication, the conditions of their own existence. Beyond this general right, several specific communication rights should be ensured in all daily interactions and interventions involving persons who have severe disabilities. These basic communication rights are as follows:

1. The right to request desired objects, actions, events, and persons, and to express personal preferences, or feelings.
2. The right to be offered choices and alternatives.
3. The right to reject or refuse undesired objects, events, or actions, including the right to decline or reject all proffered choices.
4. The right to request, and be given, attention from and interaction with another person.
5. The right to request feedback or information about a state, an object, a person, or an event of interest.
6. The right to active treatment and intervention efforts to enable people with severe disabilities to communicate messages in whatever modes and as effectively and efficiently as their specific abilities will allow.
7. The right to have communicative acts acknowledged and responded to, even when the intent of these acts cannot be fulfilled by the responder.
8. The right to have access at all times to any needed augmentative and alternative communication devices and other assistive devices, and to have those devices in good working order.
9. The right to environmental contexts, interactions, and opportunities that expect and encourage persons with disabilities to participate as full communicative partners with other people, including peers.
10. The right to be informed about the people, things, and events in one's immediate environment.
11. The right to be communicated with in a manner that recognizes and acknowledges the inherent dignity of the person being addressed, including the right to be part of communication exchanges about individuals that are conducted in his or her presence.
12. The right to be communicated with in ways that are meaningful, understandable, and culturally and linguistically appropriate.

Source. From *Guidelines for Meeting the Communication Needs of Persons With Severe Disabilities* (p. 4), by the American Speech–Language–Hearing Association (ASHA) National Joint Committee for the Communication Needs of Persons With Severe Disabilities, 1992, Rockville, MD: ASHA. Retrieved March 3, 2010, from www.asha.org/docs/html/GL1992-00201.html.

Appendix 8.F.
Principles of Universal Design (Version 2.0, April 1, 1997)

Compiled by advocates of universal design, listed in alphabetical order: Bettye Rose Connell, Mike Jones, Ron Mace, Jim Mueller, Abir Mullick, Elaine Ostroff, Jon Sanford, Ed Steinfeld, Molly Story, and Gregg Vanderheiden.

Major funding provided by The National Institute on Disability and Rehabilitation Research, U.S. Department of Education.

UNIVERSAL DESIGN

The design of products and environments to be usable by all people, to the greatest extent possible, without the need for adaptation or specialized design.

The authors, a working group of architects, product designers, engineers and environmental design researchers, collaborated to establish the following Principles of Universal Design to guide a wide range of design disciplines including environments, products, and communications. These seven principles may be applied to evaluate existing designs, guide the design process and educate both designers and consumers about the characteristics of more usable products and environments. The Principles of Universal Design are presented here, in the following format: name of the principle, intended to be a concise and easily remembered statement of the key concept embodied in the principle; definition of the principle, a brief description of the principle's primary directive for design; and guidelines, a list of the key elements that should be present in a design which adheres to the principle. (Note: all guidelines may not be relevant to all designs.)

PRINCIPLE ONE: Equitable Use
The design is useful and marketable to people with diverse abilities.

PRINCIPLE TWO: Flexibility in Use
The design accommodates a wide range of individual preferences and abilities.

PRINCIPLE THREE: Simple and Intuitive Use
Use of the design is easy to understand, regardless of the user's experience, knowledge, language skills, or current concentration level.

PRINCIPLE FOUR: Perceptible Information
The design communicates necessary information effectively to the user, regardless of ambient conditions or the user's sensory abilities.

PRINCIPLE FIVE: Tolerance for Error
The design minimizes hazards and the adverse consequences of accidental or unintended actions.

PRINCIPLE SIX: Low Physical Effort
The design can be used efficiently and comfortably and with a minimum of fatigue.

PRINCIPLE SEVEN: Size and Space for Approach and Use
Appropriate size and space are provided for approach, reach, manipulation, and use regardless of user's body size, posture, or mobility.

Please note that the Principles of Universal Design address only universally usable design, while the practice of design involves more than consideration for usability. Designers must also incorporate other considerations such as economic, engineering, cultural, gender, and environmental concerns in their design processes. These Principles offer designers guidance to better integrate features that meet the needs of as many users as possible.

Source. From *The Principles of Universal Design* (Version 2.0), by the Center for Universal Design, 1997, Raleigh: North Carolina State University. Retrieved March 3, 2010, from www.design.ncsu.edu/cud/about_ud/udprinciplestext.htm. Copyright © 1997 by NC State University, Center for Universal Design. Used with permission.

Appendix 8.G.
Guiding Questions in Selecting an Assistive Technology Device

Performance

- Does it work efficiently and effectively?
- Is it easy to learn to use this device?
- Is it compatible with other devices?
- Does this device serve only one purpose, or is it flexible?

"Elegance"

- Does this device represent the simplest, most efficient way to accomplish the task?
- Or is this device too elaborate, too complicated to be worthwhile?

Ergonomics

- Does it fit the individual?
- Is it convenient to use in the environment?
- Is the equipment portable enough to go where the user goes?
- Are different devices needed in different environments?

Reliability

- What is the manufacturer's reputation for reliability?
- Does it stand up well to normal use?
- Is it durable?

Safety

- Is it safe to use?
- What is the power source for the device? Is it safe?
- Is a margin built in for foreseeable misuse?

Practicality

- Do company sales people seem knowledgeable and helpful?
- Are the company's service people knowledgeable and helpful?
- Does the device have a warranty? How long is the device guaranteed to function?
- How available are repair services? At what cost?
- Can this device be leased?
- Is this device available for a trial period before purchase?
- Will this device soon be outdated? Is something better on the horizon?
- Will the company update the device?
- Does the manufacturer provide training in using the device?

Aesthetics

- Is this device attractive to the eye?
- Does the device fit well into the user's lifestyle?

Normalization

- Does the device assist the user with more normalized living?
- Can the user operate the device independently or with a minimum of assistance?

- Or does the device "stick out" too much and advertise the disability of the user?
- Does the equipment minimize difference or exaggerate difference?
- Does the device have the potential to increase the quantity and quality of time spent with nondisabled peers? Or does the device separate the user from others?

Cost-effectiveness

- Do the benefits the device provides justify the cost?
- Are there less expensive devices or models that serve the purpose as well?

Personal acceptance

- Is this device the user's (family's) own choice?
- Does the potential user (family) like this device and want to use it?
- Does the potential user (family) view this device as life-enhancing?
- Would the user (family) have preferred some other device or means to perform the task?
- Will using the device always be a chore or can using it become a habit?

Source. From *Family Guide to Assistive Technology* (pp. 16–17), by K. A. Kelker & R. Holt, 1997, Billings, MT: Parents, Let's Unite for Kids. Retrieved November 6, 2008, from www.pluk.org/Pubs/PLUK_ATguide_269K.pdf. Copyright © 1997 by Parents, Let's Unite for Kids. Adapted with permission.

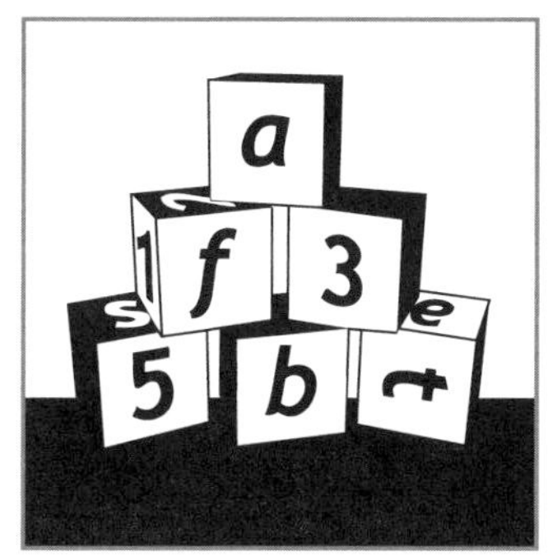

Subject Index

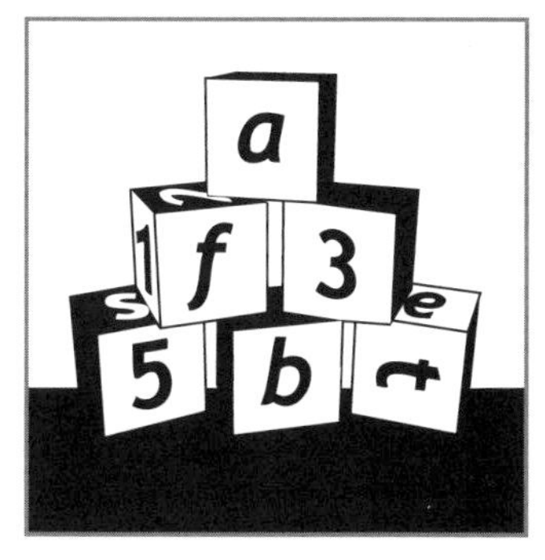

Citation Index

H

I

J

K

N

O

P

R